W0011619

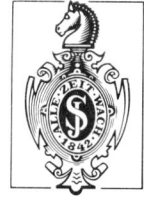

E. W. Fünfgeld (Ed.)

Rökan

Ginkgo biloba

Recent Results in Pharmacology and Clinic

With 74 Figures and 47 Tables

Springer-Verlag Berlin Heidelberg New York
London Paris Tokyo

Editor

E.W. Fünfgeld, Prof. Dr. med.
Direktor Schloßbergklinik Wittgenstein
D-5928 Bad Laasphe
Professor für Neurologie und Psychiatrie
Universitätsklinik Homburg
D-6650 Homburg/Saar

ISBN 3-540-19261-1 Springer-Verlag Berlin Heidelberg New York
ISBN 0-387-19261-1 Springer-Verlag New York Berlin Heidelberg

© Springer-Verlag Berlin Heidelberg 1988
Printed in Germany

Typesetting: B. E. Scholz, Marburg/Lahn
Printing and binding: harschdruck, Karlsruhe
2125/3145-543210

CONTENTS

CLINIC

LIST OF CONTRIBUTORS

The numbers given below refer to the first page of each contribution and there the addresses of the respective contributors can be found.

Editorial
Dementias – A Growing Social and Medical Problem

E.W. Fünfgeld

Schloßbergklinik Wittgenstein D–5928 Bad Laasphe, FRG

The expectation of life has risen constantly in most of the industrialized countries in the last 80 years. It was shown that the over 65 year-old US-population has grown from 3 millions in 1900 to more than 27 millions in 1984. About 6% of these persons suffered from Alzheimer's disease. This group of illnesses increases with age – about 20-25% of people aged 85 years will be affected – actually more than 2 millions; in 65 years time this number will have increased to 16 million persons (G.D. Cohen 1986). B.E. Tomlinson (1986) pointed out that a world-wide collaboration and the search of subgroups with detailed analysis of cases – early onset or late onset – is required. Among the multiple aetiological factors, dementia caused by ischaemic lesions must be separated from dementias of other origin. "Our thinking about Alzheimer's disease is too restricted if we assume that chemical and neuropathological findings and aetiology have to be identical and consistent from case to case" (Tomlinson). Davison (1982) pointed out that "functional deficits are greater than they would be expected from the neuropathological changes".

Glucose consumption was significantly reduced in patients with the primary degenerative type of dementia (S. Hoyer 1983), but this author could not find a significant influence of age on cerebral bloodflow and oxidative metabolism (1982). With the technique of positron emission tomography (PET) a decrease in bloodflow and glucose metabolism was found which "were related only to the duration and the severity of mental impairment, but not to the type of dementia" (W.D. Heiss et al. 1985). But there is not only a loss of cortical neurons but also a loss in some subcortical structures such as locus coeruleus, substantia nigra, substantia innominata, hippocampus, nucleus amygdala and a loss of the acetylcholine – synthesising enzyme choline acetyltransferase causing a significant reduction in acetylcholine synthesis, but other transmitters such as serotonin are equally involved (A.N. Davison 1986).

Rökan (Ginkgo Biloba). Recent Results in Pharmacology and Clinic
Edited by E.W. Fünfgeld
© Springer-Verlag Berlin Heidelberg New York 1988, pp. 11-16

We have to face the following facts:

1. The so-called normal ageing of the brain depends on very different conditions of brain's grisea and of their specific development in an individual case during the lifespan (Pathoclise C. and O. Vogt 1937).
2. The diminution of function in one grisea, e.g. of the nucleus niger in Parkinson's disease, causes an imbalance in other grisea (primary or secondary) accompanied by some repairing functions of these or other grisea.
3. A disturbed nerve cell function can be attributed to a membrane rigidity – one of the theories of ageing (A. Sun and G.Y. Sun 1979; G. Calderini et al. 1983; M. Hershkowitz 1983; J. Rotrosen 1986).
4. The permeability of the blood-brain barrier to neuropeptides in ageing and in dementias "is poorly studied and is complex" (W.A. Banks and A.J. Kastin 1986).
5. Different alterations on basis of neurotransmitter-receptor system in Alzheimer's disease (P.J. Whitehoese and K.S. Au 1985) will affect different systems with up-regulations and down-regulations and a compensator denervation supersensitivity may occur at the same time.
6. Special molecular aspects – calcium influences and others – have some actions not yet determined sufficiently in Alzheimer's type (F.E. Bloom 1986; Montarolo et al. 1986)
7. External influences such as toxic amounts of aluminium (Wisniewsky et al. 1985), stress recovery (measured in corticosterone titers in young and old rats, R.M. Sapolsky and B.S. McEwen 1986), free radicals (O_2) (D.M. Bowen and A.N. Davison 1986), exitotoxins (B. Winblad et al. 1986) and genetic factor (L.J. Whalley et al. 1985, J. Constantinides 1985; L. Amaducci and B.S. Schoenberg)

Causes and levels of disturbances in dementias are very different. Even the diagnostic aids by a number of new techniques such as computerized tomography and proton NMR-imaging have given rather disappointing results (B. Winblad et al. 1986). Compared to the variety of the disorder possibilities the clinical pictures and the changes obtained by different technical equipment are much more uniform: multiple causes and defects are reduced to a few clinical syndromes!

This situation might be compared with common conditions in the field of internal medicine: quite different microbes causing pulmonary infections are able to produce fever: If there is no time or possibility to test the sensitivity against the pathogenic bacterium we are forced to administer a broad–spectrum antibiotic. Concerning the ageing processes – in spite of the new techniques, we are only able to distinguish the different causes and levels of brain disturbances under experimental conditions (E.W. Fünfgeld 1987).

Until now the only way in humans is to observe the clinical result of a given drug after some weeks or months preferably by using standardised tests or questionnaires.

Concerning the drugs in use they may have a selective action (e.g. the calcium blocking agent Nicergolin, E.W. Fünfgeld [10] or – compared with the conditions concerning the antibiotics – compounds possessing a broader spectrum. About brain diseases the latter condition is certainly the case if we use the Ginkgo biloba extract, which has an influence on different levels of the nerve cells, vessels and tissues.

In this volume broad experimental studies and some clinical results are shown:

The Ginkgo biloba extract exerts an antiradical effect, and an inhibition of membrane lipid peroxidation was also observed (J. Pincemail and C. Deby; C. Deby and J. Pincemail), furthermore a protective influence on cytotoxic or vasogenic oedema and ischaemia (A. Etienne, F.H. Hecquet, F. Clostre; B. Spinnewyn, N. Blavet and F. Clostre) especially on membrane and ionic pumps (F. Clostre) and on oedema after radiotherapy (D. Hannequin, A. Thibert and Y. Vaschalde)was also noted. In addition a protective effect was found on the blood-brain barrier (P.E.Chabrier and P. Roubert), some protective influence on normobaric hypoxia and on the sequences of ligation of the carotid artery (J.R. Rapin and M. Le Poncin-Lafitte), and a specific effect on the noradrenergic system and on beta-receptors (G. Racagni, N. Brunello and R. Paoletti) but above all an increase of the muscarinic receptor population in the hippocampus (J.E. Taylor) was reported. From these extensive experimental studies one can assume that positive clinical results may occur. As reported by I. Hindmarch in a double-blind, cross-over study including 8 healthy female volunteers in an acute and ascending trial one hour after 600 mg Ginkgo biloba extract, there was a significant improvement of the short term memory which was not seen at the doses of 120 mg or 240 mg. J. Taillandier et al. published a double-blind longitudinal multicenter trial versus placebo with 166 patients, mean age 82.1 years; 80 patients received Ginkgo extract and 86 patients placebo over a period of 1 year. Each three months the investigators estimated the clinical status using the Geriatric Clinical Evaluation Scale (GCES). After three months the verum group was significantly ameliorated compared to the placebo group; the relative improvement after one year was 17.1 % in the verum group and 7.8 % in the placebo group. B. Pidoux derived the EEG in 14 senile patients – mean age 85 years – and carried out power spectrum analysis after the medication of the Ginkgo extract using different doses (120, 240 and 600 mg). He observed a dose-related activation of the alpha-rhythm, most prominent after 120 minutes in the dosage of 600 mg in occipital and frontal regions, and furthermore the occurrence of a state of hyperalertness. In more than 20 articles other special observations and influences of Ginkgo extract were described – on vertigo, tinnitus, myocardial ischaemia, arteriolar spasmus, arteritis etc.

Our own experiments with Ginkgo biloba are based on the infusion therapy in 20 patients. Using a more sophisticated computerised-neurophysiological technique, the Dynamic Brain Mapping (method T. Itil), we observed favourable acute and long term results (10 infusions over 10 days with 200 mg Ginkgo extract each). As one example of these observations we published the CEEG findings of a 74 year-old patient suffering from Parkinson's disease and from signs of SDAT – memory loss, lack of drive and occasional delirious states. The initial CEEG revealed strong differences between the two hemispheres; but after 10 infusions less difference was seen between the two hemispheres and clinically there was more alertness and drive (E.W. Fünfgeld and D. Stalleicken 1987).

No doubt this new technique opens up big advantages in the clinical and therapeutic field: Acute evidence of bioelectric changes – or not – and the possibility of multiple follow-up controls.

As a consequence time and money will be saved by using this technique, drugs not causing a change in the composition of the bioelectric waves could be stopped immediately.

For prevention and treatment of dementias we have quite clearly an advance in two directions:

1. a special and natural drug possessing a very broad spectrum of efficacy and
2. a highly sophisticated computerised neurophysiological method – Dynamic Brain Mapping™ – which can give immediate and long-term information on the reactions of the brain. This method opens a new chapter of applied clinical therapy and research into the causes of dementias.

Without doubt more trials in different conditions and stages of dementias with different dosages are necessary, but – even with our present knowledge – the Ginkgo biloba extract could be included in the list of therapeutics of SDAT established by C.A. Bagne et al. (1986).

References

1. Amaducci, L., Schoenberg, B.S.: Analytic Epidemiology and Risk Factors in Alzheimer's disease. *In:* Neurology, Proceed. XIIIth World Congress Neurol. eds. K. Poeck, H.J. Freund and H. Gänshirt, p. 85-91. *Springer-Verlag,* Berlin-Heidelberg-New York-Tokyo 1986.

2. Bagne, C.A., Pomara, N., Crook, T., Gershon, S.: Alzheimer's Disease: Strategies for treatment and research. *In:* Treatment development strategies for Alzheimer's Disease, eds. T. Crook, R. Bartus, S. Ferris, S. Gershon, p. 585-636. *Mark Pawley Ass.,* Madison, Conn. 1986.

3. Banks, W.A., Kastin, A.J.: Aging, peptides and the blood-brain barrier: Implications and spectulations. *In:* Treatment development strategies for Alzheimer's Disease, eds. T. Crook, R. Bartus, S. Ferris, S. Gershon, p. 245-266. *Mark Pawley Ass.,* Madison, Conn. 1986.

4. Bloom, F.E.: Molecular diversity and neuronal function. *In:* Molecular aspects of neurobiology, eds. R.L. Montalcene, P. Calissano, E.R. Kandel, A. Maggi, p. 188-192. *Springer-Verlag,* Berlin-Heidelberg-NewYork-Tokyo 1986.

5. Bowen, D.M., and Davison, A.N.: Can the Pathophysiology of Dementia Lead to Rational Therapy? *In:* Treatment Development Strategies for Alzheimer's Disease, eds. T. Crook, R. Bartus, S. Ferris, S. Gershon, p. 34-66. *Mark Pawley Ass.,* Madison, Conn., 1986.

6. Calderini, G., Bonetti AC, Battistella A. et al.: Biochemical Changes of Rat Brain Membranes with Aging. *Neurochemical Res. 18:* 483-92 (1983).

7. Cohen, G.D.: Foreword. *In:* Treatment Development Strategies for Alzheimer's Disease, eds. T. Crook, R. Bartus, S. Ferris, S. Gershon. *Mark Pawley Ass.,* Madison, Conn., 1986.

8. Constantinidis, J.: Genetics of Vascular and Degenerative Dementias: The Geneva Studies. *In*: Modern Approaches to the Dementias, ed. F.C. Rose – *Interdiscipl. Topics Geront., vol. 19,* pp. 1-11, KArger, Basel 1985.

9. Davison, A.N.: Dementia. *In*: Disorders of Neurohumoral Transmission, ed. T.J. Crow, p. 341-369. London, New York etc. Academic Press 1982.

10. Fünfgeld, E.W.: Neue therapeutische Möglichkeiten für Parkinson-Patienten. *Praxis-Kurier 25,* Nr. 37, 25-28 (1987).

11. Fünfgeld, E.W.: Editorial: Multitherapie der Parkinson-Krankheit und der senilen Demenz vom Alzheimer Typ. *Therapiewoche 37,* 4521-4522 (1987).

12. Fünfgeld, E.W., Stalleicken, D.: Dynamic-Brain-Mapping. *TW Neurol.Psychiatr. 2,* 136-142 (1987).

13. Heiss, W.D., Pawlik, G., Herholz, K., Szelies, B., Beil, C., Wienhard, K.: Investigation of Regional Cerebral Blood Flow and Metabolism in Dementia. *In*: Senile Dementia of the Alzheimer Type, eds. J. Traber and W.H. Gispen, p. 134-147. *Springer-Verlag,* Berlin-Heidelberg-New York-Tokyo 1985.

14. Hershkowitz, M.: Mechanisms of Brain Ageing – The Role of Membrane Fluidity. *In*: Aging of the Brain, eds. W.H. Gispen and J. Traber, p. 85-99. *Elsevier,* Amsterdam-New York-Oxford 1983.

15. Hoyer, S.: Circulation and Oxidative Metabolism in the Normally and Abnormally Aging Brain. *In*: Aging of the Brain, eds. W.H. Gispen and J. Traber, p. 151-165. *Elsevier,* Amsterdam-New York-Oxford 1983.

16. Itil, T.M., Shapiro, D.M., Eralp, E., Akman, A., Itil, K.Z., Garbizu, C.: A new Brain Function Diagnostic Unit, Including the Dynamic Brain Mapping of Computer Analyzed EEG, Evoked Potentials and Sleep (a new Hardware/Soft-

ware System and its Application in Psychiatry and Psychopharmacology). *New trends in exp. and clin. psychiat. 1*, 107-177 (1985) – Basic Publication –.

17. Krüger, G., Haubitz, I. and Hoyer, S.: Organic Psychiatric Disease in Young Adults and Aged Patients. *In*: The Aging Brain – Exper. Brain Research Supp. 5, ed. S. Hover, p. 236-242. *Springer-Verlag*, Berlin-Heidelberg-New York 1982.

18. Montarolo, P., Schacher, S., Castelucci, V.F., Hawkins, R.D., Abrams, T.W., Goelet, P., Kandel, E.R.: Interrelationships of cellular mechanism for different forms of learning and memory. *In:* Molecular aspects of neurobiology, eds. R.L. Montalcene, P. Calissano, E.R. Kandel, A. Maggi. p. 1-14. *Springer-Verlag*, Berlin-Heidelberg-New York 1986.

19. Sapolsky, M., and McEwen, B.S.: Stress, Glucocorticoids, and Their Role in Degenerative Changes in the Aging Hippocampus. *In:* Treatment Development Strategies for Alzheimer's Disease,eds. T. Crook, R. Bartus, S. Ferris, S. Gershon, p. 150-171. *Mark Pawley Ass.*, Madison, Conn. 1986.

20. Sun, A., Sun, G.Y.: Neurochemical Aspects of the Membrane Hypothesis of Aging. *In:* Interdisciplinary Topics in Gerontology. 15: CNS Aging and Its Neuropharmacology, ed. W. Meier-Ruge, p. 34-53, *Karger*, Basel 1979.

21. Tomlinson, B.E.: The Dementias: A view to the future. *In*: Neurology, Proceed. XIIIth World Congress Neurol. eds. K. Poeck, H.J. Freund and H. Gänshirt, p. 131-137. *Springer-Verlag*, Berlin-Heidelberg-New York-Tokyo 1986.

22. Vogt, O., Vogt, C.: Sitz und Wesen der Krankheiten im Lichte der topistischen Hirnforschung und des Variierens der Tiere. *J.A. Barth*, Leipzig 1937 und 1938.

23. Whalley, L.J., Wright, A.F., and Clair, D.M. St.: Genetic Factors in Down's Syndrome and Their Possible Role in the Pathogenesis of Alzheimer's Disease. *In*: Modern Approaches to the Dementias, ed. F.C. Rose – *Interdiscipl. Topics Geront., vol. 19*, pp. 18-31. Karger, Basel 1985.

24. Whitehouse, P.J., Au, K.S.: Neurotransmitter receptor alterations in Alzheimer's disease. *In:* Senile Dementia of the Alzheimer Type, eds. J. Traber, W.H. Gispen, p. 175-182. *Springer-Verlag*, Berlin-Heidelberg-New York-Tokyo 1985.

25. Winblad, B.G., Bucht, G., Fowler, C.J., Wallace, W.: Beyond the transmitter-based approach to Alzheimer's Disease. *In:* Treatment Development Strategies for Alzheimer's Disease, eds. T. Crook, R. Bartus, S. Ferris, S. Gershon, p. 67-97. *Mark Pawley Ass.*, Madison, Conn. 1986.

26. Wisniewski, H., Merz, G.S., and Carp., R.I.: Current Hypothesis of the Etiology and Pathogenesis of Senile Dementia of the Alzheimer Type. *In*: Modern Approaches to the Dementias, ed. F.C. Rose – *Interdiscipl. Topics Geront., vol. 19*, pp. 18-31. *Karger*, Basel 1985.

ACTIVE PRINCIPLES

Active Principles of Plant Origin: A Means for Studying Membrane Receptors

M. Plat

Faculté de Pharmacie, F 92290 Chatenay-Malabry

Summary

Ever since ancient times, considerable interest has been shown in plants for therapeutic use. Nowadays, however, studies of plant extracts are no longer based on empiricism; they provide great support to fundamental research, especially for a better understanding of the mediator/receptor couples.

This applies to the study of cholinergic (atropine, muscarine, etc.), adrenergic (yohimbine, rauwolscine, etc.), dopaminergic (apomorphine, bromocriptine, etc.), purinergic (caffeine, theophylline, etc.), opiate (morphine), GABA (strychnine, muscimol, bicuculline, etc.), cardiac glycosides (gitaloxin, digitoxin), and PAF-acether receptors (ginkgolides from Ginkgo biloba).

The art of healing dates back to the most ancient times, and the treatment of human diseases has led in the course of time to the creation of a large number of remedies. These latter make use of more or less complex substances originating from the various kingdoms. In particular, during the evolution of civilizations, close relationships have always existed between man and plants with the result that many biologically active compounds have been originated from them. They are, most of the time, the forerunners of pharmacological classes or models for molecular manipulations.

Mandragora (*Mandragora officinarum*, Solanaceae) was used by the Egyptians, and according to the Bible, by Jacob. Ginseng (*Panax ginseng*, Araliaceae) has been pescribed for 4,000 years in Chinese medicine, and Ginkgo (*G. biloba*, Ginkgoaceae) has figured in the therapies of the same country since 2800 B.C. (according to Chen Nung Pen T'sao).

The source of these remedies and their description stem from ancient times, and are, even now in traditional medical practice, passed down verbally without any scientific foundation. Current research on drugs of plant origin is based on a variety of criteria (routine tests, chemotaxonomic or ethnopharmacological considerations). An extraction procedure appropriate to both the nature of the plant and its active principles is selected in order to guarantee the stability of the latter: At the crude extraction stage, carried out on each part of the plant, a polyvalent pharmacological

Rökan (Ginkgo Biloba). Recent Results in Pharmacology and Clinic
Edited by E.W. Fünfgeld
© Springer-Verlag Berlin Heidelberg New York 1988, pp. 19-31

test is performed in order to provide a qualitative and quantitative assessment of its original activity. On the basis of this activity, fractionation, purification, and isolation of the active principle or principles then follows (through selective pharmacological testing). Plant substances continue to supply an increasingly vast basis for the discovery of new active principles(36).

This type of research has permitted and still permits basic research to advance. This has value in particular for the development of molecular pharmacology and information about the mediator-receptor pair. Thus, the discovery of ligands of plant origin and of their agonist or antagonist effects has most often been prior to that of the endogenous ligand (pilocarpine, arecoline, muscarine, with respect to acetylcholine; morphine with respect to enkephalines), and it is remarkable to find that the sensitivity of the human receptors to xenobiotics is identical, or even superior if antagonists are involved(10), to that manifested by their specific mediator. Although these drugs possess too general, too fleeting, or too toxic an activity, their structural and conformational study, as well as that of the parent compounds, make it possible to deduce, if not the structure of the receptor protein, at least the stearic, electrostatic, and hydrophobic requirements which might lead to the synthesis of a compound devoid of all or a portion of the aforementioned deficiences, the mediator owing its lack of toxicity to rapid metabolism.

Historical summary

It is perhaps to the physician-philosopher-theologian from Zurich, the inventor of laudanum, Paracelsus (Théophrast Bombast von Hohenheim, 1493-1541), that we owe a first test of the rationalization of the therapeutic use of plants through the comparison which he made between the organs in the human body and their environment (the well-known signatures theory) and the intuitive notion of the necessary presence of a receptor in order that the action of drugs might be manifested.

It was again by studying the antagonistic activities of two alkaloids, atropine and pilocarpine, that, 200 years later, Langley was led to conclude that they must be combined with a receptor substance on the basis of their concentrations and their chemical affinity for this substance. As early as 1900, Paul Ehrlich gave the details of the function, the general mechanism of effect, the specificity (key/lock or screw/nut model) of the receptors and refined the work of Langley by giving definitions which are still valid today: labile and reversible drug/receptor interaction, presence on the drugs of common anchorage points, presence on the drugs of toxophores*, differentiating the activity.

---

* Translator's Note: See Ehrlich's side-chain theory.

He thus also lays the foundation for structure/activity relationships. It could be said that there is practically no (exogenous) ligand or natural product which does not have a determined receptor as target.

Cholinergic receptors

Two sub-types of these may be distinguished: muscarinic and nicotinic receptors, both activated by the same mediator, acetylcholine, a flexible compound.

The muscarinic receptor has as agonist and antagonist rigid molecules of plant origin, muscarine and the tropane alkaloids respectively. The derivatives of ellipticine, another substance of plant origin, also shows antagonist activity(1) as elliptinium. The left conformer of choline, with respect to the rigid skeleton of muscarine, possesses very similar intra-atomic distances and therefore seems to be the conformation most probably involved in binding to the receptor(3). The antagonist presents a similar spatial arrangement(34). The quarternary ammonium group is responsible for the agonist activity. Beckett conceived a receptor possessing an anionic center separated from two cationic centers by 3 Angstrom units and 5-7 Angstrom units respectively. Grassy et al.(23) determined the chart of electrostatic potentials of the active conformation of acetylcholine hydroxide. These results make it possible to establish a receptor model by specifying the position of the anionic site and the cationic sites in respective relationship to the quarternary ammonium and the oxygen atoms of the ester function and acetylcholine. This is still a general model which does not explain the heterogeneity of this receptor which certain authors propose to divide into sub-types(5). Atropine in fact inhibits intestinal motility without abolishing secretion. Does it have central receptors (M_1) and peripheral receptors (M_2)? Are there sites with strong and weak affinity? Are there different localizations (with access by different routes) for the same receptor? Atropine here again would be a good pharmacological reagent to elucidate these problems(17). Easily purified by affinity chromatography, the muscarinic receptors found in various peripheral organs have a molecular weight of 80,000 daltons, and the central receptor has a weight of 70,000 daltons.

The nicotinic receptor is best known since it can be isolated in substantial quantities from the electric organs of Gymnotidae. The sequence of each of the five subunits of which it is composed has been determined. It is paired with a cationic cavity included in its structure. The human receptor present on the periphery only at the level of the neuromuscular plate where it is best defined and of the ganglion, is less well known because of structural divergences between peripheral and central receptors. The quarternary ammonium groups appear to be essential for its activation. Protonated nicotine behaves as an agonist, and curares as antagonists. The curares are foamy extracts prepared from the bark of trees belonging to the genera *Strychnos* (Loganiaceae) or *Chondrodendron* (Menispermaceae). The first are the "tube" curares, the second are the "gourd" curares. Both contain bis-quarternary alkaloids, toxiferins, and tubocurarines, as well as their derivatives.

These voluminous compounds react by forming a screen for the mediator. The nicotinic receptor, unlike the muscarinic receptor, does not have a hydrophobic surface.

Lehn conceived an artificial receptor to acetylcholine. This is a rigid macro-cyclic compound, named "cryptant," containing acetylcholine in its cavity and forming electrostatic interactions with it through its anionic groups (deriving from tartaric acid) and hydrophobes with its aromatic groups. This receptor still lacks selectivity, and complexes produced with acetylcholine are less stable than the natural complexes. Its improvement is in the course of development.

Adrenergic receptors

Since subdivision of the adrenergic receptor into alpha and beta sub-types, it does not seem that until the present the vegetable world has supplied agonists or antagonists for the beta receptors, themselves subdivided into β_1 and β_2. In retrospect, several alkaloids have been shown to be antagonists of alpha receptors, now divided into sub-types α_1 and α_2(45): corynanthine, as an α_1 blocker, yohimbine and rauwolscine as α_2 antagonists.

Corynanthine and rauwolscine are diastereoisomers, with similar physicochemical properties (notably with respect to lipophiler), which makes them valuable pharmacodynamic agents for differentiating the mechanisms interacting with the α_1 or α_2 receptors.

Yohimbine, in addition to its use as a pharmacological reagent, has enjoyed a reputation as an aphrodisiac, which today seems out of date. These compounds, although possessing a rigid framework, have not, unlike what was said above concerning the cholinergic receptors, contributed anything to knowledge of the conformational requirement for the activity of drugs and the structure of the receptor. They are no longer being developed for therapeutic purposes.

An endogenous substance devoid of amino acids, very hydrophobic, and positively charged, recently isolated from calf brain, was found to be capable of displacing rauwolscine and yohimbine from the membranes(2). It is believed to play a role in central regulation of blood pressure. Ergot alkaloids (ergotoxine group and their dihydrogenated derivatives) also behave as antagonists of the alpha receptors, but their action is complex and would be exerted according to an intermediary mode between the alpha and beta adrenergic modes. Through hemisynthesis, it has been possible to obtain new derivatives, more active and more specific.

Dopaminergic receptors

It now appears(41) that there must be two types of dopaminergic receptors: D_1, linked to activation of adenylcyclase in the nerve tissue, and D_2, hypophyseal, not linked, even inhibitors of adenylcyclase.

Also, at the level of the cardiovascular and renovascular peripheral systems, two DA-1 and DA-2 receptors have been identified, which are more and more often being compared with D_1 and D_2 respectively. However this may be, these receptors are very sensitive to the stereo-isomerism of the agonists and antagonists, and here again it is due to an agonist with rigid structure, derived from vegetable origin, apomorphine (of which only the enantiomer R (−) is active) that it was possible to conceive the active preferential conformation of the alpha rotamere dopamine (itself devoid of a center of assymetry). Seeman was thus able to suggest for the D_2 receptor a structure in which an anionic site (linked to the nitrogen of dopamine) is separated by a distance of approximately 7 Angstrom units (occupied by hydrophobic surface) from a pair of sites (one principal, the other accessory) connecting some hydrogen bonds with the phenol functions of dopamine. Ergot derivatives (bromocryptine, pergolid) also have agonist activity(22).

Among the numerous drugs of natural origin currently studied in China, tetra-hydropalmatine, isolated from *Corydalis ambigua* (Fumariaceae) acts as a dopaminergic blocker.

Purine receptors

It has been known for some years(42) that at the same time as the usual neuro-mediators and neuromodulators, stimulation of the autonomic nervous system releases adenosine and adenosine triphosphate, activating two purinergic receptors, P_1 and P_2 respectively. The P_1 receptor is subdivided, according to the effects of adenosine on adenylcyclase, into sub-types A_1 (inhibitor) and A_2 (activator).(15) The methylxanthines (caffeine, theophylline, theobromine) are selective antagonists of the P_1 receptors.

Quinidine is an antagonist of the P_2 receptor. Quinidine, as well as dihydroquinidine (vinyl group saturation derivative) owe their antiarrhythmic properties (these are the only antiarrhythmics of natural origin still being used) to their specific activity on a membranal receptor linked to the "h-gates", gateways for inactivation of the sodium canals.(29)

Receptors for opiates

Morphine, the major alkaloid from opium, because of its exceptional analgesic activity and the multiplicity of its toxic and habituation side effects, has for a long time been used to produce synthetic or hemisynthetic derivatives, resulting in the establishment of numerous structure/activity relationships and the demonstration of stereochemical imperatives. This led, 30 years ago, to envisaging the existence of a receptor and to postulating its structure. The original model includes a hydrophobic surface linking the aromatic ring, an anionic site linking the amine, a depression to imbed the carbons.

Other sites were later added in order to take into consideration the interconversion of conformations linking agonists or antagonists. The improved model cannot explain all of the facts observed by comparing with each other the activities of each of the agonist or antagonist compounds; it has therefore been necessary again to envisage the existence of μ, σ, χ, ε, δ sub-types (this latter being perhaps exclusively opioid). Morphine is the typical agonist of the μ receptor. The existence of these stereospecific receptors has been shown in cerebral structures by "binding"(35, 40, 43) or by autoradiography after fixation of the tritiated substances(47). The presence, in all vertebrae, of opiate receptors has quickly led to acknowledgement of their biological importance as well as the necessary presence of endogenous ligands. These ligands were soon characterized as peptides, then isolated(27). Pentapeptidic encephalines are involved:

Try – Gly – Gly – Phe – Met: Met. encephaline
Try – Gly – Gly – Phe – Leu: Leu. encephaline.

These compounds are not more or less heavy fragments of β-lipotropine from Li, but distinct entities emanating from different neurons(6). Endorphins with high molecular weight, but containing the preceding sequences would then be extracts from the hypophysis(13):

α endorphin: 16 amino acids
γ endorphin: 17 amino acids
β endorphin: 31 amino acids.

The Met-encephalin and the β-endorphin are linked to the μ receptor, the Leu-encephalin to the δ receptor, Dynorphine to the χ receptor, β-endorphin to the ε receptor, while the σ receptor ligand is not known with certainty.

As a result of numerous nuclear magnetic resonance or fluorescence studies, the spatial configuration of Met-encephalin in solution has been established. This has made it possible to establish analogies with morphine and its derivatives involving notably the area encircling this phenolic nucleus and the nitrogen atom, as well as the distance, approximately 10 Angstrom units, between the phenol and a lipophilic zone.

These investigations are the origin of the synthesis of a large number of peptide analogs, making it possible to observe the modifications which selectivity brings with respect to various receptors, maximal activity, stability toward peptidases. In this latter field in particular, the synthesis of specific inhibitors of encephalinase should be noted.

GABA and cycline receptors

Glycine and GABA are inhibitory neurotransmitters in mammals. No "glycinergic" agonist of vegetable origin is known, but several antagonists are, principally strychnine and also its derivative brucine, and extracts of *Strychnos nux vomica* (Loganiaceae)(14), which owe their convulsant activity to this mechanism.

Numerous "gabaergic" agonists and antagonists of vegetable origin are known.

Muscimol(29), extract of *Amanita muscaria,* is a very potent agonist and has been used as basic structure for the development of synthetic agonists. It has a structure very similar to that of GABA, rendered partially rigid by the presence of an isoxazole ring (to be compared with the related acetylcholine/muscarine mentioned above). This is a toxic product, and its toxicity does not originate solely from its gabaergic activity.

Bicuculline and narcotine (noscapine), extracted from opium, are both of vegetable origin(7, 32). The stereoselectivity of the action is great, the (+) bicuculline being much more active than its optical antipode. Picrotoxin (9) is extracted from cocculus indicus, *Anamirta cocculus,* Menispermaceae.

The tritiated GABA agonists and antagonists have been used by many authors to mark the GABA receptor site(4, 32, 44). Muscimol acts on the same population of receptors as GABA, whereas the "binding" of bicuculline reveals a difference in conformation between the sites of antagonist and agonist recognition.

Guidotti et al.(24) acknowledge the existence of two different affinity sites, and Hill and Bowery(26) demonstrate the existence of types of receptors, one sensitive to bicuculline ($GABA_A$), the most widespread, and the other insensitive ($GABA_B$).

The $GABA_A$ receptors alone are associated with chlorine canal and postsynaptics. The $GABA_B$ receptors are thought to have a role in regulation of the other mediators, principally noradrenergic. Picrotoxin would act at the level of the ionophore canal (with Cl^-) of the receptor and not at the level of the site of GABA recognition. Costa(12) showed the association of the GABA receptor with the benzodiazepine receptor which would activate gabaergic transmission by increasing the affinity of the receptors for GABA (competition with GABA-moduline(24), which would be the endogenous ligand of the benzodiazepinic receptor and the regulator of the GABA receptor affinity). Another endogenous ligand, DBI (Diazepam-binding inhibitor), also polypeptidic, would produce effects opposite to those of the benzodiazepines.

Here again, the plant kingdom acts as a source of benzodiazepine antagonists, by producing hallucinogenic and convulsant compounds with a β-carboline framework, encountered in particular in *Peganum harmala* (Zygophyllaceae), *Bannisteria caapi* (Malpighiaceae), *Haemadictyon amazonicum* (Apocynaceae), and serving for preparation of hallucinogenic drinks (Caapi, yagé, ayahuasca). Their actions originate, however, from several mechanisms. The derivatives having the strongest affinity for the benzodiazepines receptor are those which possess an acid, ester, or carboxylic amide residue at position 3 (R = COOH, COOR, CONHR). Substitution at 1 diminishes activity, whereas substitution at 9 annuls it. The development of these series could lead not to other antagonists but to new types of anticonvulsant substances and/or anxiolytics.

Receptors linked to a membranal enzyme

These receptors, thus named by analogy, must rather be considered as groups of specific binding sites.

Receptor for cardiotonic glucosides

The use of digitalis, *Digitalis purpurea*, Scrofulariaceae, was reported at the beginning of the 13th century by a Welsh pharmacopoeia, "Meddygon myddmai". The leaf of the plant was administered either dried and crushed, or in infusions (foxglove tea). But it has mainly been since Withering, two centuries ago, that its usage in cardiac insufficiency (with ascites = dropsy) was systematized, its toxicity recognized. The use of digitalis then spread to Europe and America at the end of the 18th century.

The therapy was highly successful, and the extracts were neither more toxic nor less effective than the glucosides currently pescribed. The substance responsible for the activity of the aqueous extracts had to be gitaloxin, more soluble in water than digitoxin, major constituent.

Their inotropic activity is based on interaction with the Na^+/K^+ pump (Na^+/K^+ ATPase Mg^{++} dependent) of the myocardial cell membrane, resulting in its inhibition, accompanied by a transitory increase in intercellular Ca^{++}. The myocardial ATPase was purified. It is composed of two polypeptide sub-units of approximately 95,000 daltons, of one sub-unit of 55,000 daltons, combined phospholipid and glycoprotein in nature (1/3 of the weight of the enzyme) necessary for activity.

The enzyme occupies the entire thickness of the cellular membrane. Its internal surface includes the hydrolytic site, while the external surface presents the digitalic "receptor" (37, 38). Structure/activity relationship studies(19, 39) show that the total length of the site is 1.9 Angstrom units, that only one of three digitoxin sugars, the one that is linked to genin, is involved; the A/Bcis junction of the genin rings is necessary for activity. The electrostatic potential chart of genin has been determined, showing that it was dipolar. The negative potentials are linked to the butenolide group and to the alcohol functions.

It is the butenolide "head' which is conducted to the interior of the receptor through electrostatic attraction. Hydrophobic interactions are less determinant, since the strength of the bond with ouabaine (extract of Strophanthus gratus, Apocynaceae), much less lipophilic than digitoxin, is identical. All these data agree with a diagram showing the various sites of drug/receptor interaction. The complex formed produces an allostearic effect by rearrangement of the receptor leading to inhibition of the enzyme.

According to Mulvany, there would be interaction at the level of the K+ sites of ATPase, resulting in partial opening of the calcium canals. The existence of two categories of receptor sites has also been demonstrated, both inhibitors, one with weak affinity and the other with strong affinity(18, 33). Is the last responsible for the cardiotoxic activity and the other for toxicity?

These ideas, added to the hypothesis according to which the sodium pumps could, in the normal state, not function at the maximum (since they must be stimulated), allow the suspicion that they may be partially inhibited by an endogenous inhibitor(30). Such a compound has been purified and named cardioginine(20). It is produced in the hypothalamus. Its molecular weight is 431, and it might be sterolic in nature(11, 16, 25). But its exact nature, curiously, is still unknown(46).

PAF receptor

The PAF acether, produced by the eosinophils, the human macrophages, the polymorphonuclears, and the cells of the vascular endothelium, is a phospholipidic ether endowed with potent platelet-aggregating, bronchoconstrictive, and hypotensive activity. Its total synthesis was carried out by Godfroid et al.(21). It seems to act via a hypothetical receptor coupled to a phosphodiesterase inositolphospholipid(29).

This receptor would have hydrophobic interaction sites with the PAF alkyl chain and an oxygen recognition site with which it would enter into an oxonium bond. This site would be sensitive to chiralite at 2 and therefore principally responsible for the activity.

These deductions, resulting from synthesis of numerous PAF derivatives, seem to be corroborated by the antagonistic activity of several compounds related to the lignanes (Kadsurenone), isolated from Piper kadsura, Piperaceae, or from polycyclic lactones (Gingkolide B), isolated from Ginkgo biloba(8, 31).

It is probably occupation of the oxygen receptor site by the furan ring which is responsible for antagonism. Studies directed towards refining the structure of the receptor, to describing precisely the mechanism of action, and thus to developing a new series and establish structure/activity relationships are still in progress.

Conclusion

Whether physiological mediators are discovered before or after natural agonists or antagonists, plants are and always will be a source of varied structures possessing this activity. First used in the form of more or less purified extracts (in which the combined substances sometimes act in a synergistic manner, cf. digitalis), compounds of vegetable origin, in addition to their sometimes unique and irreplacable therapeutic role, would assist in expanding knowledge of the biochemical phenomena involved and will serve as a model for simpler and more easily obtainable synthetic compounds. Study of vegetable extracts may therefore open a way to significant scientific perspectives and help break away from the idea that one must carry out a traditional phytotherapy.

References

1. Alberici G.F., Bidart J.M., Moingeon P., Pailler S., Mondesir J.M., Goodman P.A., Bohuon C.: Ellipticine derivatives intarct with muscarinic receptors. *Biochem. Pharmacol.*, 1985, *34*, 1701-1704.

2. Atlas B., Bustein Y.: Isolation of an endogenous clonidine-displacing substance from rat brain. *Eur. J. Biochem.*, 1984, *144*, 287-293.

3. Baker R.W., Clothia C.H., Pauling P., Petcher T.F.: Structure and activity of muscarinic stimulants. *Nature*, 1971, *230*, 439-445.

4. Beaumont K., Chilton W.S., Yamamura H.I., Enna S.J.: Muscimol binding in rat brain: association with synaptic GABA receptors. *Brain. Res.*, 1978, *148*, 153-162.

5. Birdsall N.J.M., Hulme E.C.: Muscarinic receptor subclasses. *TIPS*, 1983, *4*, 459-463.

6. Bloom F., Battenberg E., Rossier J., Ling N., Guillemin R.: Neurons containing β-endorphin in rat brain exist separately from those containing enkephalin: immunocytochemical studies. *Proc. Nat. Acad. Sci.*, USA, 1978, *75*, 1591.

7. Bowery N.G., Collins J.F., Cryer G., Inch T.D., McLaughlin N.J.: *In:* Gaba-Biochemistry and CNS functions, Mandel P., De Feudis F.V. Eds., *Plenum Press*, 1979, 339.

8. Braquet P., Spinnewyn B., Braquet M., Bourgain R.H., Taylor J.E., Etienne A., Drieu K.: BN 52021 and related compounds: a new series of highly specific PAF-acether receptor antagonists isolated from Ginkgo biloba. *Blood and Vessels*, 1985, *16*, 558-572.

9. Brookes N., Werman R.: The cooperativity of γ aminobutyric action on the membrane of locust muscle fibers. *Mol. Pharmac.*, 1973, *9*, 571-579.

10. Burgermeister W., Klein W.L., Nirenberg M., Witkopf B.: Comparative binding studies with cholinergic ligands and histrionicotoxin at muscarinic receptors of neural cell lines. *Molec. Pharmacol.*, 1978, *14*, 751-767.

11. Cloix J.F., Miller E., Pernollet M.G., Devynck M.A., Meyer P.: Purification d'un inhibiteur endogène de la sodium-potassium-ATPase. *C.R. Acad. Sci.*, 1983, 296, Série III, 231-216.

12. Costa E., Rodbard D., Pert C.: Is the benzodiazepine receptor coupled to a chloride anion channel? *Nature*, 1979, *277*, 315.

13. Cox B.M., Opheim K.E., Teschemacher H., Goldstein A.: A peptide-like substance from pituitary that acts like morphine. I. Isolation. *Life Sci.*, 1975, *16*, 1771-1775.

14. Curtis D.R., Hosli L., Johnston G.A.R., Johnston I.H.: Glycine and spinal inhibition. *Brain Res.*, 1967, 5, 112.

15. Daly J.W.: Adenosine receptors: targets for future drugs. *J. Med. Chem.*, 1982, *25*, 197-207.

16. Delva P., Wauquier I., Devynck M.A.: Chronic salt-loading and circulating inhibitor of renal NA^+, K^+ Atpase in rats. *C.R. Acad. Sci.*, 1984, *299*, Série III, 867-870.

17. Ehlert F.J., Roeske W.R., Yamamura H.K.: Muscarinic cholinergic receptor heterogeneity. *TINS*, 1982, *15*, 336-338.

18. Erdman E., Werdan K., Brown L.: Multiplicity of cardiac glycoside receptors in the heart. *TIPS*, 1985, *6*, 293-295.

19. Fullerton D.S., Griffin J.F., Rohrer D.C., From A.H.L., Ahmed K.: Computers: using computer graphics to study cardiac glycoside-receptor interactions. *TIPS*, 1985, *6*, 279-282.

20. Godfrain R.: Withering 200 years is not enough. *TIPS*, 1985, *6*, 360-363.

21. Godfroid J.J., Heymans F., Michel E., Redeuilh C., Steiner E., Benveniste J.: Platelet activating factor (Paf-acether): Total synthesis of 1-0-Octadecyl 2-0-acetyl SN-Glycero-3-Phosphoryl Choline. *FEBS Letters*, 1980, *116*, 161-164.

22. Goldberg L.I., Komli J.D.: *In:* Apomorphine and other dopaminomimetics, Vol I.: Basic Pharmacology, Gessa G.L., Corsini G.V. Eds., *Raven Press*, New-York, 1981, 273.

23. Grassy C., Bonnafous M., Loiseau P., Adam Y.: Vizualization of molecular electronic effect. *TIPS*, 1985, *6*, 57-59.

24. Guidotti A., Toffano G., Costa E.: An endogenous protein modulates the affinity of GABA and benzodiazepine receptors in rat brain. *Nature*, 1978, *275*, 553-555.

25. Henning G., Cloix J.J.: Chromatographie d'affinité pour la détection d'un inhibiteur endogène humain de la Na$^+$K$^+$ ATPase. *C.R., Acad. Sci.*, 1983, 297, Série III, 295-298.

26. Hill D.R., Bowery N.G.: ^{3}H-baclofen and ^{3}H-GABA blind to biuculline insensitive GABAH$_B$ sites in rat brain. *Nature*, 1981, *290*, 149-152.

27. Hughes J., Smith T.W., Kosterlitz H.W., Fothergill L.A., Morgan B.A., Morris H.R.: Identification of two related pentapeptides from the brain with potent opiate agonist activity. *Nature*, 1975, *258*, 577.

28. Johnston G.A.R.: *In:* GABA in nervous system function, Roberts E., Chase T.N., Tower D.B. Eds., *Raven Press*, New-York, 1976, 395.

29. Katz A.M., Franck M.D., Messineo C., Herbette L.: Ion channels in membranes. *Circulation*, 1982, *65*, 12.

30. La Bella F.S.: Is there an endogenous digitalis ? *TIPS*, 1982, *3*, 354-355.

31. Lachachi H., Plantavid H., Simon M.F., Chap H., Braquet P., Douste-Blazy L.: Inhibition of transmembrane movement and metabolism of platelet activating factor (PAF-acether) by a specific antagonist, B N 52021. *Biochem. Biophy. Res. Commun.*, 1985, *132*, 460-466.

32. Mohler H., Okada T.: Properties of gamma-aminobutyric acid receptor binding with (+)-^{0}3H bicuculline methiodide in rat cerebellum. *Mol. Pharmacol.*, 1978, *14*, 256-265.

33. Noël F., Godfraind T.: Heterogeneity of Ouabain specific binding sites and Na$^+$K$^+$-atpase inhibition in microsomes from rat heart. *Biochem. Pharmacol.*, 1984, *33*, 47-53.

34. Pauling P., Datta N.: Anticholinergic substances a single consistent conformation, *Proc. Nat. Acad. Sci. U.S.A.*, 1980, *77*, 708-712.

35. Pert C.B., Snyder S.H.: Opiate receptor: Demonstration in nervous tissu. *Science*, 1973, *179*, 1011-1014.

36. Philipson J.D.: Natural products as a basis for new drugs. *TIPS*, 1979, *1*, 36-38.

37. Repke K.R.H., Dittrich F.: Thermodynamics of information transfer from cardiotonic steroids to receptor transport ATPase. *TIPS*, 1980, *1*, 398-402.

38. Repke K.R.H., Schönfeld W.: Na^+K^+ ATPase as the digitalis receptor. *TIPS*, 1984, *5*, 393-397.

39. Repke K.R.H.: New developments in cardiac glycoside structure-activity relationship. *TIPS*, 1985, *6*, 275-279.

40. Simon E.J., Hiller J.M., Edelman I.: Stereospecific binding of the potent narcotic analgesic (3H), Etorphine to rat-brain homogenate. *Proc. Nat. Acad. Sci. USA*, 1973, *70*, 1947-1949.

41. Stoof J.C., Kebabian J.W.: Two dopamine receptors: biochemistry, physiology and pharmacology. *Life sci.*, 1984, *35*, 2281-2296.

42. Su C.: Purinergic neurotransmission and neuromodulation. *Ann. Rev. Pharmacol. Toxicol.*, 1983, *23*, 397-411.

43. Terenius L.: Stereospecific interaction between narcotic analgesics and a synaptic plasm a membrane fraction of rat cerebral cortex. *Acta Pharmacol. Toxicol.*, 1973, *32*, 317-320.

44. Ticku M.K., Olsen R.W.: Interaction of barbiturates with dihydropicrotoxinin binding sites related to the GABA receptor-ionophore system. *Life Sci.*, 1978, *22*, 1643-1651.

45. Timmermans P.B., Van Zwieten P.A.: Alpha 2 adrenoceptors: classification, localization, mechanisms. *J. Med. Chem.*, 1982, *25*, 1389-1401.

46. Wilkins M.R.: Endogenous digitalis: a review of the evidence. *TIPS*, 1985, *6*, 286-288.

47. Wood P.L.: Multiple opiate receptors: support for unique mu, delta and kappa sites. *Neuropharmacology*, 1982, *21*, 487-497.

Preparation and Definition of Ginkgo Biloba Extract

K. Drieu

Centre de Recherche I.H.B. - I.P.S.E.N., 17, Avenue Descartes. F 92350 Le Plessis Robinson

Summary

Ginkgo biloba extract is a well-defined and complex product prepared from green leaves of Ginkgo biloba. The leaves are harvested from trees growing in plantations in South Korea, Japan, and France. The mode of culture, harvesting, and extraction are perfectly standardized and controlled. Analysis of Ginkgo biloba extract makes it possible to confirm that undesirable substances have been eliminated and to measure the amount of active principles. The extract contains flavonoid substances, such as the Ginkgo-flavone glycosides and terponoids which are characteristic of Ginkgo and have a unique structure (ginkgolides, bilobalide).

Nature is an inspired "chemical engineer" whose creations should be exploited, but the quality of a vegetable extract and the consistency of its composition depend upon the rigor observed in all stages of its production, from culture of the trees up to the finished product.

Culture and Harvest

The still green leaves of Ginkgo biloba are harvested in Japan and in South Korea from plantation trees. For two years, most of the leaves necessary for fabrication of the extract have been harvested in a plantation located near Bordeaux. From production sites in both France and in the Far East, an agrocultural engineer permanently manages the plantations, the harvest conditions, drying and preparation of the bales for transport. He controls the use of fertilizers and absence of chemical treatment of the plants. The leaves are picked green, at the most favorable period, determined on the basis of the results from assays of the principal constituents in the leaves. The harvested leaves are dried as collected, in a programmed temperature dryer, and lose 3/4 of their weight in water. Then they are pressed into bales so as to prevent any reentry of humidity and risk of fermentation.

The leaves are shipped, stored, and treated at the factory for production of extract.

Rökan (Ginkgo Biloba). Recent Results in Pharmacology and Clinic
Edited by E.W. Fünfgeld
© Springer-Verlag Berlin Heidelberg New York 1988, pp. 32-36

Fabrication of the Ginkgo biloba extract

The factory producing Ginkgo biloba extract (EGb 761), meets the standards of the Food and Drug Administration.

The dried leaves are subjected to a continuous extraction process with an acetone-water mixture, under partial vacuum. After elimination of the organic solvent, several successive treatment phases make it possible, first, to eliminate useless or undesirable substances, and, second, to concentrate the extract of active principles. The final phase of the process consists of continuous evaporation of the concentrated extract solution in a microwave tunnel oven.

Analytical control of the finished Ginkgo biloba extract includes an ensemble of determinations which make it possible to assure the consistency of the composition and the quality of the manufacture. Absence of the solvents used and of their possible degradation products is verified, as well as the absence of manufacturing adjuvants. Investigation for undesirable products which must be eliminated during the extraction process is carried out, and verification is performed by two-dimensional thin-layer chromatography and high-pressure liquid chromatography for the presence of constituents in the extract, which is thus "calibrated" by comparison with a reference extract. Assays of the primary constituents in the active principles are carried out.

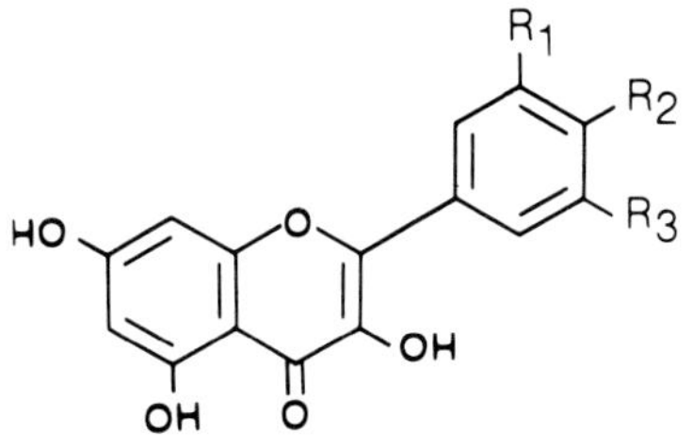

	R_1	R_2	R_3
KAEMPFEROL	H	OH	H
QUERCETINE	OH	OH	H
ISORHAMNETINE	OCH_3	OH	H

Figure 1: The structure of aglycones from Ginkgo-flavone glucosides (flavonols).

Chemical composition

Ginkgo biloba extract contains two classes of major components, flavonoids and terpenes.

Flavonoid substances

Ginkgo biloba extract is standardized at 24% flavonoid glycosides (ginkgo-flavone glucosides). These are compounds whose aglycone is a flavonol (quercetine, kaempferol, or in a smaller concentration, isorhamnetine) (*Figure 1*). These are monoglucosides or diglucosides, the glucosidic constituents of which are glucose and rhamnose.

There are thus several groups of three glycosides, with quercetine, kaempferol, or isorhamnetine as aglycone. At the end of unpublished studies (1980), some chemists of our group isolated and established the structure of a group of characteristic Ginkgo biloba glycosides. Mass spectrometry and proton and carbon 13 nuclear magnetic resonance analyses made it possible to identify coumaric esters of quercetine and of kaempferol glucorhamnoside, the structures of which are indicated in *Figure 2*. These two substances are quantitatively the most important in the group of glycosides.

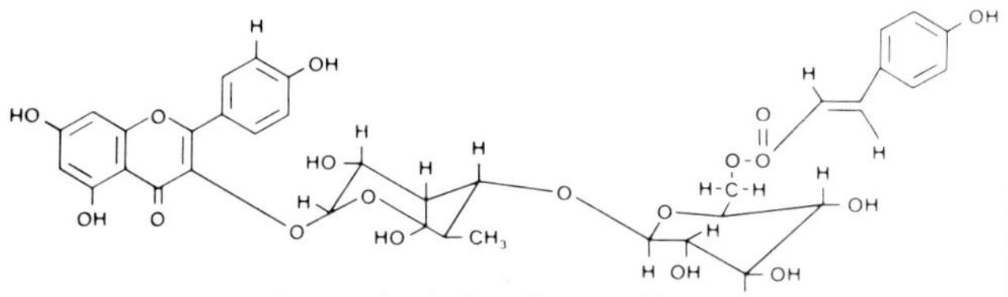

1. Coumaric ester of kaempferol glucorhamnoside

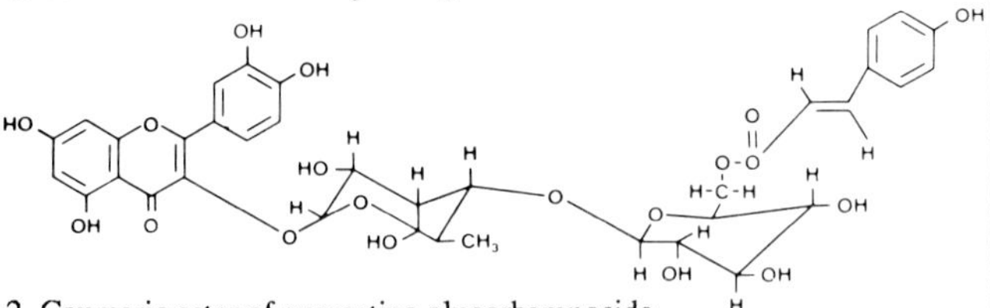

2. Coumaric ester of quercetine glucorhamnoside

Figure 2: Characteristic glycosides of Ginkgo biloba extract: (1) coumaric ester of kaempferol glucorhamnoside; (2) coumaric ester of quercetine glucorhamnoside.

In addition to ginkgo-flavone glucosides, Ginkgo biloba extract contains proanthocyanidines in more or less condensed form (dimers or polymers). The base elements of these proanthocyanidines are ionized flavonols, delphinidine and cyanidine.

The biosynthesis of flavonoids by the plant is accomplished in the course of primary metabolism, from "acetate units" and a phenylpropanoic intermediate(1). Condensation of these various elements is mediated by enzymatic reactions. This origin was determined by use of tagged precursor products, and it is necessary to compare these observations with the study of distribution of tagged Ginkgo biloba extract in animals: we have actually obtained a Ginkgo biloba extract, the flavonols of which were tagged with ^{14}C by incorporation of ^{14}C acetate into twigs cultivated in phytotron(3).

Terpene substances

A group of diterpenes, the ginkgolides, and a sesquiterpene, bilobalide, are the compounds which give Ginkgo biloba extract its bitterness (*Figure 3*). Isolated first from the roots, but also present in the leaves, their structures were determined by the studies of Japanese investigators(2, 4). These substances possess an extremely novel structure, encountered until the present only in Ginkgo biloba. The spatial representation of ginkgolides gives the molecule the form of a "cage" they possess three lactone functions and a tertiary butyl group, unique in the vegetable kingdom. The three ginkgolides present in Ginkgo biloba extract (GKA, GKB, GKC) differ by the presence of 1, 2, or 3 hydroxyl functions. Bilobalide is also a trilactone possessing a tertiary butyl group. The biosynthesis of ginkgolides by the plant was studied by measuring the incorporation of tagged precursors after their addition into the culture medium. The incorporation of ^{14}C-mevalonate led to the terpenoic structure of the ginkgolides, and the incorporation of ^{14}C-methionine explains the formation of the tertiary butyl group(5). These substances, which are remarkably specific for Ginkgo biloba, are extracted from leaves when the extract is prepared and represent 6% of it.

Other constituents in the extract

Other less novel substances are included in the composition of the extract, in particular a certain number of organic acids (hydroxykinurenic, kinurenic, protocatechic, p-hydroxybenzoic, vanillic, etc.). These substances give the extract an acidic character and play a role in its water solubility. It is, in fact, interesting to note that the different active principles, flavonoids and terpenes, are insoluble in water, but that the chemical environment in which they exist in the Ginkgo biloba extract makes them soluble.

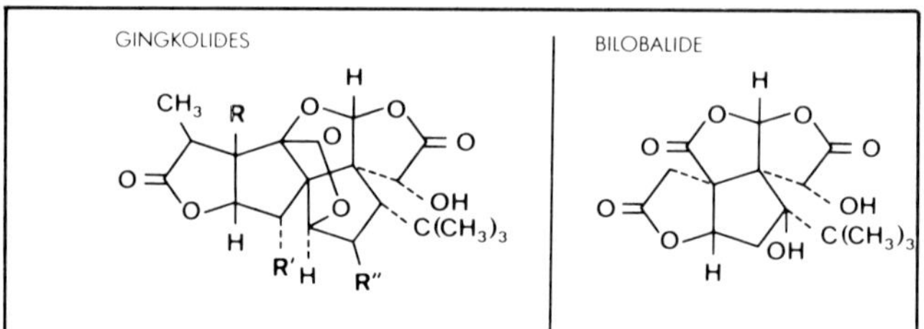

	R	R'	R"
GINGKOLIDE A	OH	H	H
GINGKOLIDE B	OH	OH	H
GINGKOLIDE C	OH	OH	OH

Figure 3: Terpenes (ginkgolides, bilobalide).

References

1. Halbrock K., Grisebach H.: Biosynthesis of Flavonoïds. *In:* The Flavonoïds, Harborne J.B., Mabry T.J., Mabry H. Eds., *Chapmann and Hall,* 1975, 866-915.

2. Maruyama M., Terahara A., Itagaki Y., Nakanishi K.: The Ginkgolides. *Tetrahedron letters,* 1967, *4,* 299-319.

3. Moreau J.P., Eck C.R., McCabe J., Skinner S.: Absorption, distribution et élimination de l'extrait marqué de feuilles de Ginkgo biloba chez le rat. *Presse Méd.,* 1986, *15,* 1458-1481.

4. Nakanishi K., Habagushi K., Nakadaira Y., Wood M.C., Mariyama M.: Structure of bilobalide, a rare tertbutyl containing sesquiterpenoid related to the C20 ginkgolides. *J. Am. Chem. Soc.,* 1971, *93,* 3544-3546.

5. Nakanishi K.: Biosynthesis of Ginkgolide B, its diterpenoid nature and origine of the tertbutyl group. *J. Am. Chem. Soc.,* 1971, *93,* 3546-3547.

Absorption, Distribution, and Excretion of Tagged Ginkgo Biloba Leaf Extract in the Rat

J.P. Moreau, C.R. Eck, J. McCabe, S. Skinner

Biomeasure, Hopkinton, Massachussetts, U.S.A.

Summary

The absorption, distribution and elimination of a radiolabelled ^{14}C extract prepared from Ginkgo biloba leaves have been studied in rats. Following oral administration, expired ^{14}C-CO_2 represented 16% of the administered dose excreted within the first 3 hours post-dose out of a total of 38% after 72 hours. An additional 21% of the administered dose was eliminated in the urine. The absorption of the radiolabelled Ginkgo biloba extract was at least 60%.

The pharmacokinetics of the drug, based on blood specific activity data versus time course, were characteristic of a two-compartment model with an apparent first-order phase and a biological half-life of approximately 4.5 h.

During the first 3 hours, radioactivity was primarily associated with the plasma, but through a gradual uptake after 48 h. The specific activity in erythrocytes matched that of plasma. A site of absorption in the upper gastrointestinal tract is suspected since specific activity in blood peaked after 1.5 hours. Glandular and neuronal tissues and eyes showed a high affinity for the labelled substance. These results provide the first tentative link between the therapeutic effectiveness of Ginkgo biloba extract and the biological fate of some of its constituents.

The preparation of an extract from Ginkgo biloba leaves, according to a patented process, yields a complex mixture of substances including terpenes, proanthocyanidines, and flavonoid glycosides. The therapeutic use of Ginkgo biloba extract (EGb 761, Rökan®, Intersan) in treatment of vascular and cerebral disorders is well established.

However, no precise information concerning the biological fate of the principal constituents of EGb could be obtained up to the present because of methodological difficulties. The realization of a radioactive extract tagged with ^{14}C has made it possible to study absorption, distribution, and excretion of the product administered orally in the rat.

Rökan (Ginkgo Biloba). Recent Results in Pharmacology and Clinic
Edited by E.W. Fünfgeld
© Springer–Verlag Berlin Heidelberg New York 1988, pp. 37-45

Material and Methods

Study product

The tagged substance was prepared from leaves from branches of Ginkgo biloba placed in a phytotron at the University of Heidelberg and growing in a synthetic medium enriched with ^{14}C-acetate. An extract was prepared from these leaves according to a process similar to the industrial process. The extract had a specific radioactivity of 0.23 µCi/mg.

Animals, treatment, collection of samples

Male and female Sprague-Dawley rats (230-290 g), fasted for 16 hours, received by intubation approximately 20 µCi of ^{14}C-EGb in suspension (or 380 mg/kg).

Drinking water was supplied *ad libitum* and they received nourishment three hours after administration of the product.

Three groups of rats, I, II, and III, were sacrificed at 72, 48, and 3 hours respectively.

The rats were placed individually in metabolism cages. The urine and feces were collected at the following time intervals: 0-3, 3-6, 6-12, 12-24, 24-48, and 48-72 hours. The expired carbon dioxide was collected on appropriate material.

The blood samples were collected by an incision of the caudal vein at the following times: 0, 0.25, 0.50, 0.75, 1, 1.5, 3, 6, 12, 24, and 48 hours.

After the last samplings, the rats were sacrificed, the principal organs removed, dissected, and washed in physiological serum. The following organs were removed: Central Nervous System: cerebral cortex, hippocampus, striated body, hypothalamus, mesencephalon, brain stem, cerebellum, spinal cord; Cardiovascular System: aorta, portal vein, heart, lungs, kidneys; Gastrointestinal Tract: stomach, small and large intestines, liver; Eyes: crystalline lens, vitreous humor, retina; Endocrine System: thyroid, adrenal glands, spleen, gonads; Skeletal Muscles (quadriceps, femoral); Skin; Carcass.

Measurement of radioactivity

The liquid and solid samples were handled according to the procedure published by Mahin and Lofber(3) for liquid scintigraphy counting in a Packard 300 D spectrophotometer. All of the samples were analyzed twice. Counting was done in comparison with an external reference, using a calibration curve. A control was used for each type of tissue removed from the control animals. The results were processed by computer in order to calculate the percentage of dose administered in each sample, expressed as equivalents of tagged substance administered.

Results

Balance of urinary, fecal, and respiratory elimination

The respiratory route represents a significant route of elimination, on the order of 16%, during the first three hours. In Group I (72 hours), the radioactivity eliminated in the form of ^{14}C-CO_2 (38%) exceeds that excreted in the urine (21.7%) and the feces (29.4%); only 2.55% of the dose was found in the tissue and carcass samples after 72 hours, a negligible portion of which was in the gastrointestinal tract. *Figure 1* represents the distribution of total radioactivity at the three sampling times.

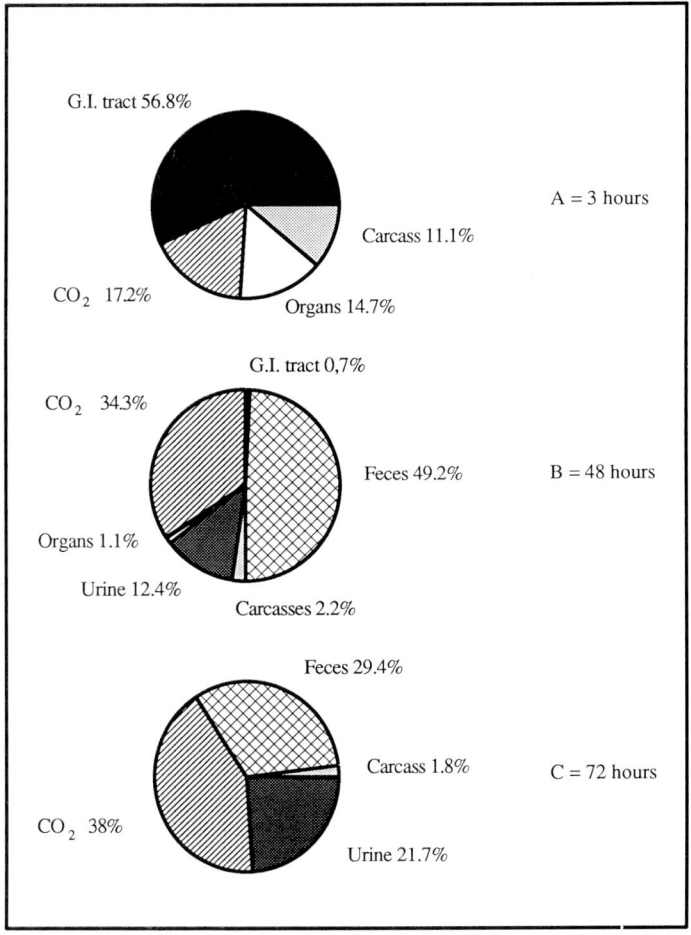

Figure 1: Distribution of ^{14}C-EGb administered orally in the rat. Tissue retention and respiratory, urinary, and fecal elimination.

Excretion profile

Exhalted CO_2: the results obtained for Group I show that the maximal quantity of
$^{14}C\text{-}CO_2$ was exhaled during the first three hours, and elimination was practically
completed at 12 hours. In the first approximation, these values correspond to a
one-compartment model with a regression coefficient of 0.927. The elimination
constant is 0.105 hours, and the biological half-life is 6.5 hours. Fecal and urinary
excretion: in Groups I and II, no feces were collected between 0 and 12 hours,
intestinal transit having been slowed because of the large dose administered(5). The
largest quantity of radioactivity eliminated fecally was from 12 to 24 hours (*Figure*
2). The elimination constant (0.097 h $^{-1}$) from urinary excretion in Groups I and II
corresponds to a biological half-life of 7 hours.

Renal clearance: calculated from the cumulative curve of the equivalents excreted
in the urine and in the area under the blood concentration curve as a function of time,
renal clearance was estimated at 7.9 L/hour.

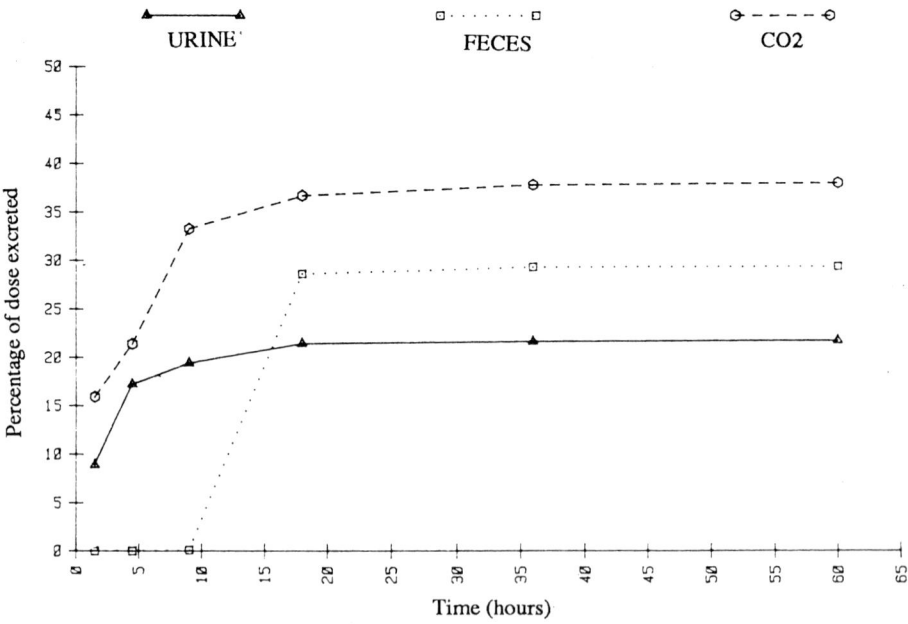

Figure 2: Respiratory, urinary, and fecal excretion in a rat treated with Ginkgo biloba
extract orally (380 mg/kg).

Blood pharmacokinetics

The blood pharmacokinetics of the radioactivity expressed as nanoequivalents of Ginkgo biloba extract administered corresponds to the characteristics of a two-compartment model with an absorption phase on the order of 1.

The low number of samples (six from 0 to 3 hours and four from 6 to 48 hours) makes it possible to establish a rather precise profile of the curve from 0 to 6 hours, but approximate for the second part (6 to 48 hours).

In addition, the values measured represent the overall ^{14}C radioactivity, and the exchanges between the metabolites of the tagged substances with the biological constituents increase the life duration of the blood radioactivity.

A first radioactivity peak is observed at 1.30 hours (Tmax) with a mean concentration of 22.5 nEq/mg of blood (Cmax). After decreasing with a minimum observed at 6 hours, a second peak is observed at 12 hours (12.8 nEq/mg), perhaps related to the existence of an enterohepatic cycle or to absorption of the metabolites formed by enzymatic hydrolysis by the intestinal flora. The half-life measured graphically on the curve from 0 to 6 hours has a value of approximately 4 1/2 hours.

Tissue distribution (Figure 3)

The tissue samples were taken from Groups III, II, and I, at 3, 48, and 72 hours after treatment, times selected so as to correspond closely to the time of maximum blood level, the middle of the excretion phase, and the end of the study.

As anticipated for a plant extract containing numerous constituents, radioactivity was broadly but not uniformly distributed. The tissues which show a more rapid rate of elimination than that observed in the plasma are the stomach and the small intestine. The high specific radioactivity measured at three hours in these two organs suggests that they constitute the principal site of absorption. The radioactivity in the large intestine, carcass, and kidneys, was eliminated at a rate identical to that of the plasma. It decreased more slowly in the liver and whole blood.

The tissues presenting a distinctly lower specific activity than that of the plasma are the cerebral cortex, the mesencephalon, the brain stem, the cerebellum, the erythrocytes, and the muscles. The spinal cord, vitreous humor, retina, gonads, spleen, lungs, heart, and skin retained the radioactivity in a manner equivalent to that of the plasma. Finally, the hippocampus, the striated body, the hypothalamus, the crystalline lens, the thyroid, the adrenal glands, and the portal vein retain and concentrate radioactivity.

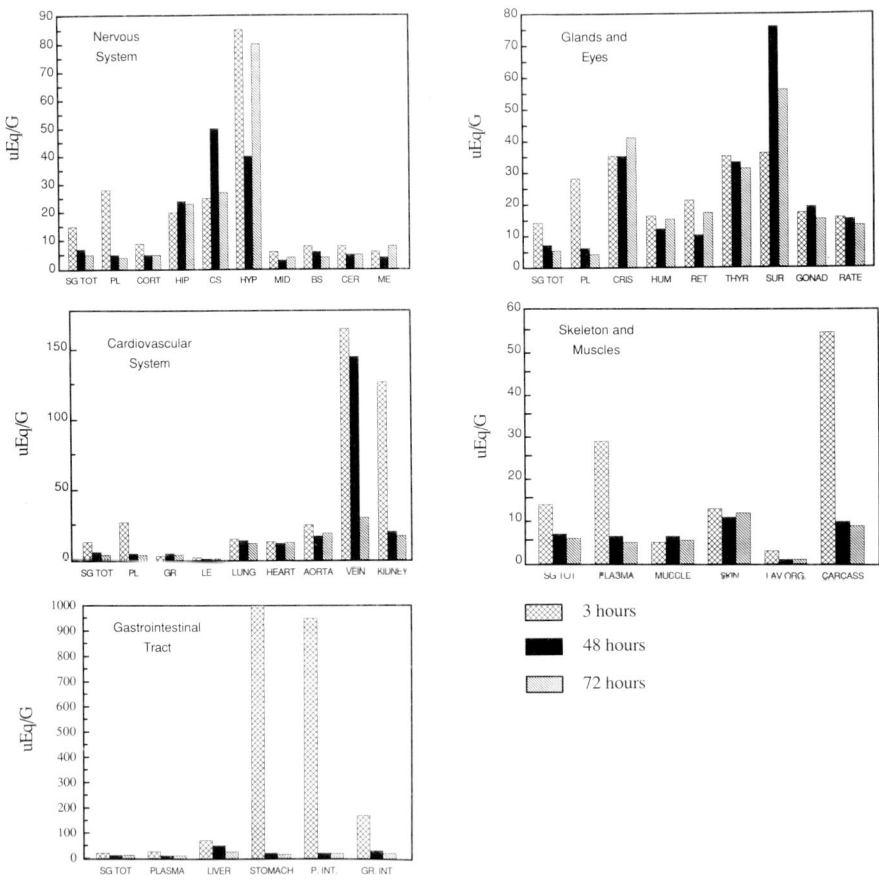

Figure 3: Distribution of radioactivity in the tissues and organs after administration of ¹⁴C-EGb. Abbreviations: total blood, SG TOT; plasma, PL; cerebral cortex, CORT; hippocampus, HIP; striated body, CS; hypothalamus, HYP; mesencephalon, MID; brain stem, BS; cerebellum, CER; spinal cord, ME; crystalline lens, CRIS; vitreous humor, HUM; retina, RET; thyroid, THYR; adrenal glands, SUR; erythrocytes, GR; erythrocyte lavage, LE; small intestine, P.INT.; large intestine, GR.INT.

Discussion

Studies of absorption, distribution, and excretion of EGb were made difficult by technical difficulties related to biosynthesis of tagged extract. The analytical study of tagged extract showed that the ^{14}C radioactivity was not uniformly distributed among the various constituents of the extract. The incorporation of the radioactivity in the Ginkgo biloba extract originating from ^{14}C-acetate took place principally in the constituents which originated from the biosynthesis depending on the acetate route: in this case, some flavonoids which are represented in EGb by two groups of constituents, the flavonoid glycosides and the proanthocyanidines. No radioactivity was found in the terpenes, nor in the principal sugars after hydrolysis of the glycosides. Despite these limitations, the administration of tagged EGb made it possible to gain access to the fate of the extract in the body. Because of the small quantity of tagged product available and the relatively weak incorporation of ^{14}C, this test was limited to three groups of two rats sacrificed at 3 hours, 48 hours, and 72 hours after oral administration of 20 µCi (380 mg/kg) of extract.

The CO_2 expired during the first three hours represents 16% of the dose administered, and 38% after 72 hours. In fact, at 12 hours, respiratory elimination was practically completed. The biological half-life for the ^{14}C-CO_2 was 6.5 hours. Parallely, the quantity of ^{14}C excreted in the urine represents 21% of the dose. Consequently, absorption of the tagged EGb can be estimated at 60%.

Blood radioactivity as a function of time corresponds to a two-compartment model with a first-order absorption phase. The relatively small number of blood samples makes it possible to observe a maximum concentration peak (Cmax) at 1.5 hours and to measure a biological half-life of approximately 4.5 hours. The existence of a second blood concentration peak at 12 hours suggests the existence of an enterohepatic cycle or absorption of flavonoid metabolites after enzymatic fission by the intestinal flora.

According to the results obtained by measuring distribution in the tissues, blood radioactivity is principally associated with the plasma during the first three hours, but through progressive uptake in the erythrocytes, it is equilibrated at 48 hours between erythrocytes and plasma. These observations show both similarities with and differences from the results obtained by Harmand and Blanquet(1), who examined the biological fate of flavonoid oligomer (OFT) extracts of *Vitis vinifera*, in the rat.

After intravenous injection of tagged OFT, elimination of the radioactivity from the cellular compartment is slower than that from the central compartment. In the case of ^{3}H-Diosmine, a flavonoid glycoside, a slow decrease in radioactivity in the general circulation has been reported(4). The existence of an enterohepatic cycle has been suggested to explain the slow clearance of the radioactive product transported in the blood after intravenous injection of ^{14}C-OFT or of ^{3}H-Diosmine. In the case of Diosmine, there is the possibility of isotopic exchange of tritium with water, which would modify the metabolic situation, and, in the case of OFT, the erythrocytes and the liver would be the compartments limiting the excretion rate.

From our study, a single absorption site may be suspected, because of the delay in appearance of a maximum peak at 1 hour or 1.5 hours, although a second maximum might perhaps be discerned at 12 hours.

However, the large dose of EGb (380 mg/kg) can slow gastrointestinal transit and disturb absorption, which may be corroborated by the absence of feces during the first 12 hours(5). The rapid appearance of radioactivity in the blood following oral administration of EGb suggests that the gastric mucosa and, to a lesser degree, the jejunum and ileum are the absorption sites, without taking into consideration the existence of an enterohepatic cycle, which has not been identified. Retention and possible concentration of radioactivity in compartments with high affinity and weak metabolic activity can explain the slow elimination from the blood.

The decrease in specific activity in the liver is approximately one third slower than that estimated for the plasma. This suggests a limiting effect in the liver perhaps because of biotransformation of phenolic compounds into sulfo-conjugates or glycuro-conjugates. The renal clearance rate is identical to that of the plasma, with nevertheless four times higher concentration of radioactivity. Thus the kidneys are not a limiting factor for elimination, although retaining tagged substances, perhaps through affinity for the rich renal vascular bed.

An affinity of tagged substances has been observed for organs rich in conjunctive tissues, such as the aorta, the skin, and the lungs. Similar fixation has been reported with OFT by Harmand and Blanquet, but the specific activity here does not show a peak as for these authors. Nevertheless, in these tissues, the radioactivity is two or three times higher than that in the plasma and decreases little over the course of time. The distribution profile in the portal vein shows significant accumulation (20 times the plasma level) maintained for 48 hours, followed by rapid decrease. In the heart, specific activity retained is twice that retained in the skeletal muscles.

Glandular and nerve tissues and eyes show a strong affinity. In the cerebral cortex, the brain stem, and the cerebellum, the radioactivity level is low in comparison with the hippocampus and the striated bodies, which show at 72 hours radioactivity five times greater than that of the plasma. Fixation in the hypothalamus is even higher. This selective fixation in certain cerebral areas is similar to results from the circulation improvement observed after ischemia due to embolization in the rat(2).

As a whole, these results supply a first test of the relationships between therapeutic efficacy of EGb and the biological fate of its constituents.

References

1. Harmand M.F., Blanquet P.: The fate of total flavonolic oligomers (OFT) extracted from "Vitis vinifera L." in the rat. *Eur. J. Drug Met. Pharma.,* 1978, *1,* 15-30.

2. Le Poncin-Lafitte M.C., Rapin J., Rapin J.R.: Effects of Ginkgo biloba on changes induced by quantitative cerebral microembolization in rats. *Arch. Int. Pharmacodyn,* 1980, *243,* 236-244.

3. Mahin D., Lofber R.: A simplified method of sample preparation for determination of Tritium, Carbon-14, or Sulfur-35 in blood or tissue by liquid scintillation counting. *Anal. Biochem.,* 1966, *16,* 500.

4. Oustrin J., Fauran M.J., Commanay L.: A pharmacokinetic study of ^{3}H-Diosmin. *Arzneim. Forsch./Drug Research,* 1977, *27,* 1688-1691.

5. Viswanathan S., Thirugnama P., Bapna J.A., Kameswaran: Flavonoïd-induced delay in the small intestinal transit: possible mechanism of action. *Arch. Int. Pharmacodyn,* 1984, *270,* 151-157.

PHARMACOLOGY

Is There a Pharmacological Model of Aging?

Y. Christen

IPSEN. 30, Rue Cambronne. F 75015 Paris

Summary

The development of experimental models to study general or cerebral ageing comes up against great obstacles of a methodological nature. However, due to recent progress, tests can already be made on theoretical or even global models. As for Alzheimer's disease for which no natural animal model is known, new studies which involve surgical or chemical destruction of the cholinergic pathways leading to the cortex seem to be particularly promising for a better comprehension of degenerative processes in the neo-cortex.

When the center of gravity of the age pyramid tends to alter at the expense of the youngest fractions of the population, the study of aging becomes a priority which is both sociological and medical.

From the experimental standpoint, understanding aging, and the study of possible therapeutic methods capable of influencing it, present particular difficulties: difficulty in maintaining animals throughout their life span and difficulty in applying to man (notably because of individual differences) the results obtained.

The problem can nevertheless be the subject of certain approaches which are of two types: direct studies of the elderly subject or of a model of aging, or theoretical studies as a function of various hypotheses of the mechanisms of senescence.

Aging Models

Hypothesis of the mechanisms of senescence

There are numerous theories about aging which are not mutually exclusive(6, 12).

Genetic hypotheses

The existence of genetic programming establishing life span is at least probable. It is this which probably accounts for the fact that the maximal duration of life of humans is about 120 years.

Rökan (Ginkgo Biloba). Recent Results in Pharmacology and Clinic
Edited by E.W. Fünfgeld
© Springer–Verlag Berlin Heidelberg New York 1988, pp. 49-56

Very sensitive to certain agents which accelerate aging, particularly radiation, DNA is naturally protected from degradation by repairing enzymes which are absent in certain diseases (this is the case with *Xeroderma pigmentosum*).

Evolutionist hypotheses

It is logical to think that the force of natural selection decreases with age. Having gone beyond their reproductive period, living beings "are no longer involved" in this essential mechanism of evolution.

Immunological hypotheses

The very early involution of the thymus, the fact that elderly subjects frequently become victims of infectious diseases and of changes in the activity of the cells implicated in immune reactions, particularly the T-lymphocytes(8), plead strongly in flavor of these hypotheses. However it is still difficult to say to what extent these changes constitute causes of senescence(4).

Physiological and hormonal hypotheses

Abundant data (for example, the fact that early ablation of the hypophysis is accompanied, in rats receiving a steroid supplement, by an increase in life span) suggest that the hypothalamus and hypophysis could function as a veritable clock, intervening not only in growth and sexual maturation, but also in aging.

The hormonal hypotheses are only several of the physiological hypotheses of senescence.

Cellular hypotheses

The discovery by Léonard Hayflick of the fact that culture cells divide only a limited number of times largely contributed to launching experimental gerontology. It has been shown that this number of cellular divisions was even lower when the age of the cell donor was high. It is also reduced in diseases accompanying early aging (progeria, mongolism, etc.). These discoveries obviously fit very well with the hypotheses indicating intervention of genetic programming for aging.

Hypothesis of the succession of errors

In 1963, Orgel postulated the hypothesis according to which an accumulation of errors among the principal proteins of the organism could be the major factor responsible for aging. It now seems that the errors are less frequent than was then supposed.

Free radicals hypothesis

This biochemical hypothesis should be considered separately, since it currently has strong support(11). The free radicals, because of their great chemical appetite, attack the principal cellular constituents: membranes, nucleic acids, and macroproteins of the cytoplasm. These are in theory good candidates for life attrition agents.

Certain experiments suggest that treatments with free radical scavengers could increase the length of existence and that there would be a relationship between the level of superoxide dismutase, the cellular enzyme trapping the superoxide radical, and the life expectancy of each species(5).

Can we hope to act on aging?

Most of the various hypotheses which we have just examined suggest that there is no hope. In reality, all of them contain a theoretical possibility for manipulation.

Genetic and evolutionist hypotheses

Although genes contribute to establishing life expectancy, it is through the intermediary of the synthesis of certain proteins. We could therefore in theory hope to manipulate either the genes in question directly, or the proteins which they synthesize (finding, for example, inhibitors linked specifically to the receptor at the level at which they act).

Immunological hypotheses

Immunomanipulation is already a reality. The use of interleukines or of other mediators exerting an effect on the immune mechanism could therefore contribute to manipulation of aging.

Physiological hypotheses

The fact that ablation of the hypophysis, accompanied by the administration of potent steroids, increase life expectancy, clearly inicates the possibility for mani-pulation in this field.

Also, nutrition would exert a considerable effect on life expectancy. A slightly deficient diet has made it possible to notably increase the life duration of the rat. A moderate decrease in temperature would exert the same effect.

Biochemical hypotheses

Among these hypotheses, it is those relating to the free radicals which give the best possibility of a therapeutic approach. In fact, we know of several substances capable of scavenging free radicals (one of which is Ginkgo biloba extract).

It appears that all of the hypotheses relative to the mechanisms of senescence accommodate, at least theoretically, the possibility of therapeutic intervention.

Study models

Global study models

The most directly usable model is that consisting of studying animals throughout their lives(3). Thus it has been possible to show that subnutrition(16), the use of substances scavenging free radicals(8), or thermal modifications may increase the mean life duration. Although apparently easy to interpret, studies of this type encounter various methodological problems. Thus, since sub-nutrition increases the duration of life, the use of products which decrease food consumption could exert an indirect effect. It is therefore necessary to verify that the treated animals consume as much food as the control group animals.

Another drawback concerns the long duration of the experiments to be undertaken, which practically prohibits any possibility of exhaustive screening, at least on the usual small laboratory animals: mice live for two years, rats for three years, and guinea pigs for eight years. It is possible to use strains of rats or mice genetically selected for their short life expectancy. Toshio Takeda and his co-workers thus obtained a strain of mice presenting with a 100% incidence of amyloidosis as early as six months of age, and another with a 70% rate of cataracts at 16 months, as well as, in an overall manner, a 26% decrease in life expectancy in comparison with a series of animals qualified as senescence-resistant(13).

It is also possible to use very different animal species with very brief life spans: amoeba, paramecia, worms (nematodes in particular), fruit flies, ants, wasps, bees, and fish with a short life span (in particular *Cynolebias bellottii* of Brazil), sparrows, etc. But the problem is obviously that, generally speaking, the shorter the life span, the less similar the animal species is to us, and the more difficult will be the evaluation of a possible therapeutic benefit.

In vitro models

Cell culture (fibroblasts, but also hepatocytes and lymphocytes) constitutes a model of choice, but more in order to study the mechanisms of senescence or the metabolism of drugs as a function of age or of pathological condition of the donor than their impact on overall aging.

Theoretical models

These are those which directly concern the various hypotheses of senescence and not, strictly speaking, aging. Thus various models studying the scavenging of free radicals could be considered as approaches for the study of the impact of a product on aging.

Models of cerebral aging

Cerebral aging, and particularly Alzheimer's disease, are currently the subject of many studies oriented both toward understanding the mechanisms of the pathological processes responsible and to develop possible therapies.

Overall study models

There is no model reproducing senile dementia of Alzheimer type in animals. The injection of aluminum induces the formation of neurofibrillar structures(10) in rabbits, which are similar to those found in the patient, but the filaments are not twinned exactly as in the case of Alzheimer's disease, likewise the administration of alcohol, whereas the scrapie virus agent induces in the cortex of mice the appearance of plaques similar to human senile plaques. But the meaning of these observations is still difficult to interpret, since these models seem rather distant from clinical reality. The transplantion of the cortex of subjects suffering with Alzheimer's disease into a rat occipital cortex would produce changes more in keeping with the situation in man, but without constituting an easily usable model(14).

Behavioral studies

Behavioral changes in the elderly animal have been the subject of very numerous studies, in particular with respect to the capacities for memorization in the aging rat. As in man, the situation appears to be less simple than was previously thought: the decline in memorization capacities is not as dramatic as anticipated, and only certain components of animal intelligence seem to be affected(9).

More recently, studies conducted on a simple animal memorization model, the marine mollusk *Aplysia,* also have demonstrated an evolution of memorization with age which is similar to that noted in mammals. It would therefore be feasible to test drugs on this animal(2).

Biochemical studies

The biochemical abnormalities observed in the elderly human subject are found in all aging rodents. This is true for changes involving nucleic acids, proteins, particularly those in the glial cells, the metabolism of catecholamines, and in a more debatable manner, for the effect on the cholinergic pathways, the role of which in Alzheimer's disease is often emphasized.

The study of drugs on the receptors and neuromediators, notably in the aged animal, is of obvious value.

In vivo models can combine biochemical and behavioral changes. Recently Flicker et al. showed that performances in passive avoidance tests are considerably modified in the rat after injection of ibotenic acid, which destroys the magnocellular basal nucleus (equivalent in rodents to Meynert's basal nucleus, essential source of cholinergic cerebral innervation in man)(7).

Other studies have shown that the injection of the neurotoxin AF64A, which eliminates acetylcholine at the level of the hippocampal and frontal cortex, considerably modifies the animal performances in the labyrinth test, again emphasizing the relationships between the cholinergic system and the memorization faculties(15). Although it is not completely certain that AF64A affects only the cholinergic system, the use of rats suffering with lesions of the magnocellular basal nucleus may be considered as a valuable model mimicking the lesions of the cholinergic system encountered in Alzheimer's disease(1).

Conclusion

The development of models aimed at testing the effect of a substance on life span or on cerebral aging is hampered by numerous difficulties. Studies involving the entire life span of the animal present, in addition to various methodological obstacles, the disadvantage of a long duration which excludes any possibility of exhaustive screening. The other models are more indirect. As to Alzheimer's disease, there is still no animal model which is strictly identical to it, but certain tests constitute valuable approaches. It appears that the data obtained from basic research warrant new types of approach, for the moment mainly related to the hypotheses relative to the mechanism of general or cerebral aging. The development of more encompassing and easily applicable models seems to be well under way and should constitute a significant advance.

The author thanks Miss Agnes Cordier for her effective collaboration.

References

1. Archer T., Fowler C.J.: Towards an animal model for the cholinergic lesion in Alzheimer's disease. *TIPS*, 1985, *6*, 61.

2. Bailey C.H., Castelluci V.F., Koester J., Chen M.: Behavioral changes in aging Aplysia: a model system for studying the cellular basis of age-impaired learning, memory, and arousal. *Behavioral and Neural Biology*, 1983, *38*, 70-81.

3. Brunaud M.: La gérontologie, Essai d'abord expérimental. *Act. Pharmacol.*, 1971, *24*, 1-26.

4. Christen Y.: Immunologie et vieillissement. *In:* Progressi in geritria, Illuminati L., Riondino G., Scattaretico P. Eds, *Societa Editrice Napoletana*, Naples, 1980, 3-14.

5. Cutler R.G.: Superoxide dismutase, longevity and specific metabolic rate. *Gerontology*, 1983, *29*, 113-120.

6. Cutler R.G.: La biologie du vieillissement et de la longévité. *Gerontologica Biomedica Acta*, 1985, *1*, 7-33.

7. Flicker C., Dean R.L., Watkins D.L., Fisher S.K., Bartus R.T.: Behavioral and neurochemical effects following neurotoxic lesions of a major cholinergic input to the cervical cortex in the rat. *Pharmaco. Biochem. Behav.*, 1983, *18*, 973-981.

8. Hendricks L., Heidrick M.L.: Greater susceptibility of T-cells than B-cells to free radical damage with time. *Gerontologist*, 1983, *23*, (special issue), 248.

9. Ingram D.K.: Analysis of age-related impairments in learning and memory in rodent models. *Ann. N-Y. Acad. Sci.*, 1985, *444*, 312-331.

10. Klatzo I., Wisniewski H., Streicher E.: Experimental production of neurofibrillary degeneration. *J. Neuropath. Exp. Neurol.*, 1965, *24*, 187-199.

11. Pryor W.A.ed.: Free radicals in biology. *Academic Press*, Orlando, 1984.

12. Robert L.: Mécanismes cellulaires et moléculaires du vieillissement. *Masson Ed.*, Paris, 1983.

13. Takeda T., Hosokawa M., Takeshita S., Trino M., Higuchi K., Matsushita T., Tomita Y., Yasuhira K., Hamamoto H., Shimizu K., Ishii M., Yamamuro T.: A new murine model of accelerated senescence. *Mechanisms of Aging and Development*, 1981, *17*, 183-194.

14. Van den Bosch de Aguilar P., Langhendries-Weverberg C., Goemaere-Vanneste J., Flament-Durand J., Brion J.P., Couck A.M.: Transplantation of human cortex with Alzheimer's disease into rat occipital; a model for the study of Alzheimer's disease. *Experienta,* 1984, *40,* 402-403.

15. Walsh T.J., Tilson H.A., DeHaven D.L., Mailman R.B., Fisher A., Hani I.: *Brain Res.,* (in print).

16. Weindruch R., Walford R.L.: Dietary restriction in mice beginning at 1 year of age: effect on life-span and spontaneous cancer incidence. *Science,* 1982, *215,* 1415-1418.

Oxygen Toxicity, Free Radicals, and Defense Mechanisms

C. Deby, J. Pincemail

Laboratoire de Biochimie Appliquée, Unité de Biologie de l'oxygène
Université de Liège. Sart-Tilman, 4000 Liège. Belgique.

Summary

Oxygen is essential for the life of aerobic organisms as the terminal acceptor of electrons. Due to its high affinity for lone electrons it fosters radicalar reactions and opposes recombinations of radicals after rupture of covalent linkages. Lipoperoxydation processes then occur, attacking the cellular membranes. These radicalar reactions are at the origin of many pathological phenomena.

A complex arsenal of endogenous protective agents is normally present in all cells to face up to the danger of lone electron structures in oxygenated media.

Food and natural or synthetic pharmacological agents compensate for the deficiencies.

That oxygen can be toxic is an idea that is difficult to accept, as this element seems to us to be essential for life, and unconditionally beneficial!

Nevertheless, various harmful effects from prolonged exposure to hyperoxic oxygen (100%) have been described: severe retinal lesions in newborns subjected to oxygen therapy for too long a time, the inexorable death of rodents breathing pure oxygen continuously for more than 70 hours.

The principal beneficial effect of oxygen lies in the fact that it is the universal acceptor of electrons, at the end of the cellular respiratory chain. Its deleterious action, when it is manifested, is due to the property of this element for fostering radical reactions occurring within the tissues, while inhibiting the prompt disappearance of undesirable free radicals.

Toxicity of free radicals

Birth of organic free radicals

In the molecules which constitute living matter, the atoms are linked to each other by covalent bonds. This type of linkage is based on the sharing, between neighboring atoms, of electrons with antiparallel spins, which pair up in a particularly stable match.

Rökan (Ginkgo Biloba). Recent Results in Pharmacology and Clinic
Edited by E.W. Fünfgeld
© Springer-Verlag Berlin Heidelberg New York 1988, pp. 57-70

Electronic spin is a vector representing the magnetic field induced by the rotation of the electron, an electrically charged particle. The electronic pairing, basis of covalence, occurs between electrons with opposite spins, which reciprocally cancels their magnetic field. Through an adequate supply of energy (radiant, thermal, or more often chemical), the electronic bond may be broken, and the magnetic field of each "free" electron may be manifested. The molecules or atoms bearing such "free" electrons or *lone* electrons present remarkable paramagnetic properties, but they are very unstable, since they are "impatient" to recouple with their lone electrons. These molecules or atoms with nonpaired electrons are designated by the expression "free radicals".

The avid search for electrons in order to recouple their lone electron and cancel its magnetic field make free radicals formidable aggressors. The electron is most often matched, with the hydrogen atom to which it is electrically linked, to a nearby carbon chain. Rupture of the covalent bond is produced at the level of a carbon atom; the newly formed free radical in its turn starts on the hunt and so on; a chain reaction process is put into motion, threatening integrity.

In most cases ultra-rapid phenomena are involved, with a duration on the order of 10^{-4} second. Usually the chain reaction stops very quickly, either through the presence of protective substances called radical scavengers, or through the phenomenon of recombination, in the course of which two more or less identical radicals or two radicals separated by the energy supply combine again by re-pairing their free electrons:

$$
\begin{array}{ccc}
\text{H} \ \ \text{H} & & \text{H} \\
\overset{\cdot\cdot}{-:\text{C}}\overset{\cdot\cdot}{:\text{C}}:- & \xrightarrow{\ \text{energy}\ } & -:\overset{\cdot\cdot}{\text{C}}\overset{\cdot\cdot}{:\text{C}}:- + \text{H}\!\uparrow \\
\text{H} \ \ \text{H} & & \text{H} \ \ \text{H}
\end{array}
$$

$$
\text{or:} \quad \text{R}\,\overset{\nearrow}{\underset{\swarrow}{:}}\,\text{H} \xrightarrow{\ \text{energy}\ } \text{R}^{\nearrow} + \text{H}\searrow \xrightarrow[\text{recombination}]{\hspace{3cm}} \text{R}:\text{H}
$$

In most cases, the pairs of free radicals formed on saturated chains, by passage of protons or of particles, immediately recombine. This is not true if the chain is unsaturated. Double bonds, such as exist in polyunsaturated fatty acids, constitute escape routes for the lone electron, because of the nature of the π bonds which double the σ bonds that assure the simple covalent bonds. In these molecules, the electron is delocalized(8, 10), and a possible partner would have all the more difficulty in meeting it when double bonds are numerous. Such delocalized lone electron radicals are much more stable than the others, and because of this, less reactive. Certain of these can exist for several hours. Nevertheless, everything changes if molecules of oxygen are present.

The radical states of oxygen(5, 8)

The oxygen that we breathe, which is in the basic state, is a diradical. Its molecule includes two lone electrons and is very stable; it can be represented in a very simplified manner, showing only its covalent electrons:

$$O_2 \text{ or } \overset{\uparrow}{\underset{\cdot\cdot}{\overset{\cdot\cdot}{O}}} : \overset{\cdot\cdot}{\underset{\cdot\cdot}{\overset{\cdot\cdot}{O}}} \overset{\uparrow}{} \text{ or } \cdot \overset{\cdot\cdot}{\underset{\cdot\cdot}{O}} : \overset{\cdot\cdot}{\underset{\cdot\cdot}{O}} \cdot \text{ or } \cdot O - O \cdot$$

Quantum mechanics demonstrate that the presence of two lone electrons on a small molecule such as O_2 prohibits spontaneous chemical reactions of the diradical with nonradical molecules, which are in great majority in living matter. Through acquisition of an electron, and thanks to an outside energy source, oxygen can couple one of its free electrons by acquiring a negative charge.

$$\cdot \overset{\cdot\cdot}{\underset{\cdot\cdot}{O}} : \overset{\cdot\cdot}{\underset{\cdot\cdot}{O}} \cdot + e^- \xrightarrow[\text{energy}]{} \left[: \overset{\cdot\cdot}{\underset{\cdot\cdot}{O}} : \overset{\cdot\cdot}{\underset{\cdot\cdot}{O}} \cdot \right]^- \text{ or } O_2^-$$

This is the superoxide anion, O_2^-. In this symbol, the "minus" sign stands for the electrical charge, and the period, the existence of a lone electron.

The energy necessary to overcome the unreactivity of O_2 is generally of enzymatic origin (activity of xanthine-oxidase of milk, for example). The superoxide anion, a simple radical, is spontaneously reactive, and can take part in various reactions of destruction of organic molecules. The superoxide anion was for a long time considered as a particularly deleterious oxidating factor(7), but it acts directly only through its nucleophilic properties(5); this reactivity is manifested only in proton-free media (H^+). Such *aprotic* areas are encountered within the phospholipidic double layers constituting the cellular membranes; here, O_2^- can destabilize the phospholipoproteic structure by releasing, through de-esterification, the fatty acids constituting phospholipidic molecules.

But in proton-containing media, the existence of O_2^- is very short, since the presence of H^+ ions permit the *dismutation* phenomenon, in the course of which an O_2^- molecule gives up its electron (to become O_2 again), to another of its kind.

Dismutation is therefore a process of oxidation/reduction between molecules of the same type. It forms basic oxygen and hydrogen peroxide H_2O_2:

$$O_2^- \longrightarrow O_2$$
$$\Big\downarrow e^-$$
$$O_2^- \longrightarrow O_2^= \; ; \; O_2^= + 2H^+ \longrightarrow H_2O_2$$

Hydrogen peroxide H_2O_2 presents no more lone electrons, but in presence of ferrous iron Fe^{2+}, it undergoes a Fenton reaction, in the course of which it decomposes into a common OH^- ion, and an $^{\cdot}OH$ hydroxyl radical, an extremely reactive oxidizer type, capable of attacking the most stable organic structures. This potent reagent permits hydroxylation of benzene at ordinary temperature and pressure, the attack and dehydrogenation of alkanes (aliphatic saturated fat chains), etc.(5, 7)

$$HO:OH + Fe^{2+} \xrightarrow{\quad e^- \quad} Fe^{3+} + [:OH]^- + {}^{\cdot}OH$$

$$Fe^{3+} + O_2^- \longrightarrow Fe^{2+} + O_2$$

The destructive effect of O_2^- is exerted essentially *indirectly* in proton-containing media: through spontaneous dismutation or enzymatically accelereated dismutation, it produces hydrogen peroxide, which in presence of divalent iron, produces $^{\cdot}OH$; it enters into the Fenton reaction by reducing Fe^{3+} into Fe^{2+}.

The entire phenomenon (dismutation of O_2^- producing $H_2O_2^-$, the decomposition of which into OH through the intervention of Fe^{2+} and regeneration of the latter by O_2^- constitutes the Haber-Weiss cycle(5). The coexistence of O_2^- and H_2O_2 in biological media (inevitably containing iron) is dangerous. In absence of iron (a rare circumstance, since iron is a universal contaminant) or even if this atom is "paralyzed" by the presence of a chelator, H_2O_2 decomposes spontaneously, but slowly, into water:

$$2H_2O_2 \rightarrow 2H + O_2$$

Oxygen and free radicals(10)

Although oxygen is practically inert with respect to substances with paired electrons, it reacts energetically with free radicals (facile reaction of diradicals with monoradicals). Even in the case of free radicals stabilized by resonance, oxygen easily finds the "lost" lone electron in order to pair it with one of its two free electrons, forming a new radical, the peroxide radical:

$$R^{\cdot} + O^{\cdot} - O^{\cdot} \longrightarrow R:OO^{\cdot} \text{ or } ROO^{\cdot}$$

The peroxide radical can be recombined, but it then forms an extremely unstable tetroxide bridge:

$$ROO^{\cdot} + ROO^{\cdot} \longrightarrow ROO{:}OOR$$

which fragments, releasing singlet oxygen, all of whose electrons are paired:

$$\overset{\cdot\cdot \;\; \cdot\cdot}{\underset{\cdot\cdot \;\; \cdot\cdot}{:O:O}}$$

and which, because of this, reacts *spontaneously,* and as vigorously as the hydroxyl radical, with the most stable organic structures.

The peroxide radical takes away hydrogens in the medium where it appears, starting radicalar reaction chains:

$$ROO^{\cdot} + R_1{:}H \longrightarrow ROOH + R_1^{\cdot}$$

$$R_1^{\cdot} + R_2{:}H \longrightarrow R_1{:}H + R_2^{\cdot} \longrightarrow \cdots$$

It is by inhibiting the recombination of newly formed radicals that oxygen exerts its toxic effect. This property is well demonstrated by radiobiology: living organisms are much more altered by Y, X, and particulate radiations administered in an oxygen atmosphere than in presence of an inert gas such as nitrogen or argon. The free radicals appearing through rupture of covalent bonds easily recombine in inert atmosphere, whereas the peroxides formed with oxygen are the origing of successions of radical reactions.

Lipid autoxidation

Polyunsaturated fatty acids are capital elements in cellular architecture. They participate in the constitution of lipoproteic membranes, conferring upon them their physicochemical characteristics. The presence on their chain of several double bonds (there are respectively two and four of these for linoleic and arachidonic acids, for example) facilitates the appearance of stable free radicals, through electronic delocalization.

In *Figure 1*, we see that the rupture of a covalent bond may occur through the intervention of a newly formed free radical (an $^{\cdot}OH$ formed by a Fenton reaction, for example). But this phenomenon may also be produced by a high-energy particle or photon, or by the presence of an appropriately complexed ferrous atom, which very easily captures a hydrogen equipped with its electron. The radical stage undergoes the conjugation process (two double bonds separated by a single bond), which permits from then on electronic resonance between four carbons, and, consequently, the delocalization of the lone electron. The latter would be stable enough to await the arrival of an oxygen molecule. At that time, an irreversible process is launched: the peroxide radical (stage B), takes from an intact unsaturated chain a hydrogen and its electron, becoming a lipidic hydroperoxide ROOH (stage C), while a new lipidic radical (stage A) can begin a new cycle. The ROOH lipidic hydroperoxides are nearly nonreactive, but in presence of Fe^{2+} (universal biological contaminant), they undergo a strong Fenton reaction which converts them into alkoxyl radicals $RO^{\cdot}$, agents as "terrible" as the hydroxyl radical:

$$ROOH + Fe^{2+} \longrightarrow RO^{\cdot} + OH^- + Fe^{3+}$$

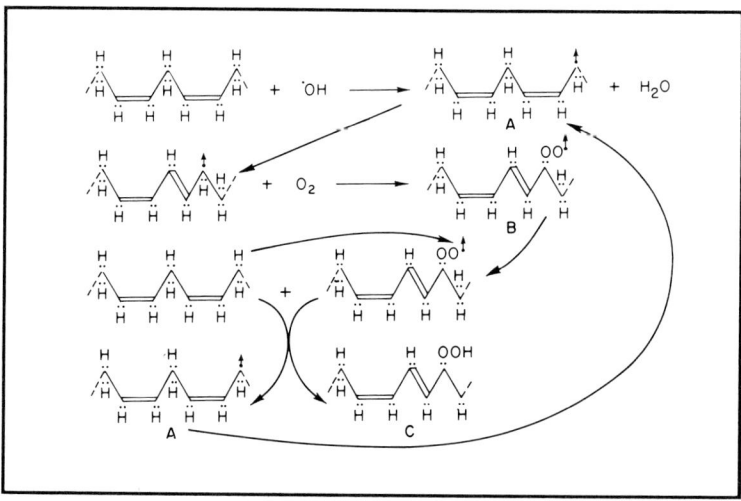

Figure 1. Lipidic auto-oxidation cycle. A polyunsaturated fatty acid, of which we see only a part of the carbon chain, is converted into a lipid radical (stage A), by taking over an H· : initiation. After altering the position of the double bonds, the lipid radical combines with an oxygen molecule to form the peroxide radical (stage B). The latter is in the process of taking an H· with a new intact molecule of polyunsaturated fatty acid, which in its turn becomes a radical (stage A) while the peroxide radical becomes a lipidic hydroperoxide (stage C). The arrows represent the electronic spins of the lone electrons.

Origin of free radicals in living tissues(3)

It appears increasingly probable that the threat of creation of free radicals is permanent in living matter, through the ubiquity of iron and oxygen.

Iron, and other metals called "transition" metals, have the capacity to play, in some way, the role of radical agents, when they are complexed by certain organic compounds (adenosine-diphosphoric acid, or ADP, for example), as well as by certain phosphates(1). By oversimplifying, one could write (R:H being a polyunsaturated fatty acid):

$$\text{COMPLEX} - Fe^{3+} + R{:}H \longrightarrow$$
$$\text{COMPLEX} - Fe^{2+} + R^{\cdot} + H^{+}$$

It requires only the intervention of an oxygen molecule:

$$R^{\cdot} + O_2 \longrightarrow ROO^{\cdot}$$

to start up a lipoperoxidation chain.

Various enzymes produce the superoxide anion: this is true of xanthine-oxidase of milk; but xanthine-dehydrogenase, which plays a part in purine catabolism to form uric acid, under certain abnormal conditions can behave as xanthine-oxidase, causing the appearance of O_2^- in the tissues. In presence of suitably complexed iron, sustained production of $^{\cdot}OH$ is obtained (Haber-Weiss cycle). The hydroxyl radical, in turn, can initiate lipidic auto-oxidation cycles, according to the diagram in *Figure 1*. Another route of induction for the lipoperoxidation chain is therefore opened in this manner.

A third cause for the massive appearance of free radicals within the cells is due to disturbances of electron transport in the respiratory chain. Under normal conditions, the electrons conducted to the last link in the chain, cytochrome-oxidase, instantly and completely reduce the oxygen molecules arriving at the level of this enzyme:

$$O_2 + 4e^- + 4H + \frac{\text{CYTOCHROME}}{\text{OXIDASE}} \longrightarrow 2\,H_2O$$

Through a mechanism which is still poorly understood, not only does cytochrome-oxidase remove the energy barrier preventing the spontaneous reduction of oxygen, but all of the steps in reduction (O_2^-, H_2O_2) are instantaneously passed through. The appearance and coexistence of O_2^- and H_2O_2 is avoided, preventing the formation of $^{\cdot}OH$.

Various circumstances can block the flow of electrons ahead of the cytochromes, such as the action of poisons such as antimycine, and mainly anoxia, followed by return to normoxia(9). The oxygen then climbs to the level of ubiquinone, a revolving platelet in the respiratory chain. Here, each of the O_2 molecules is reduced by a single electron; superoxide anion is produced, with the succession of events resulting in ˙OH. Ischemic tissue undergoes a process of lipoperoxidation at the time of reoxygenation by reestablishment of circulation(9).

Another important source of cyto-destructive agents, free radicals, and potent oxidizing species, is found in the activated polymorphonuclear leukocytes and macrophages(2). Stimulation of these white cells occurs principally at the time of activation of the alternate route of the complement, by C_3 and C_5 fractions; it constitutes one of the principal elements in the inflammatory process. The most obvious biochemical fact, at the time of leukocytic activation, is acceleration of oxygen consumption, which has been designated by English-speaking people by the picturesque term "respiratory burst". In the course of the phenomenon, leukocytic metabolism is oriented toward *massive production of superoxide anion* by a membrane enzyme, NADPH-oxidase, which requires a very considerable supply of reduced NADPH coenzyme: this supply is assured by initiation of shunting of hexosemonophosphates, also called pentose cycle, major producer of NADPH. The superoxide anion is thus emptied into the phagosomes, where the phagocytic elements are imprisoned by the activated leukocytes, and institutes various cellular destruction processes, notably de-esterification of membranal phospholipids. At the same time, a significant quantity of H_2O_2 is formed by dismutation of O_2; hydrogen peroxide is then taken over by an enzyme present in the phagosome, myeloperoxidase.

This curious enzyme, very similar to that which allows fixation of iodine on proteins in the thyroid, converts hydrogen peroxide into hypochlorous acid(11) in presence of Cl-B ions:

$$H_2O_2 + Cl^- \longrightarrow HOCl + OH^-$$

HOCl, reacting with H_2O_2 produces singlet oxygen, the superactive type of O_2, mentioned above:

$$H_2O_2 + HOCl \longrightarrow HCl + \overset{..}{\underset{..}{O}} : \overset{..}{\underset{..}{O}} + H_2O$$

Finally, HOCl can form strongly oxidizing chlorinated amines, similar in activity to the chloramines of Dakin's liquor:

$$R - NH_2 + HOCl \longrightarrow R - \overset{H}{\underset{Cl}{N}} + H_2O$$

R — NH_2 are amines such as glucosamine, taurine, etc.
Another reaction may occur with the NH_4^+ ion:

$$NH_4^+ + HOCl \longrightarrow NH_2Cl + H_2O + H^+$$

The NH_2Cl amine chloride is a strongly oxidizing type, attacking particularly the thiol groups, by transforming them into sulfoxides, which definitively prevents any participation of the –SH in oxidation/reduction processes. Substances of major importance, such as glutathione, are thus reduced. Also, H_2O_2 in presence of iron produces ˙OH.

In summary, activated leukocytes produce O_2^-, ˙OH, singlet oxygen, and chloramines, a group of reagents eminently aggressive toward organic structures.

The action of these destructive agents may be limited to the content of phagosomes, and henceforth play a helpful role by facilitating bacteriolysis and cytolysis of cells in the process of degeneration, which have been phagocytized.

But, by a process of exocytosis, the content of the phagosomes may be released into the exterior medium, hence inevitable biochemical wastes will occur. For example, remarkable cooperation is established between the chloramines (formed from HCl and animated molecules, or from the NH_4^+ ion), and the proteases simultaneously released by the activated leukocytes. Normally, the action of these proteases is inhibited by the presence in the plasma and the interstitial spaces, of antienzymes such as α_1-antiprotease. The chloramines, irreversibly oxidizing the thiol functions of α_1-antiprotease, render this agent inactive for the struggle against the proteases, and notably elastase, destroyer of elastin fibers.

Defense against free radicals

Various arguments therefore support the hypothesis that free radicals may be formed continuously within living tissues. What are the means of endogenous protection which the cells have available in the face of these attacks? Can diet help our organism to fight against the deleterious effect of free radicals? Are there therapeutic methods to combat them?

We have seen how an auto-oxidation cycle of polyunsaturated fatty acids can be induced by the hydroxyl radical (OH˙), this being produced by the coexistence of the superoxide anion (O_2^-) and hydrogen peroxide (H_2O_2), in presence of traces of iron. In *Figure 2*, representing an auto-oxidation cycle, various existing methods to combat the effect of free radicals are indicated in Roman numerals.

Endogenous defense methods

The first natural defense method is constituted by the superoxide dismutases (SOD), enzymes which accelerate the rate of dismutation of O_2^- into H_2O_2 by approximately a thousand times (*Figure 2, I*), which prevents these two oxygenated species from coexisting and consequently from engendering $OH^.$(7). Two superoxide dismutases are known in mammals, one being localized in the mitochondria, the other in the cytoplasm. Mitochondrial SOD is a manganese metalloprotein; cytoplasmic SOD contains copper and zinc.

At present, certain clinical cases in which the presence of free radicals is suspected (cardiac or renal ischemia) are treated by injection of SOD with encouraging results.

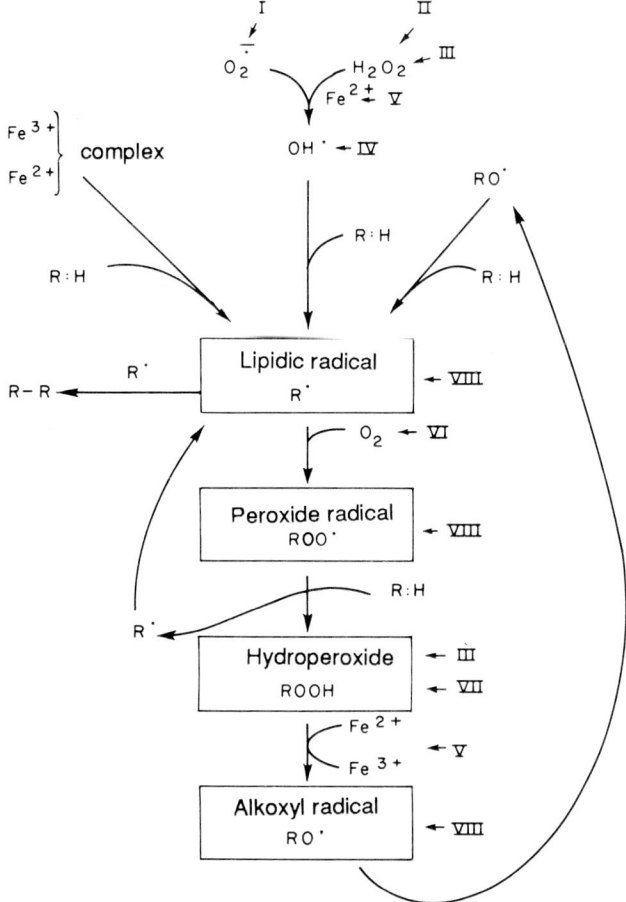

Figure 2: Auto-oxidation cycle of polyunsaturated fatty acid and protection methods. I: superoxide dismutase (SOD); II: Catalase; III: Glutathion peroxidase (GPO); IV: Uric acid, Ginkgo biloba extract, Vitamin E, P vitamins; V: Ginkgo biloba extract, P vitamins, ceruleoplasmin; VI, VII, and VIII: Vitamin E.

A second important enzyme is catalase (*Figure 2, II*), which destroys hydrogen peroxide according to the equation: $2\ H_2O_2 \longrightarrow 2\ H_2O_2 + O_2,$ thus preventing the latter from participating in the Fenton reaction.

$$(Fe^{2+} + H_2O_2 \longrightarrow Fe^{3+} + OH^- + OH^{\cdot})$$
$$\text{producing } ^{\cdot}OH$$

Catalase is localized in the cellular organoids, the peroxisomes. Another enzyme also capable of destroying H_2O_2, through a different mechanism, is glutathione peroxidase (GPO), an enzyme containing selenium distributed throughout the cytoplasm(6). It requires a hydrogen donor, reduced glutathione (GSH), and acts according to the reaction:

$$2\ GSH + H_2O_2 \longrightarrow 2\ H_2O + GS - SG$$

Two amino acids producing GSH, essential co-factor of GPO, must be supplied by the diet: these are methionine and cystine.

If despite the action of these enzymes on O_2^- and H_2O_2, the hydroxyl radical is produced and sets off an auto-oxidation cycle, the glutathione peroxidase then goes into action to limit radical propagation (*Figure 2, III*). Through a mechanism identical to that of the destruction of H_2O_2, GPO can reduce the hydroperoxides (ROOH) into hydroxylated fatty acids (ROH) according to the equation:

$$ROOH + 2\ GSH \longrightarrow ROH + H_2O + GSSG$$

Exogenous defense mechanisms

Any substance capable of quenching the hydroxyl radical would obviously play a beneficial role for the protection of polyunsaturated fatty acids (*Figure 2, IV*). In order however to be considered as a good radical quencher, a product must meet certain conditions(4):

It must give, after reaction with the radical, a nonradical product.

The rate constant between the radical quencher and the radical must be greater than that between the radical and the substrate to be protected. Thus, in the case which interests us, we would have $k_1 >>> k_2$.

$$OH^{\cdot} + quencher \xrightarrow{k_1} \text{produces nonradicalar}$$

$$OH^{\cdot} + R{:}H^{\cdot} \xrightarrow{k_2} R^{\cdot} + HOH$$

A quencher is not effective against all radicals: there is a degree of specificity explained by certain stearic incompatibilities, or even by solubility differences: the radical being lipophilic, the quencher being hydrophilic. Thus for example, uric acid is an effective quencher for the hydroxyl radical, but has no effect on lipid radicals, which are $R^{\cdot}$, $RO^{\cdot}$, and $ROO^{\cdot}$. Among other good $OH^{\cdot}$: quenchers, we list the flavonoids such as quercetine or rutin, tocopherol, mannitol, and the anthocyanidines.

Iron (*Figure 2, V*) appears to be an extremely dangerous element, since only traces of it are necessary in order to set off a Fenton reaction. Also, it also serves as initiator of the cycle transforming hydroperoxides (ROOH) into alkoxyl radicals ($RO^{\cdot}$), particularly toxic, since they can assume the role of initiator of the auto-oxidation cycle played by the $OH^{\cdot}$ radical. Complexation of this element by ligands is not necessarily a guarantee of protection. In fact, when it is complexed, iron, in its Fe^{2+} or Fe^{3+} forms, can take on two different electronic states: one (high-spin complex) promoting the deleterious activity of this element, the other (low-spin complex) rendering it harmless. When iron is combined with adenosine diphosphate (ADP) or with a chemical agent such as sodium ethylenediaminetetraacetic acid (NA_2EDTA), it is capable of directly attacking a polyunsaturated fatty acid molecule and of producing an R radical. Thus, for example, a lipid peroxidation of microsomes of rat liver may be induced within several minutes by the $FeCl_3$/ADP/NADPH system. Ceruleoplasmin, a protein complexed with copper, is often considered as a protective agent, since it oxidizes Fe^{2+} into Fe^{3+}, inhibiting the Fenton reaction. This action must be considered cautiously however, since, first, we have seen that iron could be active in both of its forms, and second, this protein is found exclusively in the plasma.

Another way to inhibit the cycle is to act at the level of oxygen. In the absence of oxygen, the $R^{\cdot}$ radical dimerizes to yield a nontoxic product according to the equation:

$$R^{\cdot} + R^{\cdot} \longrightarrow R - R$$

In summary, in presence of oxygen, $R^{\cdot}$ reacts very rapidly with oxygen to give the $ROO^{\cdot}$ peroxide radical. In order to prevent this reaction from occurring, there must be available lipophilic substances which react more rapidly than the $R^{\cdot}$ radical with oxygen. A substance may be supplied by our diet: tocopherol or Vitamin E.

The polyphenolic substances to which tocopherol and Ginkgo extract belong also play a protective role at another level. During their transformation into quinone, they can give up two hydrogen atoms and their electron to the lipoperoxides (ROOH).

With respect to the respiratory burst of the leukocytes, few medications have been suggested to control it when it begins, threatening the integrity of the tissues where the aggregated platelets come to a stop. Certain flavonoids seem to regulate the activity of NADPH-oxidase. Ginkgo biloba extract significantly decreases production of the active oxygenated species with reduction of formation of chlorine-containing species as a probable result.

Conclusions

Oxygen is necessary for the life of aerobic organisms, and as an acceptor terminal for electrons.

Because of its high affinity for single electrons, oxygen supports radical reactions and opposes the recombinations of radicals, after rupture of covalent bonds. Lipoperoxidation processes follow, attacking the cellular membranes. Incessant threats of the appearance of free radicals influence the future of the cells: the ubiquity of transition metals, particularly iron, constitutes the principal cause of creation of these dangerous entities.

Transitory ischema is also the origin of radical reactions. But a frequent danger arises from anarchic leukocytic activation; the respiratory distress syndrome in adults, a frequent complication in severe accidents with septic disorders, peritoneal infections, and pancreatitis, is a vicious circle of pathological events, the prime mover of which would be excessive activation of polymorpho-nuclear leukocytes. These cells tend to aggregate, and their masses are retained in the capillary bed of the lungs, where the discharge of oxidizing agents and of proteases produce severe lesions in the pulmonary parenchyma.

A complex arsenal of endogenous protective agents must be present in all of the cells in order to oppose the danger represented by the lone electron structures in the oxygenated milieux.

Diet can considerably aid the cells by supplying factors such as tocopherol, certain amino acids, and certain flavonoids (Vitamin P). Vitamin E acts effectively to protect the polyunsaturated acids. Let us note that in the course of the past few years dietary fashions have introduced increased consumption of polyunsaturated fatty acids, not compensated by a proportional intake of Vitamin E. The future will teach us whether this practice is healthy. The action of Vitamin C (which is not the question in this article, an absence which might perhaps have surprised the reader) is currently very controversial, as to its protective or activating effect on toxicity of oxygen; more thorough research is required in order to position the role of this vitamin exactly.

There are various pathological circumstances in which the natural defense mechanisms (endogenous and dietary) may be overwhelmed. Under such circumstances, it would be extremely useful to have available pharmacological agents which would make it possible to compensate for the natural deficiencies.

References

1. Babbs C.F.: Role of iron ions in the genesis of reperfusion injury following successful cardiopulmonary resuscitation. *Ann. Emergency Med.*, 1985, *14*, 777-783.

2. Badwey J.A., Karnovsky M.L.: Active oxygen species and the functions of phagocytic leukocytes. *Ann. Rev. Biochem.*, 1980, *49*, 695-726.

3. Borg D.C., Schaich K.M., Elmonre J.J.: Autoxidation and cytotoxicity. *In:* Oxygen and Oxy-radicals in chemistry and Biology, Rodgers M.A.J., Powers E.L., Eds., *Academic Press.*, New-York, 1985, 177-195.

4. Deby C., Pincemail J., Hans P., Braquet P., Lion Y., Deby-Dupont G., Goutier R.: Mechanisms of free radicals production in the arachidonic acid cascade and role of anti-lipoperoxidants and free radical scavengers. *In:* Cerebral Ischemia, Bes A., Braquet P., Paoletti R., Sjesjö B.K., Eds., *Excerpta Medica,* 1984, 249-258.

5. Fee J.A., Valentine J.S.: Chemical and Physical properties of superoxide. *In:* Superoxide and Superoxide Dismutases, Michelson A.M., Mc Cord J.M., Fridovich I., Eds., *Academic Press,* New-York, 1977, 19-57.

6. Flohé L.: Glutathione peroxidase: Fact and fiction. *In:* Oxygen free radicals and tissue damage, Ciba Foundation Symposium 65, *Excerpta Medica,* Amsterdam, 1979, 95-121.

7. Fridovich I.: Superoxide dismutases, *Ann. Rev. Biochem.*, 1975, *44*, 19-43.

8. Hamilton G.A.: Chemical models and mechanisms for oxygenases. *In:* Molecular mechanisms of oxygen activation, Hayashio., Ed., *Academic Press,* New-York, 1974, 405-451.

9. Hillered L., Ernster L., Afors K.E.: Brain Ischemia and oxygen radicals. *In:* Cerebral ischemia, Bes A., Braquet P., Paoletti R., Sjesjö B.K., Eds., *Excerpta Medica,* Amsterdam, 1984, 293-300.

10. Vladimirov Y.A., Olenev V.I., Suslova T.B., Cheremisina Z.P.: Lipid peroxidation in mitochondrial membrane. *Adv. Lipid. Res.,* 1980, *17*, 173-249.

11. Weiss S.J., Lambert M.B., Test, S.T.: Long-lived oxidants generated by human neutrophils: characterization and bioactivity. *Science,* 1983, *222*, 626-628.

The Antiradical Properties of Ginkgo Biloba Extract

J. Pincemail, C. Deby

Laboratoire de Biochimie Appliquée, Unité de Biologie de l'Oxygène
Université de Liège. Sart-Tilman. 4000 Liège. Belgique

Summary

The anti-radical properties of Ginkgo biloba extract have been determined on several **in vitro** *models. The product is as effective as uric acid, an anti-radical agent known to entrap the hydroxyl and diphenylpicrylhydrazyl radicals. In addition, it inactivates the formation of radicals, such as adriamycyl, which escape uric acid activity. It also inhibits membrane lipid peroxidation and, owing to its anti-radical activity exerts a stimulant effect on the biosynthesis of prostanoids.*

Various arguments support the hypothesis according to which free radicals may be formed continuously within living tissues(8). Because polyunsaturated fatty acids (PUFA) are the principal elements constituting the cellular membranes, the harmful effect which the propagation of a radical chain reaction in their midst is understandable. In fact, the cellular membrane gradually loses its semipermeable properties, which are necessary for cell life.

Normal tissues seem to be well prepared to repel the attacks of radicals which threaten them constantly. Proteins such as superoxide dismutase(14), catalase(17), and glutathion-peroxidase(12) assure enzymatic defense, while the diet can considerably aid the cells through a supply of factors such as tocopherol (Vitamin E), certain amino acids (methionine and cystine), or certain Vitamin P factors. There are however various pathological conditions in which the natural endogenous or exogenous defense mechanisms may be overwhelmed. In such cases, it would be extremely useful to have available pharmacological agents making it possible to substitute for the natural deficiencies.

Principle

In this respect, we studied *in vitro* the antiradical behavior of Ginkgo biloba extract, EGb 761, the therapeutic applications of which are becoming increasingly nume-

Rökan (Ginkgo Biloba). Recent Results in Pharmacology and Clinic
Edited by E.W. Fünfgeld
© Springer-Verlag Berlin Heidelberg New York 1988, pp. 71-82

rous(19). The antiradical property of the whole extract has been determined by its capacity for quenching three different free radicals: the hydroxyl radical (OH), the diphenylpicrylhydrazyl radical (DPPH), and the adriamycyl radical. The hydroxyl radical may be produced either by radiolysis (γ irradiation of an aqueous solution(23)), or by the Fenton reaction.(15)

The diphenylpicrylhydrazyl radical is stable at ordinary temperature and is characterized by a violet coloration. Its colorimetric assay is very easy, but it can also be measured by a physical technique: paramagnetic electronic resonance (PER). By this same technique, the adriamycyl radical produced by the hepatic microsomes of rats is very easily demonstrated.

Lastly, it is possible to study the action of free radicals on two *in vitro* models. In the first case, rat liver microsomes are incubated with a peroxidizing system composed of iron and adenosine diphosphate, which has been proved to produce hydroxyl radicals(13). These would assault the microsomial membranes by inducing a fatty acid auto-oxidation cycle described in detail previously(5, 8). The lipoperoxides formed degenerate rapidly into malonaldehyde, the assay of which would permit evaluating the magnitude of lipid peroxidation. In this system, the active species would be an iron-oxygen complex, perferryl ion(22). Both types lead in the same way to the same result: lipid peroxidation.

In the second model, an enzyme is used, cyclo-oxygenase, responsible for the biosynthesis of prostanoids, the activity of which is inhibited by various free radicals(9). *Figure 1* shows the mechanism of effect of this enzyme. In a first stage, it catalyzes the incorporation of two molecules of oxygen into arachidonic acid, a polyunsaturated fatty acid with 20 carbons and four double bonds. The result is the formation of an endoperoxide G_2 (PGG_2), characterized by a hydroperoxide function $-OOH$. PGG_2 is then converted into the endoperoxide H_2 (PGH_2), which, under the influence of other enzymes, yields the approach for synthesis of prostanoids. In the course of the conversion of PGG_2 into PGH_2 (reduction of $-OOH$ into $-OH$), radical oxygenated types are produced (OH˙, the alkoxyl radical RO˙) which inactivate cyclo-oxygenase and thus limit the production of prostanoids (cyclo-oxygenase is therefore a "suicidal" enzyme). It is therefore logical to believe that an antiradical substance would increase the production of prostanoids, since it would protect the enzyme against the free radicals produced during its activity. This hypothesis has been verified with uric acid and other antiradical factors(3, 4).

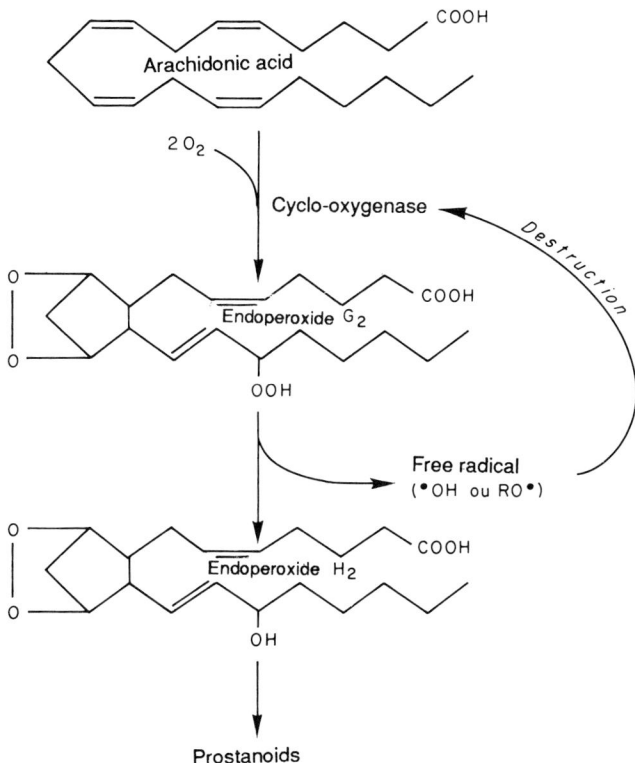

Figure 1: Biosynthesis of prostanoids by cyclo-oxygenase. Action of free radicals.

Material and Methods

Production of the OH radical

By radiolysis: Irradiation is obtained by exposure of the targets to the γ ray (0.6 MeV) from a source of ^{137}Cs; the rate per minute was 0.8 Gy, at a distance of 80 cm. In a first series of experiments, a solution of α -keto-γ -methiolbutyric acid (KMB, Sigma) dissolved in a phosphate buffer (0.15M, pH 7.4) treated with chelex, was irradiated (total dose: 10 Gy). The OH radical attacks the KMB, releasing ethylene(24). The irradiation was performed in hermetically sealed bottles with a rubber septum, permitting taking of gas samples. These latter are injected into a Porapak P column mounted on a Barber-Colman 3000 chromatograph equipped with a flame ionization detector, using argon as vector. The injection temperatures, of the column and of the detector, were respectively 170, 100, and 170°C.

In a second series of procedures, hyaluronic acid solutions (HYA) were irradiated by doses of 25 and 50 Gy. The HYA (Sigma), polyose of high molecular weight (approximately 400,000), was dissolved in a phosphate buffer (0.15M) at pH 7.4. The OH radicals depolymerize the HYA, thus bringing about a decrease in its viscosity proportional to the production of $OH^{\cdot}$(6). The loss of viscosity was measured by means of the Ostwald viscosimeter.

By Fenton reaction: Fe^{π} sulfate ($10^{-4}M$) was dissolved in a phosphate buffer (pH 7.4) in the presence of ethylenediaminetetraacetic acid ($5 \cdot 10^{-5}M$) and salicylic acid ($10^{-3}M$); the addition of hydrogen peroxide ($10^{-4}M$) produces OH radicals. These oxidize the salicylic acid present in the solution, forming dihydroxybenzoic acid, the appearance of which is followed for one hour, at ten-minute intervals, by spectrophotometry (490 nm) according to a method previously described(16).

The diphenylpicrylhydrazyl radical test

This radical presents the property of being stable at ordinary temperature and is characterized by a violet coloration with an absorption maximum at 517 nanometers. In the presence of an antiradical substance, it is possible to measure the discoloration of the radical at the wavelength indicated by spectrophotometry. The procedure is described in detail in a previous publication(6).

The adriamycyl radical

Rats received phenobarbital sodium (50 mg/kg) i.p. every day for the purpose of stimulating the P-450 cytochrome of the liver. After four days, they were sacrificed, and the hepatic microsomes were isolated according to the method of Ernster(10). The proteins were assayed by the method of Folin-Ciocalteu(18). The microsomes (2 mg of proteins per milliliter) were then incubated at 37°C under nitrogen for four minutes in a KCl-Tris-$MgCl_2$ buffer (150-20-50 mM; pH 7.4) containing glucose-6-phosphate dehydrogenase (0.67 units/mL) and adriamycin (200 µg/mL). The reaction starts following the addition of NADP (0.39 mM)(21). After transfer into a quartz cell, the signal of the adriamycyl radical is identified by paramagnetic electronic resonance (PER) on a Varian E-9-X Band spectrometer with a frequency of 9.5 GHz and a field modulation of 100 KHz.

Lipid peroxidation

Rat liver microsomes are isolated according to the method described above. The incubation medium is composed of KCl (125 mM), Tris (25 mM), pH 7.4, and microsomes (1 mg of proteins per mL). Lipid peroxidation is induced by the

NADPH/FeCl$_3$/ADP system (0.18 mM:12 μM:1 mM). After 30 minutes of constant agitation at 37°C, the lipid peroxidation is determined by assay of the malonaldehyde(1), produced by degradation of the lipoperoxides formed.

Activity of cyclo-oxygenase

Cyclo-oxygenase was isolated from the microsomes originating from the seminal vesicles of bulls(3). These microsomes were incubated at 37°C with arachidonic acid tagged with ^{14}C (7.510^{-2} μCuries/mL) in the presence of reduced glutathion (10^{-4}M). The tagged prostanoids formed (PGD$_2$ and PGE$_2$) were extracted with diethyl ether. After evaporation under nitrogen, the samples were placed on silica plates (Merck) and chromatographed with an elution medium (CHCl$_3$/CH$_3$OH/HAc/H$_2$O (90:8: 1:0.75)). After localization by autoradiography, the prostanoids were eluted and their activity was counted in a beta spectrophotometer.

In the different systems described, the antiradical effect of Ginkgo biloba extract (EGb) was studied by introduction of this substance at concentrations varying between 125 μg to 500 μg/mL. All of the tests were done in duplicate.

Results

Hydroxyl radical

EGb shows very marked anti –OH˙ properties, since in the presence of 500 μg of EGb/mL, the production of ethylene is no more than 35% of control, which represents an inhibition of reaction equal to 65%. At 250 and 125 μg/mL, the production of ethylene is respectively 46 and 65%, or inhibitions equal to 54 and 35%. By comparison, uric acid, recognized as an excellent scavenger of hydroxyl radicals, reduces the production of ethylene to 73% of control at a concentration of 10^{-3}M.

Figure 2 shows the significant decrease in the coefficient of viscosity of hyaluronic acid after γ irradiation. With doses of 25 Gy and 50 Gy, there remained respectively only 16 and 10% of the initial viscosity (100%). This decrease was significantly inhibited by uric acid at 10^{-3} (31 and 20%). A similar result was obtained by EGb at 500 μg/mL (29 and 18%). At lower concentrations, the extract still had significant activity.

In *Figure 3*, the quantity of dihydroxybenzoic acid (expressed in millimoles) formed in the course of the Fenton reaction is proportional to the reaction time. If the reaction took place in the presence of EGb at 250 μg/mL, the speed of the reaction in comparison with the control was distinctly slowed, as with 10^{-3}M uric acid. The effect of EGb on the production of dihydroxybenzoic acid confirms its OH˙-scavenging effect observed in both of the preceding experiments.

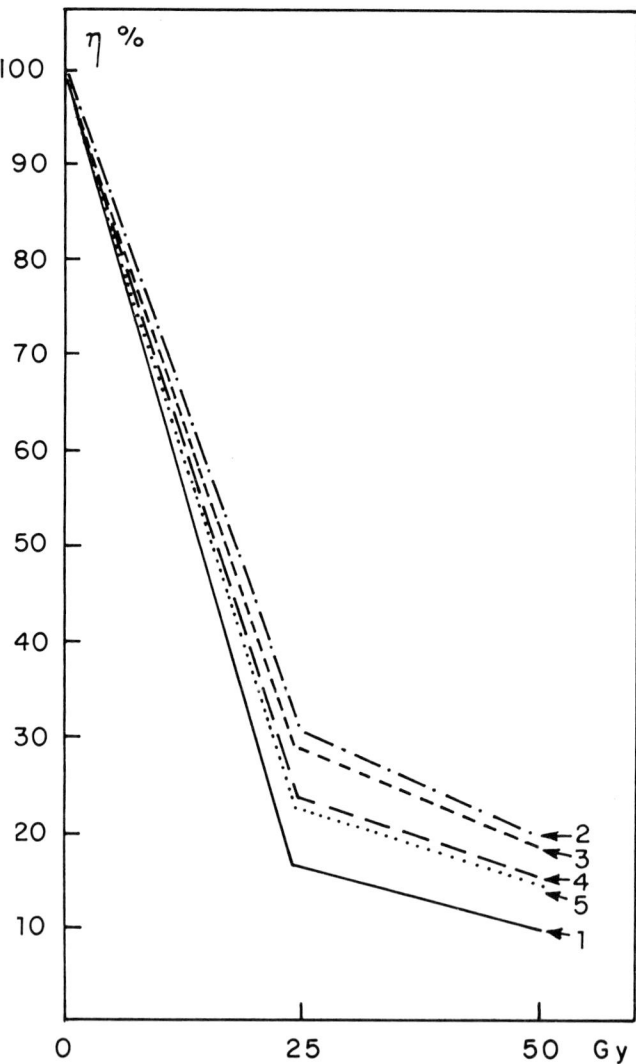

Figure 2: Inhibition exerted by EGb and uric acid on the decrease in viscosity coefficient (η) of hyaluronic acid after γ irradiation (25 and 50 Gy). Coefficient of initial viscosity before irradiation = 100%.

   1. Control;
   2. Control + uric acid 10^{-3}M;
   3. Control + EGb 500 μg/mL;
   4. Control + EGb 250 μg/mL;
   5. Control + EGb 125 μg/mL.

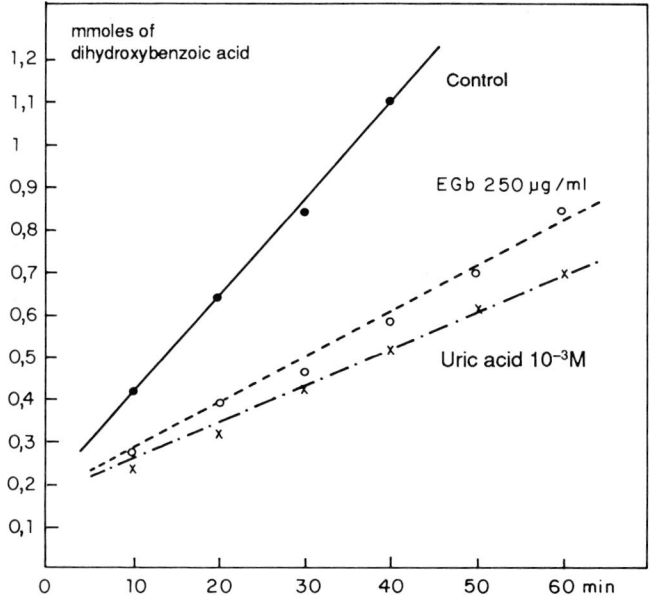

Figure 3: Inhibition of the Fenton reaction ($Fe^{2+} + H_2O_2 \rightarrow Fe^{3+} OH^-$) by EGb and uric acid.

Diphenylpicrylhydrazyl radical

EGb shows very high reactivity with the DPPH radical (*Figure 4*). At a concentration as low as 8 μg/mL, inhibition of the radical is observed equal to 20%. In the presence of 100 μg/mL, the DPPH is completely decolored, which indicates a maximum inhibition of 100%. It is interesting to note that the inhibiting effect is proportional to the concentration of EGb. Uric acid inhibits the radical 100% at concentrations of 10^{-3}M and 10^{-4}M.

Adriamycyl radical

The adriamycyl radical is easily obtained in a stable manner by incubation of adriamycin with rat liver microsomes which have been enriched with P-450 cytochrome by pharmacological stimulation. The amplitude of the PER signal is proportional to the concentration in adriamycyl radical. In comparison with control, it is reduced by approximately 50% when incubation is performed in the presence of EGb (500 μg/mL). Uric acid has no effect on the production of this radical.

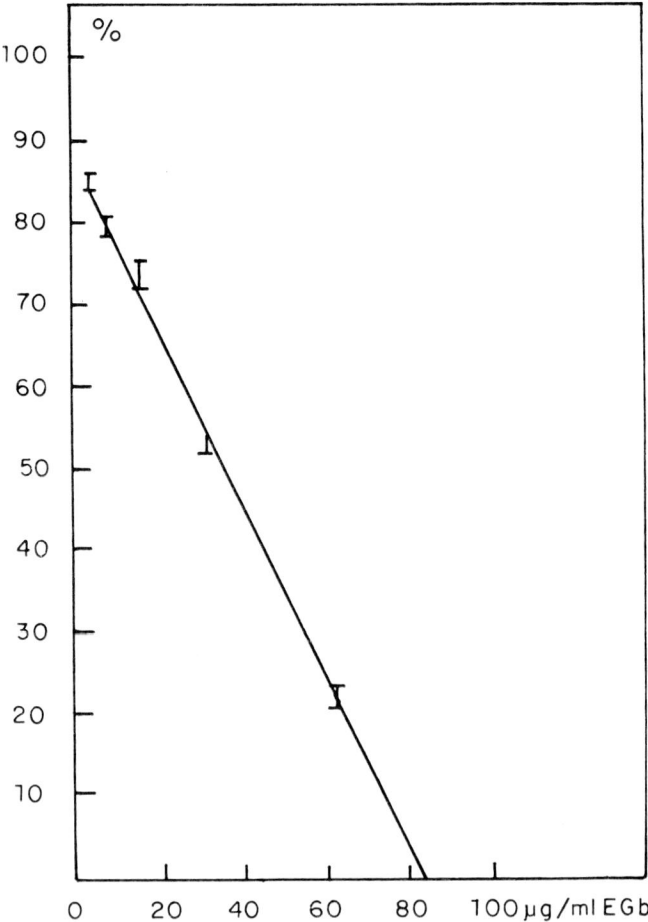

Figure 4: Effect of EGb concentration on the destruction of the DPPH radical. The results are expressed as % of control, which is the coloration of the free radical in absence of any inhibitor (=100%).

Lipid peroxidation

EGb completely inhibits the formation of malonaldehyde at concentrations of 500, 250, and 125 µg/mL. This indicates that EGb protects the lipid membrane to the maximum against the radical attack induced by the peroxidizing system $FeCl_3$ /ADP/NADPH. Controls have shown that EGb does not interfere with the assay of malonaldehyde.

Cyclo-oxygenase activity

In summary, in the presence of EGb at 250 and 125 µg/mL, the biosynthesis of prostanoids is stimulated respectively up to 129 and 140% of the control (100%) which is obtained in absence of any inhibitor of free radicals. Uric acid stimulates the production of prostanoids up to 200%.

Discussion

In our various experiments, the antiradical effects of EGb were compared to those of uric acid, considered as a typical scavenger of the OH radical(23). The concentration of this scavenger, used as reference, was established at 10^{-3}M. EGb contains notably flavonoid glycosides and proanthocyanidines, which represent 47% of the total extract. These substances may be considered as responsible for radical activity as shown by the studies in progress in our laboratory. We can attribute to them a mean molecular weight of 700, which would represent for 500 µg of extract a concentration of antiradical substances of 5.10^{-4}M, or a concentration similar to that of uric acid.

It appears from the experiments described above that EGb and uric acid have a rather similar anti-OH˙ activity, whereas, for the test with DPPH, the extract has a distinctly superior activity. Also, unlike uric acid, EGb is effective against the adriamycyl radical. This property has been confirmed *in vivo* by Etienne et al(11). It may be explained by the lipophilic character of the extract, which is unlike that of uric acid.

The antiradical properties of EGb may explain its effect on lipid peroxidation of membranes and on the biosynthesis of prostanoids.

As a remarkable inhibitor of the lipid peroxidation of membranes, EGb could participate at two levels in the experimental system used. Fong et al.(13) supplied several proofs of the formation of the OH radical in the course of lipid peroxidation of membranes by the NADPH/FeCl$_3$/ADP system, which was later confirmed by PER(2). EGb, through its anti-OH˙ properties, must therefore play a protective role. The participation of the OH radical in lipid peroxidation is, however, in doubt(5). The initiation of the radical chain would be produced by the perferryl ion which directly removes a hydrogen from a polyunsaturated fatty acid. EGb would seem therefore to act also on the formation of this species (as toxic as OH˙) by a possible complexation with iron.

On the other hand, EGb, like other good radical scavengers, stimulates the biosynthesis of prostanoids *in vitro*. We have confirmed this observation *in vivo* in a model using the rabbit sensitized to arachidonic acid, which allowed us to show that EGb would promote the production of prostacycline to the detriment of that of thromboxane A$_2$(7).

The antiradical properties of EGb must give it therapeutic potential in some pathological conditions where the free radicals are implicated. Thus, for example, it is well known that activated leukocytes produce oxygenated radical types (O_2^-, $OH^.$) which play a part in inflammatory phenomena. Recent experiments on human leukocytes activated with phorbol myristate have shown us that EGb diminishes the production of these oxygenated types.[20]

Conclusions

Ginkgo biloba extract contains chemical factors capable of trapping hydroxyl and diphenylpicrylhydrazyl radicals in a manner as effective as that of uric acid, a well-known antiradical agent. Furthermore, it also prevents the formation of radicals which escape the action of uric acid, such as the adriamycyl radical. Finally, it inhibits lipid peroxidation of membranes, and its antiradical property gives it a stimulating effect on the biosynthesis of prostanoids.

References

1. Asakawa T., Matsushita S.: Coloring conditions of thiobarbituric acid test for detecting lipid hydroperoxydes. *Lipids,* 1979, *15,* 137-140.

2. Chin-San Lai, Piette L.H.: Hydroxyl radical production involved in lipid peroxidation of rat liver microsomes. *B.B.R.C.,* 1977, *78,* 51-59.

3. Deby C., Deby-Dupont G., Noël F.X., Lavergne L.: In vitro and in vivo arachidonic acid conversions into biologically active derivatives are enhanced by uric acid. *Biochem. Pharmac.,* 1981, *30,* 2243-2249.

4. Deby C., Deby-Dupont G.: Natural factor modulating the intervention of activated oxygen in the biosynthesis of prostanoids. *Clin. Resp. Physiol.,* 1981, *17,* (Suppl.), 129-139.

5. Deby C., Deby-Dupont G., Hans P., Pincemail J., Neuray J., Goutier R.: Complementary procedures for pro- and antilipoperoxidant activity measurements. *Experientia,* 1983, *39,* 1113-1115.

6. Deby C., Magotteau G.: Relation entre les acides gras essentiels et le taux des antioxydants tissulaires chez la souris. *C. R. Soc. Biol.,* 1970, *164,* 2675-2681.

7. Deby-Dupont G., Pincemail J., Braquet P., Jeuniaux D., Deby C.: The effect of a Ginkgo biloba on lipoautoperoxidation and in vivo et in vitro prostacyclin biosynthesis. *24th International Conference on the Biochemistry of Lipids,* Toulouse, 14-15 Septembre 1983, Abstract 150 P, p 117.

8. Deby C., Pincemail J.: Toxicité de l'oxygène, radicaux libres et moyens de défense. *Presse Méd.,* 1986, *15,* 1468-1474.

9. Egan R.W., Paxton J., Kuehl R.A.: Mechanism for irreversible self-deactivation of prostaglandin synthetase. *J. Biol. Chem.,* 1976, *251,* 7329-7335.

10. Ernster L., Nordenbrand K.: *In:* Methods in enzymology. Vol. 10, Estabrook R.W., Pullman M.E., Eds., *Academic Press,* New-York, London, 1967, p. 574.

11. Etienne A., Chapelat M.Y., Braquet M., Clostre F., Drieu K., Defeudis F.V., Braquet P.: In vivo studies of free radical scavenging activity. Relation to cerebral ischemia. *In:* Cerebral Ischemia, Bes A., Braquet P., Paoletti R., Siesjö L., Eds., *Excerpta medica,* Amsterdam, New-York, Oxford, 1983, 379-384.

12. Flohé L.: Glutathion peroxidate: fact and fiction. *In:* Oxygen free radicals and tissue damage. Ciba Foundation Symposium, *Excerpta Medica,* Amsterdam, 1979, 95-121.

13. Fong K.L., Mac Kay P.B., Poyer J.L., Keele B.B., Misra H.: Evidence that peroxidation of lysosomal membranes is initiated by hydroxyl free radicals produced during flaving enzyme activity. *J. Biol. Chem.,* 1973, *248,* 7792-7797.

14. Fridovich I.: Superoxyde dismutase. *Ann. Rev. Biochem.,* 1975, *44,* 19-43.

15. Haber F., Weiss J.: The catalytic decomposition of hydrogen peroxide by iron salts. *Proc. Roy. Soc. London,* 1934, B, *147,* 332-351.

16. Halliwell B., Ahluwalia S.: Hydroxylation of p-coumaric acid by horseradish peroxidase. *Biochem.* J., 1976, *153,* 513-518.

17. Lehninger A.: Biochimie. Chapitre 18. Les enzymes d'oxydo-réduction et le transport d'électrons, *Flammarion,* Paris, 1981, p. 497.

18. Lowry O.H., Rosebrough N.J., Farr A.L., Randall R.J.: Protein measurement with the Folin phenol reagent. *J. Biol. Chem.,* 1951, 193, 265.

19. Pidoux B., Bastien C., Niddam S.: Normalization electroencephalographie activity in ageing brain by an extract of ginkgo biloba. *In:* Cerebral Ischemia, Bes A., Braquet P., Paoletti R., Siesjö K., Eds., *Excerpta Medica,* Amsterdam, New-York, Oxford, 1984, 385-388.

20. Pincemail J., Thirion A., Dupuis M., Braquet P., Drieu K., Deby C.: Ginkgo biloba extract inhibits oxygen species production generated by phorbol myristate acetate stimulated human leukocytes. *Experientia,* (sous presse).

21. Sato S., Iwaizumi M., Handa K., Tamura Y.: Electron spin resonance study on the mode of generation of free radicals of daunomycin, adriamycin and cardoquinone in NAD (P) H-microsome system. *Gann,* 1977, *68,* 603-608.

22. Sugioka K., Nakano H., Nakano M.: Less involvement of hydroxyl radical and a great importance of proposed perferryl ion complexes in lipid peroxidation. *Biochim. Biophys. Acta,* 1983, *753*, 411-421.

23. Van Caneghem P., Deby C., Bacq Z.M.: Protection par l'acide urique de l'acide hyaluronique contre la dépolymérisation par un rayonnement ionisant. *C.R. Soc. Biol.*, 1982, *176*, 391.

24. Weiss S.J., Rustaji P.K., Lo Buglio A.F.: Human granulocyte generation of hydroxyl radical. *J. Exp. Med.*, 1978, *147*, 316-323.

Effect of Ginkgo Biloba Extract on the Electrophysiology of the Isolated Diabetic Rat Retina

M. Doly[1], M. T. Droy-Lefaix[2], B. Bonhomme[1], P. Braquet[3]

(1) Laboratoire de Biophysique, Facultés de Médecine et de Pharmacie et Unité INSERM U.71,
   B.P.38. F 63001 Clermont-Ferrand Cedex.
(2) IPSEN, 30, Rue Cambronne. F 75015 Paris.
(3) Centre de recherche, I.H.B. 17, Avenue Descartes, F 92350 Le Plessis-Robinson

Summary

The purposes of the experimental work presented here were to ascertain that diabetes causes impairment of the visual function and to test the protective properties of Ginkgo biloba extract against this impairment. The experimental method selected was the isolated albino rat retina maintained in survival by perfusion. Retinal function was evaluated by electroretinographic recording in response to a light stimulus. The rats were made diabetics by injection of alloxan. After one month of diabetes the electroretinogram amplitude was significantly decreased in diabetic rats as compared with control animals. This decrease in amplitude was more pronounced after 2 months of diabetes, which confirmed that retinal function was worse. In rats treated with Ginkgo biloba extract, after 2 months of diabetes the electroretiograms had a significantly greater amplitude than that observed in untreated rats. These results are attributed to the specific role played by free oxygenated radicals on the retina of diabetic rats and to the free radical scavenger property of Ginkgo biloba extract.

The life expectancy of diabetic individuals is currently increasing, the neurovascular lesions related to diabetes becoming increasingly severe and frequent(6). However, the problem of their prevention or their treatment is still to be resolved. These vascular disorders, particularly marked in the retina, are responsible for irreversible damage to visual function.

In the retina, visual perception brings two steps into play: the first purely photochemical, the second electrophysiological in nature. The latter corresponds to actual stimulation of the retina, as excitable tissue, and produces a specific electric signal, the electroretinogram (ERG). This signal is therefore the direct reflection of

Rökan (Ginkgo Biloba). Recent Results in Pharmacology and Clinic
Edited by E.W. Fünfgeld
© Springer-Verlag Berlin Heidelberg New York 1988, pp. 83-90

retinal excitation by light and faithfully expresses the quality of visual function. Our study was carried out on the isolated retina kept alive by perfusion. This experimental technique makes it possible to study retinal function exclusively, the retina being isolated in particular from the pigmentary epithelium. Any variation in the ERG obtained on the isolated retina would therefore directly reflect an impact on the retinal metabolism.

We have tested the protective effects, against retinal damage, of Ginkgo biloba extract (EGb 761, Rökan®, Intersan)(8). The deleterious retinal effects due to diabetes are most often interpreted, in experimental models, as being at least partially related to the genesis of free radicals(2, 7, 8). Under these conditions, we wanted to test the hypothesis of a protective effect of EGb, administered orally, with respect to impact on retinal function such as appear after induction of experimental diabetes in animals.

Material and Methods

We work with the retina of albino rats(3), since this animal has almost exclusively scotopic vision, which simplifies interpretation of the ERGs obtained. After sacrifice of the animal, one of the eyes was removed, the retina was dissected and mounted as a membrane in a cell perfused with a nutritive fluid kept at 37°C and permanently oxygenated. The retina was stimulated by means of a photostimulator delivering flashes of white light: 300 lux, 1 ms. Collection of the ERGs was assured by two Ag electrodes immersed in the anterior and posterior perfusion chambers. The signal was amplified and processed by a microcomputer. We chose to quantify the ERG by measuring the amplitude of the b wave. In effect, this wave originates at the level of the internal layers of the retina(11), its amplitude reflects the quality of the intraretinal nerve transmissions and therefore of retinal metabolism.

The diabetic condition was induced in the experimental rats by administration of alloxane: intravenous injection (caudal vein) of 12 mg alloxane for a 200-g rat; one hour after injection, administration of 2 mL 5% glucose orally; for 24 hours, the bottles in the animal cages were filled with a 10% sucrose solution. The animals were monitored by determination of glycemia every 48 hours and maintaining it at less than 30 mM/L by injection of 1 I.U. or 0.5 I.U. insulin. Alloxane-induced diabetes constitutes a very widely used animal model for study of diabetes. Alloxane, in presence of ascorbate and of molecular oxygen, results in the formation of peroxide radicals that are particularly toxic for the cells. However, the target cells in which the alloxane becomes concentrated are the pancreas β cells(2). The destruction, quite specific, of these cells secreting insulin results in installation of the diabetic condition.

Treatment with EGb consists of oral administration of 100 mg/kg EGb daily. The fasted animals are gavaged in the morning. The treatment is begun 15 days before induction of the diabetes and continued throughout the duration of evolution.

We experimented with four groups of animals: a reference group (n=10); a group of diabetic rats, one month of development (n=3); a group of diabetic rats, two months of development (n=5); a group of diabetic rats treated with EGb, two months of development (n=4). Comparison of the experimental results obtained between groups was carried out by analysis of covariance.

Results

When the isolated retina of albino rats is stimulated at regular time intervals (every 5 minutes), the amplitude of the b wave on the ERG is not consistent in the course of life. The curves obtained by registering the amplitude of the b wave over time – a curve called "survival curve" – all have the same appearance (*Figure 1*): the retinal adaptation phase under experimental conditions corresponds to a systematic increase in the b wave which remains practically constant for several hours, finally to decrease steadily up to the end of survival. The mean survival curve (*Figure 1*) serves as reference for this study (control-animal group).

The mean survival curve obtained with diabetic rats having had diabetes for one month is practically identical with the control curve during the first hour of survival, but later on the amplitudes of the ERG recorded are routinely less in the diabetic rat in comparison with the controls (*Figure 2*). The difference observed between the two survival curves is definitely significant (P < 0.001 upon analysis of covariance).

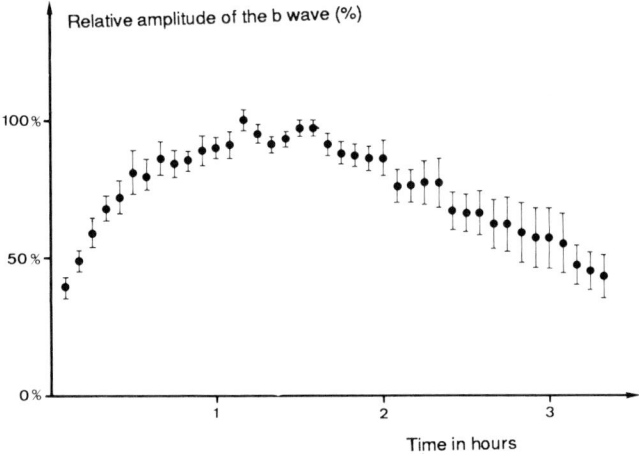

Figure 1: Evolution of the relative amplitude of the ERG b wave on isolated albino rat retina.

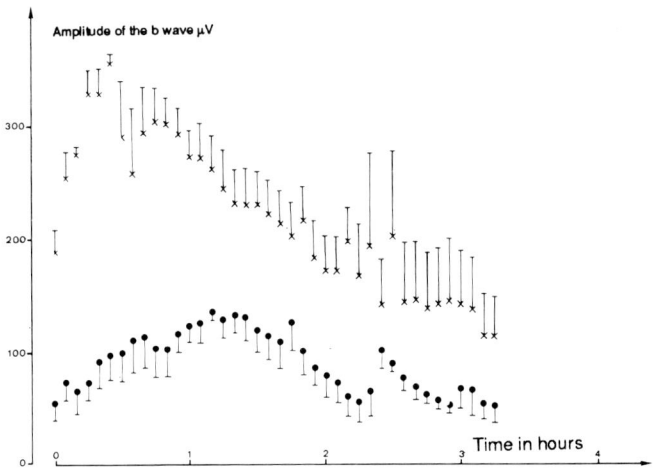

Figure 2: Comparison of the amplitude of the ERG b wave obtained in isolated retina of control rats (n=10; •———), and in diabetic rats of one month's evolution (n=3; x———).

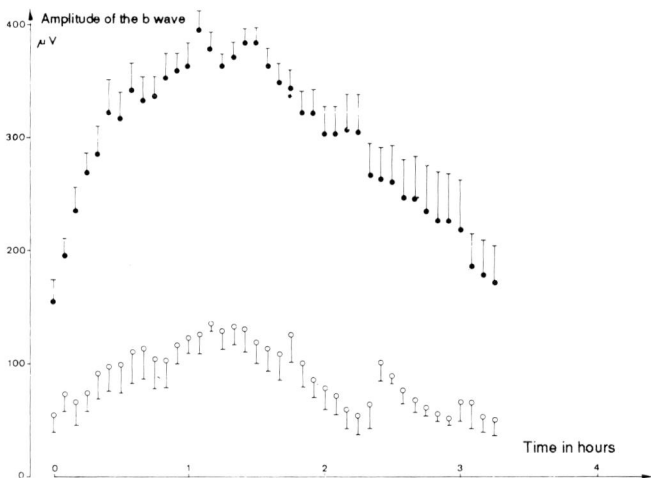

Figure 3: Comparison of the amplitude of the b wave in ERGs obtained from the isolated retina of control rats (n=10; •———), and from diabetic rats of two month's evolution (n=5; °———).

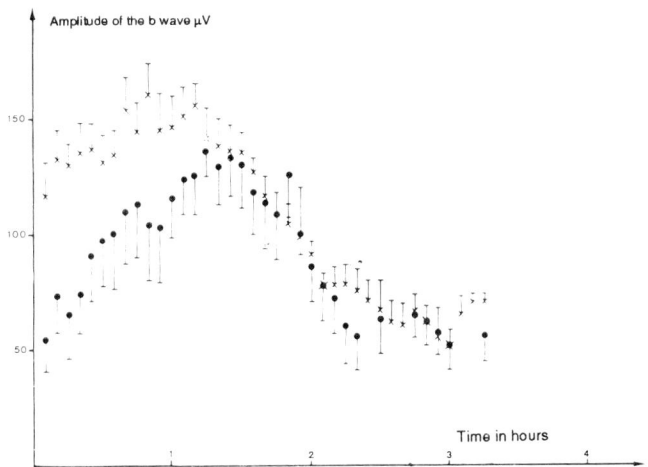

Figure 4: Comparison of the amplitude of the b wave on ERGs obtained from the isolated retina of diabetic rats of one month's evolution (n=3; ———x), and of two month's evolution (n=5; ———•).

When we compare the survival curve obtained in the diabetic rats after two months of evolution of the disease with the reference curve, we find that from the beginning of survival, the amplitude of the ERG b wave is less in the diabetic rat in comparison to the controls (*Figure 3*). The analysis of covariance shows a distinctly significant difference between the two curves (P < 0.001), the maximum amplitude in the diabetic rats on the average not exceeding a quarter of the reference value. In *Figure 4* we have reported the survival curves obtained in diabetic rats after one month and two months of evolution. A distinctly significant difference is found in amplitude of the ERG, which was confirmed by analysis of covariance (P < 0.001).

The mean survival curve recorded in the diabetic rats treated with Ginkgo biloba extract is of course very different from the reference curve. But, in order to show objectively an effect of EGb treatment, we recorded on the same graph the survival curves obtained after two months of evolution of the diabetes with and without treatment (*Figure 5*). The analysis of covariance which, in its principle, takes into consideration the entire curve, shows that there is a distinctly significant difference between the two curves (P < 0.001), the amplitude of the ERG obtained after treatment being globally significantly greater than that measured on the retinas of the untreated rats.

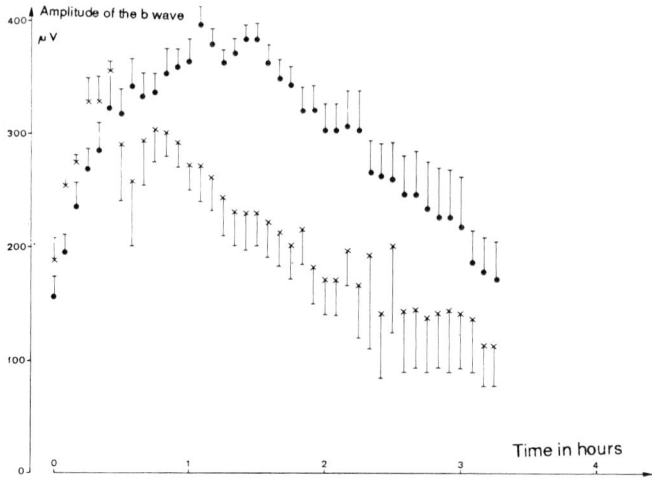

Figure 5: Comparison of the amplitude of the b wave from the ERGs obtained from the isolated retina of diabetic rats, at two months' evolution, treated with Ginkgo biloba extract (n=4; ———x), and untreated (n=5; •———) (mean ± m.s.e.).

Discussion

The primary concern of our study was to demonstrate an irreversible impact on the ERG, which was greater the longer the diabetes had been in progress. This result seems to be completely in agreement with impairment of visual function, as this also evolves with the duration of the diabetes. In fact, the electroretinogram, which originates in the photoreceptor cells, the membrane of which hyperpolarizes to light, constitutes the specific electrophysiological signal for the retina, responsible for coding visual information. Any change, even minimal, in retinal function is therefore indicated by an effect on the ERG. This is easier to show objectively when the retina is isolated from all of the other ocular milieux. However, numerous earlier studies have demonstrated only a moderate influence on the ERG *in vivo* in diabetics. In the early stages of diabetic retinopathy, the changes are essentially localized with the oscillatory potentials which appear, under certain conditions of stimulation, in the course of the ascendant phase of the ERG b wave(12). However, the intraretinal origin of these electrical accidents still being uncertain, these modifications do not explain the effects on visual function. In fact, the most marked changes in the ERG are found after treatment of the retinopathies(9). It would therefore seem that by using an isolated retina model, and having available only the neurosensorial, it would be possible to detect disturbances of visual perception even in the early stages of the diabetes.

The origin of the retinopathy is still at the present time completely obscure. Globally, at a sufficiently advanced stage of the disease, rupture of the blood-retinal barrier(1, 5) is observed, related to an increase in capillary permeability. In the alloxane-induced diabetes experimental model, these membranal changes could be due to reactivity of the oxygenated free radicals. In fact, Murata et al.(7) were the first to establish a close relationship between retinal degeneration in the diabetic rat and an increase in membranal lipoperoxidation. These experimental facts have just been confirmed by Nishimura et al.(8), who measured a significant elevation in the rate of retinal lipoperoxidation in the rat model rendered diabetic by streptozotocine. At the level of the photoreceptor cells, this lipoperoxidation, due to reactivity of the oxygenated radicals (hydroxyl and superoxide particularly) on the lipid membranes, results in irreversible functional changes shown objectively by the modifications in the ERG(4). For Nishimura et al.(6), it is prolonged hyperglycemia, induced by streptozotocine or alloxane, which is responsible for the increase in the rate of retinal lipoperoxidation. Also, the physiological mechanisms protecting against lipid per-oxidation (superoxide dismutase and α-tocopherol essentially) may also be over-whelmed under such pathological circumstances.

Particularly rich in glycosides of the benzopyrone family, Ginkgo biloba extract possesses the capacity to very actively entrap oxygenated free radicals. In this respect it may be compared with substances such as Vitamin E or butylhydroxytoluene(10). This property may be exerted wholly with respect to the retina, and the injection of EGb into the fluid perfusing the isolated retina can inhibit the deleterious effects of a peroxidizing system such as the (Fer + ascorbate) mixture(4). Under these conditions, the interpretation of the results which we are presenting would be based on the fact that after oral administration, the concentration of EGb in the retina is adequate to exert a notable free radical "trapping" activity. Thus, membranal peroxidations produced by the reactivity of these radicals would be limited, and the ERG, the genesis of which involves several membranes, would be partially preserved. Of course this hypothesis, as to the mechanism of effect of EGb in the retina, requires more ample experimental confirmation, particularly based on assay of the free radicals. However, it seems logical to us to reconcile the probable oxyradical origin of diabetic retino-pathy with the pharmacological properties of Ginkgo biloba extract.

References

1. Blair N.P., Tso M.O.M., Dodge J.T.: Pathologic studies of the blood-retinal barrier in the spontaneously diabetic BB rat. *Invest. Ophtalmol. Vis. Sci.,* 1984, *25,* 302-311.

2. Cohen, G.: Oxy-radical production in alloxan-induced diabetes: an example of an *in vivo* metal-catalyzed Haber-Weiss reaction. *In:* Free Radicals in Molecular Biology, Aging and Disease. D. Armstrong et al. Eds., *Raven Press,* New York, 1984, p. 307-316.

3. Doly M., Braquet P., Bonhomme B., Meyniel G.: Effects of lipid peroxidation on the isolated rat retina. *Ophtalmic Res.,* 1984, *16,* 292-296.

4. Doly M., Braquet P., Droy M.T., Bonhomme B., Vennat J.C.: Effets des radicaux libres oxygénés sur l'activité électrophysiologique de la rétine isolée de rat. *J. Fr. Ophtalmol.,* 1985, *8,* 273-277.

5. Ishibashi T., Tanaka K., Taniguchi Y.: Disruption of blood retinal barrier in experimental diabetic rats: an electron microscopic study. *Exp. Eye Res.,* 1980, *30,* 401-410.

6. Leuenberger P.M.: Retinopathie diabétique expérimentale: possibilités et limites. *Ophtalmologica,* 1976, *172,* 263-265.

7. Murata T., Nishida T., Eto S., Mukai N.: Lipid peroxidation in diabetic rat retina. *Metab. Pediat. Ophtalmol.,* 1981, *5,* 83-87.

8. Nishimura C., Kuriyama K.: Alterations in the retinal dopaminergic neuronal system in rats with streptozotocin-induced diabetes. *J. Neurochem.,* 1985, *45,* 448-455.

9. Palmberg P.F.: Diabetic retinopathy. *Diabetes,* 1977, *26,* 703-711.

10. Shvedova A.A., Sidorov A.S., Novikov K.N., Galushchenko I.V., Kagan V.E.: Lipid peroxidation and electric activity of the retina. *Vision Res.,* 1979, *19,* 49-55.

11. Tomita T., Yanagida T.: Origins of the ERG waves. *Vision Res.,* 1981, *21,* 1703-1707.

12. Yonemura D., Aoki T., Tsuzuki K.: Electroretinogram in diabetic retinopathy. *Arch. Ophtalmol.,* 1962, *68,* 49-54.

Effects of Ginkgo Biloba Extract on the Morphological Preservation of Vestibular Sensorial Epithelia in Mice

J. Raymond

INSERM U.254, Laboratoire de Neurophysiologie Sensorielle
U.S.T.M., Place Eugène Bataillon. F 34069 Montpellier Cedex

Summary

Oral or parenteral Ginkgo biloba extract seems to uniformly improve the ultra-structural qualities of vestibular sensorial epithelia when fixed by vascular perfusions. The improvements observed may be consequential to the effects of Ginkgo biloba extract on capillary permeability and general microcirculation, which would accelerate penetration of the fixator into vestibular tissues, and/or to more complex processes associated with cellular metabolism and membrane protective systems.

The methods for preparation of receptors in the inner ear for morphological and ultrastructural investigations vary according to the species studied, but the method for fixation of membranal structures in all cases is basically the same, whether laboratory animals are involved or human samples removed at autopsy. The goal sought for good preservation of the tissue structures is for the fixative, to come rapidly into contact with the tissues in order to avoid any ultrastructural changes induced by the effects of postmortem anoxia.

In principle, fixation by vascular perfusion fulfills these conditions by means of rapid and homogenous penetration of the fixative into all areas of the body before autolysis of the tissues at the time of prior procedures. The central nervous structures are generally fixed satisfactorily under such conditions(6, 9). It is different for the inner ear receptors. These are imprisoned in liquid compartments, and their blood supply is low and assured by extremely delicate capillary vessels(10). However, as the structures in the membranal labyrinth present only a few layers of cells, we might assume that rapid fixation by local immersion of the tissues, a technique usable only in human postmortems, permits a good genetration of the fixative. However, whatever changes are made in fixation techniques(1, 3), variability is observed in preservation of the cells of the sensorial epithelium; certain structures are particularly vulnerable

Rökan (Ginkgo Biloba). Recent Results in Pharmacology and Clinic
Edited by E.W. Fünfgeld
© Springer-Verlag Berlin Heidelberg New York 1988, pp. 91-97

to conditions of anoxia, however short this period may be. This vulnerability is even more manifest when postmortem samples are taken from man(7).

Ginkgo biloba extract (EGb 761, Rökan®, Intersan), a substance rich in specific terpenes and in flavonoid glycosides, has a major potential for trapping free radicals and has shown a beneficial activity on the vascular tree; arteries-capillaries-veins(2).

Its administration is reflected in an overall increase in tissue perfusion and an action on microvascularization, with a consequential special therapeutic indication in neurosensorial disorders in otorhinolaryngology(4, 5, 8), disorders which might be assumed in numerous cases to have an ischemic or metabolic cause. Furthermore, recent results have drawn attention to a membrane protection action which might be responsible for these effects.

This study has the purpose of observing the consequences of EGb administration on the morphological preservation of the most fragile ultrastructural elements of the vestibular sensorial epithelium at the time of fixation of this structure by vascular perfusion in mice.

Material and Methods

Twenty-four mice weighing approximately 20 g were divided into four groups:

– Group A, control, made up of six mice fixed by vascular perfusion;

– Group B, of six mice fixed under the same conditions as Group A, with the addition of EGb (1 g/100 mL) in the fixative;

– Group C, of six mice having received EGb treatment orally (2 mg/kg) for eight days preceding fixation by vascular perfusion.

– Group D, of six mice having received IPS 200 treatment (lyophilized injectable Ginkgo biloba extract) by intraperitoneal injection (40 mg/kg) for eight days preceding fixation by vascular perfusion.

After anesthesia of the animal with pentobarbital sodium(1), vascular perfusion with 100 mL fixative was carried out for approximately ten minutes through the ascending aorta by means of a cannula connected to a perfusion pump. The fixative was composed of 2.5% glutaraldehyde (TAAB) in an 0.1M cacodylate buffer at pH 7.2.

The vestibular receptors were removed separately under an operative microscope and postfixed in a 1% osmium tetroxide solution in 0.1M cacodylate buffer for one hour, dehydrated in 70% ethyl alcohol at 100°, and enclosed in Araldite. The ultrafine sections were taken with an ultramicrotome by means of a diamond knife. The sections were contrasted with uranyl acetate and with lead citrate. Alternating with the ultrafine sections, semifine sections gave, after staining with toluidine blue, a global image of the various vestibular receptors.

Results

The morphological and ultrastructural characteristics of the vestibular epithelium were analyzed by comparison in the various groups of animals. The sections were observed both in the ampullary receptors and in the utricular macula. This analysis involved essentially the ciliated sensorial cells and the adjacent nerve fibers and endings. The following points were the subject of special attention: inflation or retraction of the cytoplasm, cytoplasmic protusions on the surface of the sensorial cells, dilatation of the nerve calices around the type 1 cells; at the ultrastructural level, fine structure of the cellular and nuclear membranes, mitochondria, endoplasmic reticulum, formation of intracellular vesicles, myelin figures, afferent and efferent nerve endings.

At the time of fixations according to the classical methods (Group A), good preservation of the sensorial cells, the cellular and nuclear membranes, and of intracellular organoids is obtained, sometimes with frequent variations in the ultra-structural qualities. Thus, in *Figure 1*, variations may be observed in the electronic density of the cytoplasm with vacuolization or densification of certain cellular contents. It is also found that the nerve calices surrounding the type I sensorial cells are very dilated, sometimes with loss of their cytoplasmic content. Furthermore, the mitochondria are often split, with fragmentation of the mitochondrial crests. At the level of the fasciculus of myelinized afferent fibers under the sensorial epithelium (*Figure 2*), the histological quality is good, with retraction of certain axoplasms within the myeline sheaths, however.

In Group B, the observations do not allow a conclusion as to better preservation of the most delicate structures of the vestibular sensorial epithelium. In fact, in certain specimens retraction may be observed of the sensorial cells, accompanied by very accentuated dilatations of the nerve calices. However, very good preservation of the mitochondrial membranes was found in all cases.

In the animals in Group C (*Figures 3, 4, and 5*), a reproducible attenuation was observed in the changes induced above (Group A). Preservation of the intracellular organoids – endoplasmic reticulum, neurofilaments, mitochondria, vesicles and synaptic membranes – is very good. In general, the nerve calices were not dilated, except very slightly (*Figure 5*), and the axoplasms were never retracted within the myeline sheaths.

In Group D, preliminary observations, still inadequate in number, show that the vestibular sensorial epithelia present excellent preservation with very good definition of the dual membranes, of the mitochondrial crests, and of all of the cytoplasmic organoids (*Figure 6*).

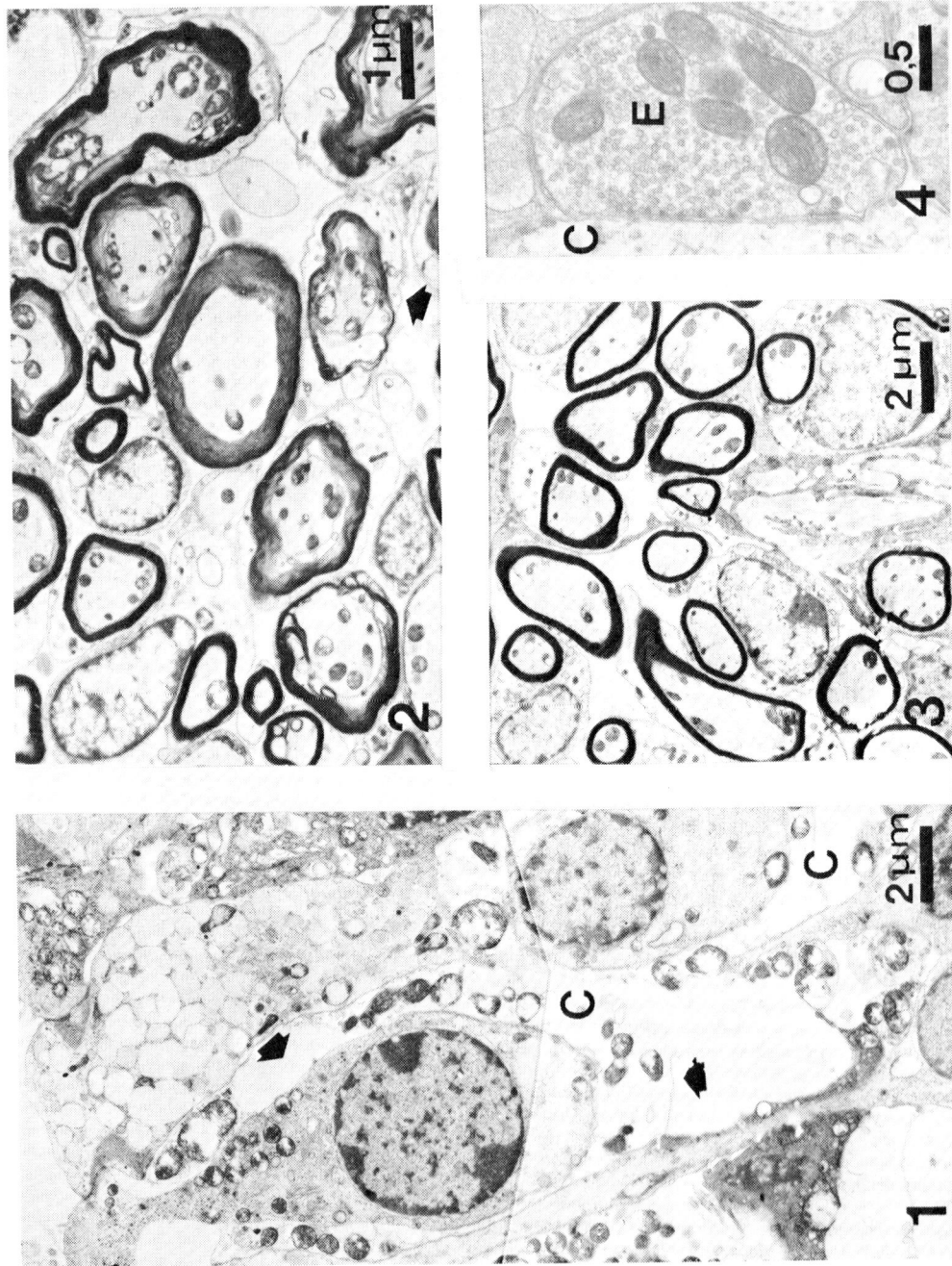

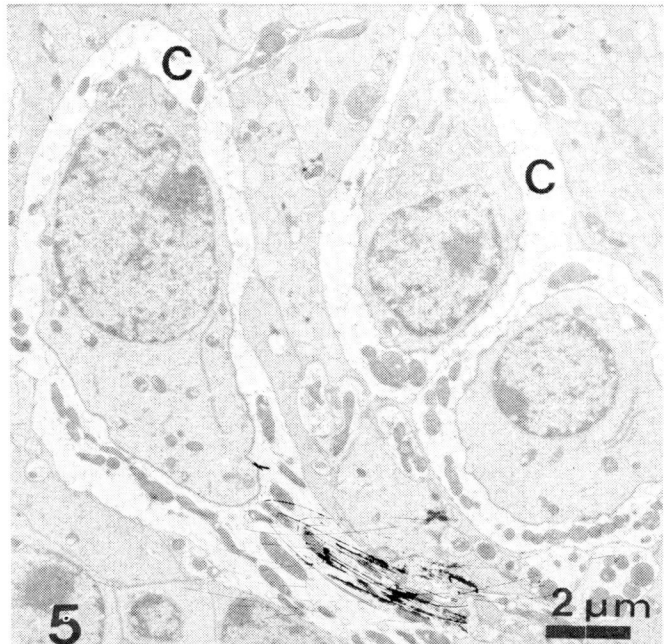

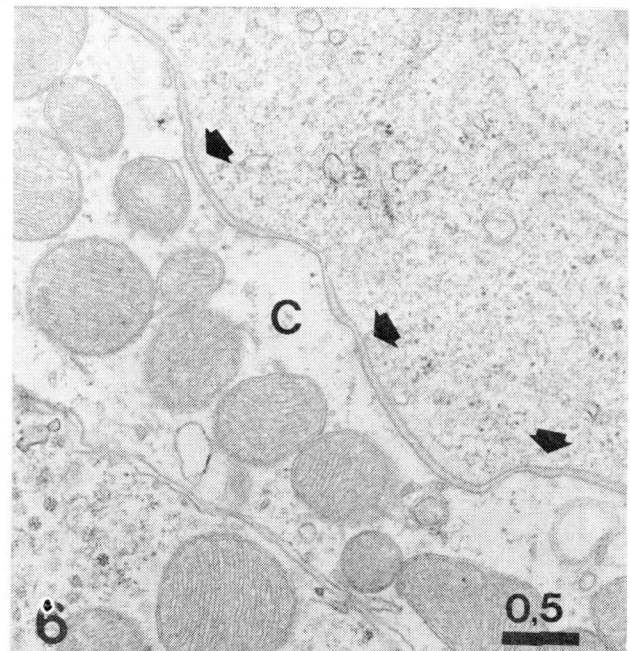

Figure:

1) Vestibular sensorial epithelium - Group A, control. Note the splitting of the nerve calices (C) and numerous mitochondria.

2) Ampullary nerve fibers – Group A, control. Certain axoplasms have retracted within the myeline sheaths, which are sometimes frayed.

3) Ampullary nerve fibers – Group C.

4) Efferent vestibular ending (E) in contact with a nerve calyx (C). Note the quality of preservation of the mitochondria and of the synaptic contours.

5) Vestibular sensorial epithelium – Group C.

6) Sensorial cell and nerve calyx – Group D. Note the precision of resolution of the membranes between the sensorial cell and the afferent calyx (C) and that of the mitochondrial crests.

Conclusion

The administration of EGb orally or by injection seems to consistently improve the ultrastructural qualities of vestibular sensorial epithelia fixed by vascular perfusion. Additional observations are in progress on very old animals where, under the usual conditions of fixation, it is sometimes difficult to evaluate whether the abnormalities observed are due to aging of the nerve and sensorial structures or to changes related to the conditions of fixation. The improvements observed may be attributed to the effects of EGb on capillary permeability and general microcirculation, which would increase penetration of the fixative into the vestibular tissues, and/or more complex mechanisms of effect of EGb related to cellular metabolism and to protection of the membranal systems.

References

1. Anniko M., Lundquist P.G.: Temporal bone morphology after systemic arterial perfusion or intralabyrinthine *in situ* immersion. I. Hair cells of the vestibular organs and the cochlea. *Micron,* 1980, *11,* 73-83.

2. Auguet M., Hellegouarch A., Delaflotte S., Baranes J., DeFeudis F.V., Clostre F., Braquet P., Drieu K.: Effects of Ginkgo biloba extract on rabbit isolated blood vessels. *In:* Cerebral Ischemia, Bes A., Braquet P., Paoletti R., Siesjö B.K., Eds., *Excerpta Medica,* Amsterdam, 1984, 347-354.

3. Favre D., Sans A.: Technical proposition for a better ultrastructural preservation of nerve endings in the vestibular sensory epithelium. A.T.E.M. and X-ray micro-analysis study. *Micron Micr. Acta,* 1983, *14,* 319-327.

4. Guerrier Y., Basseres F., Artières J.: Le Tanakan dans le traitement des vertiges. A propos de 26 observations. *Cahiers O.R.L.,* 1978, *13,* 421-428.

5. Igounet J., Negrevergne M.: Le Tanakan dans les troubles vasculaires de l'oreille interne. Insuffisances circulatoires et vasorégulation artérielle, capillaire et veineuse. *Colloque pluridisciplinaire (Paris) GG. Ed.,* 1976.

6. Karlsson U., Schultz R.L.: Fixation of the central nervous system for electron microscopy. I. Preservation with aldehyde perfusates versus direct perfusion with osmium tetroxide with special reference to membranes and the extracellular space. *J. Ultrastruct. Res.,* 1965, *12,* 160-186.

7. Nadol J.B., Burgess B.: A study of post-mortem autolysis in the human organ of Corti. *J. Comp. Neurol.,* 1985, *237,* 333-342.

8. Post A.: Troubles neurosensoriels d'expression otologique: apport de l'extrait de Ginkgo biloba. A propos de 255 cas. Thèse. Université Paris VII - Faculté de Médecine Xavier Bichat, 1978.

9. Schultz R.L., Case N.M.: A modified aldehyde perfusion technique for preventing certain artefacts in electron microscopy of the central nervous system. *J. Microsc.*, 1970, *92*, 69-84.

10. Wersall J.: Studies on the structure and innervation of the cristae ampullares in the genuinea pig. *Acta Otolaryngol.* (Stockh.), 1956, Suppl. *126*, 1-85.

Variations in Neuromediators in Cerebral Aging
Effect of Ginkgo Biloba Extract

G. Racagni, N. Brunello, R. Paoletti

Istituto di Farmacologia et Farmacognosia, Centro di Neurofarmacologia
Universita di Milano, Via Balzaretti 9.20133 Milano, Italy

Summary

Ginkgo biloba extract exerts a specific effect on the noradrenergic system and on beta-receptors. No variation was found in alpha 2-receptors and serotonin uptake. These findings provide the first evidence of central effects of a drug acting on cerebral ageing, connected specifically to reactivation of the noradrenergic system in the cerebral cortex.

During the past few years, our knowledge about the metabolism of neuromediators in physiological or pathological aging has been amplified considerably.

Physiological aging

Experiments made on animals have demonstrated a diminution in choline acetyltransferase (CAT) related to age.

In parallel, elderly subjects have a lower number of acetylcholine receptor sites of muscarinic type.

Numerous studies have demonstrated a reduction in activity of the catecholamines in the brain of aged rats and in tyrosine hydroxylase in elderly rats and man(5, 8). Since the activity of tyrosine hydroxylase is the step which limits the synthesis of catecholamines, its reduction in relation with age suggests special interactions.

Research conducted postmortem in man have demonstrated reduced levels of dopamine (DA) and noradrenalin (NA) related to age(6). Attempts to establish a correlation between the serotonin (5HT) level and aging have given contradictory results. In man (although an increase has been shown in levels of 5HT in the cerebral brain stem) they decrease with age in the cortical areas(6). Studies conducted in our laboratory have demonstrated that the molecular complex for uptake of 5HT is

Rökan (Ginkgo Biloba). Recent Results in Pharmacology and Clinic
Edited by E.W. Fünfgeld
© Springer-Verlag Berlin Heidelberg New York 1988, pp. 98-102

modified during aging. In fact, a decrease is found in bonding sites for ^{3}H-imipramine(3). The latter data is related to the results found in the cerebral cortex in elderly humans. The correlation of the level of homovanillic acid (HVA) with age is null or inadequate. The correlation between 5-hydroindolacetic acid (5-HIAA) and age is positive in the caudate nucleus, in the hippocampus, in the cortex, in the *Gyrus cinguli,* and in the cerebellum. In the cerebrospinal fluid, the correlation between age and HVA and 5-HIAA metabolites is positive.

It has been demonstrated that the activity of monoaminoxidases (MAO), the principal catabolic enzyme for the monoamines, increases with age(6). It seems that the correlation between age and the activity of MAO, evaluated with β-phenylethylamine as substrate (MAO-B) is greater than with serotonin as substrate (MAO-A). There is also an age-related increase in MAO activity of the platelets(9).

GABA receptors in the rat brain diminish with age, particularly in the cerebellum, in the *Substantia nigra,* in the hypothalamus, and in the striated body, whereas they are modified less markedly in the cerebralcortex, in the hippocampus, in the spinal cord, in the pons, and in the medulla. In all of the cerebral regions, the decrease is due to the reduction in total density of the sites for recognition of GABA.

Alzheimer-type senile dementia

Numerous studies have demonstrated that in Alzheimer-type senile dementia, there is a reduction in CAT activity(4). No reduction in the number of muscarinic receptors has been found in subjects suffering with this disease. However, it seems that in them, the cholinergic system is particularly modified at the presynaptic level. Even if from a pathogenic point of view the alterations in the acetylcholinergic system are very significant in senile dementia of Alzheimer type, it seems improbable that there is only one neuromediator concerned, bearing in mind the extent of the cerebral degeneration of these patients. It is now known that other mediator systems are also altered. Thus, several authors(1, 7) have demonstrated that the concentration of the principal metabolite of dopamine, HVA, is reduced in the basal ganglia of subjects suffering with Alzheimer's disease. It is known that the concentrations of HVA are related to the severity of the dementia: the more serious the intellectual deterioration, the lower the HVA levels. The HVA concentrations are not reduced in dementia due to multiple infarctions, nor in control subjects. Also, the concentrations of dopamine (DA) and noradrenalin (NA) are also found to be decreased in certain areas of the brain in patients suffering with Alzheimer's disease in comparison with normal subjects of the same age. On the contrary, the final metabolite for metabolism of NA, 3,4-methoxyl-hydroxyl-phenylglycol, seems increased in subjects suffering with Alzheimer's disease. The cerebrospinal fluid from these subjects contains much lower levels of HVA than of 5-HIAA in comparison with controls of the same age(7).

The hypothesis according to which senile deterioration and dementia would be related to a deficiency in folic acid and Vitamin B_{12}(11) has been suggested. The stage which limits the rate of synthesis of catecholamines and of serotonin is in fact hydroxylation of an amino acid, a chemical reaction the folate of which is the coenzyme. A folate insufficiency could therefore induce a disturbance in "turn-over" of monoamines. However, the observations made on senile dementia(10) suggest that it is improbable that in these patients the folate deficiency is such that it could bring about a disturbance in metabolism of monoamines.

In subjects suffering with Alzheimer's senile dementia, the enzymatic activities such as MAO and superoxide-dismutase increase in the cerebral tissue. Such an increase could probably reflect changes in the cerebral tissue capable of having pathogenic importance. It should, however, be noted that the increase in activity of MAO in Alzheimer's senile dementia appears not only in the cerebral tissue but also in the platelets. This indicates that a generalized alteration is involved.

In conclusion, study of variations in the cerebral neuronal systems, of the properties of the receptors and of the processing of information in the brain are assuming major importance for better understanding of the gradual functional loss due to age and to the pathogenesis of age-related diseases.

Effect of Ginkgo biloba

These data on variations in the levels and "turn-over" of cerebral neuromediators in the course of normal and pathological aging emphasize the importance of identification of nontoxic therapeutic methods which would be active permanently on these systems.

Recent research done in our laboratory(2) demonstrated that purified Ginkgo biloba extract (EGb 761, Rökan®, Intersan) used clinically in syndromes related to cerebral aging increases turn-over of cerebral NA in the cortex of adult rats, but only after prolonged treatment (one to two months).

We show here (*Table I*) that the effect is specific on the noradrenergic system and on the β receptors, since no variations were observed in the α_2 receptors nor in serotonin uptake. This is the first demonstration of the central effects of a therapy active in cerebral aging, which appears to be linked specifically to reactivation of the noradrenergic system in the cortex.

Table 1

Effects of long-term treatment with Ginkgo Biloba extract (EGb) on the concentrations of normetanephrine (NMN) and on the activity of the cerebral receptors (number of animals: 10 in each group)

| | | NMN | Binding of ^{3}H.DHA | |
| | | | K_D | Bmax |
Treatments		(pmol/mg/pr)	(nm)	(fmoles/mg/pr)
Physiological saline solution		0.43 ± 0.08	3.03 ± 0.21	237.3 ± 19.4
EGb (100 mg/kg)	7 days	0.34 ± 0.04	2.91 ± 0.19	248.1 ± 16.8
	14 days	2.13 ± 0.20	–	–
	30 days	–	2.31 ± 0.18	133.4 ± 12.1
	60 days	–	2.60 ± 0.22	167.6 ± 10.4

References

1. Adolfsson R., Gottfries C.-G., Roos B.E., Winblad B.: Post mortem distribution of dopamine and homovanillic acid in human brain, variations related to age, and a review of the literature. *J. Neural. Transm.*, 1979, *45*, 81-105.

2. Brunello N., Racagni G., Clostre F., Drieu K., Braquet P.: Effects of an extract of Ginkgo biloba on noradrenergic systems of rat cerebral cortex. *Pharmacol. Res. Comm.*, 1985, *17*, 1063-1072.

3. Brunello N., Riva M., Volterra A., Racagni G.: Age-related changes in 5HT uptake and ^{3}H-imipramine binding sites in rat cerebral cortex: *Eur. J. Pharmac.*, 1985, *110*, 393-394.

4. Davies P., Maloney A.J.F.: Selective loss of central cholinergic neurons in Alzheimer's disease. *Lancet*, 1976, *2*, 1403-1405.

5. Finch C.E.: Catecholamine metabolism in the brains of ageing male mice. *Brain Res.*, 1973, *52*, 261-276.

6. Gottfries C.G.: Monoamines and their metabolites and monoamine oxidase activity related to age and to some dementia disorders. *In:* Drugs and the Elderly. Perspective in geriatric clinical pharmacology, J. Crooks, I.H. Stevenson, Eds., Proceed. of a symposium held in Ninewells Hospital University of Dundee 13 and 14 September 1977, *MacMilliam*, London, 1979, 189-197.

7. Gottfries C.G., Ross B.E.: Acid monoamine metabolites in cerebrospinal fluid from patients with pre-senile dementia (Alzheimer's disease). *Acta Psychiatry Scand.*, 1973, *49*, 257-263.

8. McGeer E.G.: Aging and brain enzymes. *Exp. Gerontol.*, 1971, *6*, 391-396.

9. Robinson D.S., Nies A., Davis J.N., Bunney W.E., Davis J.M., Colburn R.W., Bourne H.R., Shaw D.M.: Ageing, monoamines and monoamines oxidase levels. *Lancet*, 1972, *1*, 290-291.

10. Shaw D.M.: Folate and amine metabolites in senile dementia: a combined trial and biochemical study. *Psycho. Med.*, 1971, *1*, 166-171.

11. Shulman R.: A survey of vitamin B_{12} deficiency in an elderly psychiatric population. *Br. J. Psychiatry*, 1967, *113*, 241-251.

Binding of Neuromediators to Their Receptors in Rat Brain
Effect of Chronic Administration of Ginkgo Biloba Extract

J. E. Taylor

Biomesure Inc., 11-15 "E" Avenue, Hopkinton, MA 01748. USA

Summary

The present data confirm the results of others that post-synaptic receptor changes may contribute to the decline in brain cholinergic function in ageing and dementia. We have also shown that chronic oral treatment with an extract of Ginkgo biloba increases the apparent muscarinic receptor population in the hippocampus of the aged Fisher 344 rat. The possible effect on (^{3}H) kainic acid binding to the kainate-excitatory amino acid site is also interesting because of the proposed association of neurodegenerative disease and excessive excitatory amino neurotransmission.

Numerous studies have been made of changes in activity of the neuromediators of the central nervous system, associated, it seems, with the process of senescence(7, 14). Certain of these changes, among the most important and the most frequent, occur essentially at the level of the muscarinic cholinergic systems. Thus, a significant diminution in choline acetyltransferase has been observed in several areas of the brain of patients suffering with Alzheimer's disease(1, 3, 12). The same observation was made in the brain of aged rodents(1). Despite a certain number of negative results(1), several authors have also discussed a weakening of binding with the muscarinic receptor in the cerebral cortex and hippocampus in subjects suffering with Alzheimer's disease and in aged rats(1, 8, 10, 11, 13). Others have discussed changes affecting the binding of the adrenergic receptors and those for opiates, as well as binding of the receptors for somatostatin and glutamate (2, 5, 14).

We are examining here the *in vitro* effects of long-term administration of Ginkgo biloba extract (EGb 761, Rökan®, Intersan) on the binding of several receptor/neuromediator pairs in the brains of Fisher 344 rats, young and old.

Rökan (Ginkgo Biloba). Recent Results in Pharmacology and Clinic
Edited by E.W. Fünfgeld
© Springer-Verlag Berlin Heidelberg New York 1988, pp. 103-108

Methods

Medical treatments and preparation of the tissues

The male Fisher 344 rats (Charles River) received Ginkgo biloba extract (EGb) in the drinking water at the rate of 100 mg/kg/day for 28 days. The rats were sacrificed by decapitation 24 hours after ingestion of the last dose. The areas of the brain rich in specific receptors were then removed and placed at a temperature of $-80°C$. The samples of tissues were thawed and homogenized in a buffer solution kept in the cold, using a Brinkman polytron (6 to 15 seconds). After two centrifugations of the homogenized substance at the rate of 39,000 x G for ten minutes, the sediment containing the crude membrane preparations was placed in a buffer solution, then immediately used to study the binding of the receptors. The homogenized substance, meant for tests for (^{3}H) kainic acid, was washed three times by centrifugation, whereas the membranes meant for testing for dopamine$_2$ with 5-HT$_2$ and with the opiate μ group, were preincubated at 37°C being centrifuged a second time.

Experiments with receptor bindings

Aliquot portions of the washed membrane preparations were placed in glass test tubes (12 x 75 mm) containing the ligand (^{3}H). After incubation the thermal equilibrium, then rapid filtration through Whatman GF/B filters, under low pressure, each tube and each filter was immediately washed three times with 5 mL of the aliquot portions of the buffer, and the radioactivity of the filters was measured by liquid scintillation spectrometry. All of the tests were done twice. Specific binding was defined as the difference between certain factors bound to the ligand (^{3}H) and these same factors placed in the presence of a saturated concentration of ligand of an undetermined receptor (*Table 1*). The linear regressions of the Scatchard curves were used to determine the dissociation constants of apparent equilibrium (Kd), as well as the maximal number of binding sites (Bmax). The binding curves from the (^{3}H) kainic acid tests were analyzed by nonlinear regression techniques(9), and statistical analysis of the data was done with the Student t-test.

Table 1

Parameters used in tests on binding of radioligands to their receptors

Receptor	(^{3}H) Ligand	Concentration	Area of the brain	Incubation (min/°C)
α_1-adrenergic	WB4101	Phentolamine (1 μM)	Cerebral cortex	30/25
α_2-adrenergic	Clonidine	Phentolamine	Cerebral cortex	30/25
β-adrenergic	DHA	(±) Propanol (1 μM)	Cerebral cortex	30/25
Dopamine$_2$	Spiperone	(+) Butaclamol	Striate body	15/37
5-HT$_2$	Spiperone	5-HT	Frontal cortex	15/37
Opiate, μ	Naloxone	Levallorphan	Mid-brain	60/25
Kainic acid	Kainic acid	Kainic acid	Cerebral cortex	60/0-4
Musarinic	QNB	Atropine	Hippocampus	60/37

Results

The effects of chronic administration of EGb on the binding of (^{3}H) QNB to the muscarinic cholinergic receptors of the hippocampus are shown in *Table 2*. Comparison with the control group shows a significant diminution (−20%) in Bmax of the elderly animals in comparison to the younger animals. These results confirm the data previously reported, according to which the number of muscarinic receptors situated in the brain of rodents decreases with age.(6, 8, 10, 11, 14)

Table 2

Effects of long-term administration of Ginkgo Biloba extract (EGb) on specific binding of (^{3}H) QNB to the muscarinic cholinergic receptors in the hippocampus

Animal	(n)	Bmax (fmol/mg tissue)
Control, 3 months	8	133.7 ± 4.2
Control, 24 months	5	108.8 ± 6.8*
+ EGb, 3 months	6	140.9 ± 3.5
+ EGb, 24 months	6	127.6 ± 3.7

*Significant difference from the 3-month controls, 3-month EGb, and 24-month EGb.

A slight increase in the number of muscarinic receptors was observed, regardless of age, following long-term treatment with EGb base. This increase, more marked in the elderly animals, may be considered as statistically significant. The Bmax value in the 24-month EGb group is similar to that observed in the 3-month control group, which suggests that long-term administration of EGb to elderly animals normalizes the density of the muscarinic receptors.

With respect to the effects of long-term administration of EGb on the other neuromediator receptors in the brain (*Table 3*), it was found that the number of beta-adrenergic receptors decreases, whereas the bonds involving (^{3}H) kainic acid increase with age. The last observation is interesting if we refer to the recent report by Geddes et al.(4), who observed an increase in binding relative to (^{3}H) kainic acid in the hippocampus of patients suffering with Alzheimer's disease, as well as in an animal model of neurodegeneration (denervation of the entorhinal cortex induced by lesion). The EGb treatment had no effect on beta-adrenergic binding. However, in elderly animals treated with EGb, an increase was noted – not statistically significant, it is true – in bonds involving (^{3}H) kainic acid. Let us add that no changes were noted, related to age or to administration of EGb, in binding of the radio-ligands with the alpha-adrenergic and μ-opiate receptors, or with receptors for dopamine D_2 or the 5-HT_2 group.

Table 3

Effects of long-term administration of Ginkgo Biloba extract (EGb) on the adrenergic, serotonin$_2$, opiates (μ), and kainic acid receptors

Recptors	Bmax (fmol/mg tissue)			
	Control (3 months)	Control (24 months)	+ EGb (3 months)	+ EGb (24 months)
α_1-adrenergic	8.9 ± 0.3	9.0 ± 0.6	9.7 ± 0.5	8.4 ± 0.9
α_2-adrenergic	5.6 ± 0.3	4.9 ± 0.6	6.0 ± 0.1	5.3 ± 0.4
β-adrenergic	8.1 ± 0.6	6.7 ± 0.3[a]	9.3 ± 0.5	6.7 ± 0.9[a]
Dopamine$_2$	16.1 ± 1.9	13.7 ± 1.0	12.0 ± 0.7	15.1 ± 0.7
5-HT_2	12.1 ± 1.2	11.0 ± 1.2	12.7 ± 1.1	11.5 ± 1.3
Opiate, μ	6.7 ± 0.5	6.7 ± 0.06	8.2 ± 0.9	10.9 ± 1.1
Kainic acid	0.51 ± 0.14	2.6 ± 0.9	[b]	1.5 ± 0.7

[a] Significantly different from time 3 months, P < 0.05.
[b] Not tested.

Discussion

Numerous and very reliable indices, drawn from experiments made *in vivo* and *in vitro*, have already supported the thesis according to which the decline in cholinergic muscarinic activity could play a part in certain mnesic and cognitive deficits related to age(1, 3, 7). The present data confirm the fact that changes in the postsynaptic receptors may contribute to the decline in cholinergic function of the brain in elderly subjects and in those suffering with senile dementia. We have also noted that long-term oral treatment with Ginkgo biloba extract increases the apparent population of muscarinic receptors in the hippocampus of elderly Fisher 344 rats. The possible effect of (^{3}H) kainic acid binding to the site bearing the kainate-excitatory amino acid is also interesting because of the suggested association between neurodegenerative diseases and excessive neurotransmission of the excitatory amino acid(15). More thorough research in this field is amply justified at present. The clinical meanings of these changes occurring in the receptors are difficult to determine, but they can contribute, in part, to the therapeutic actions of EGb.

References

1. Bartus R.T., Dean IIIR.L., Beer B., Lippa A.S.: The cholinergic hypothesis of geriatric memory dysfunction. *Science, 1982, 217,* 408-417.

2. Beal M.F., Mazurek M.F., Tran V.T., Chattha G., Bird E.D., Martin J.B.: Reduced number of somatostatin receptors in the cerebral cortex in Alzheimer's disease. *Science, 1985, 229,* 289-291.

3. Davis K.L., Yamamura H.I.: Cholinergic under-activity in human memory disorders. *Life Sci., 1978, 23,* 1729-1734.

4. Geddes J.W., Monaghan D.T., Cotman C.W., Lott I.T., Kim R.C., Chui H.C.: Plasticity of hippocampal circuitry in Alzheimer's diseases. *Science, 1985, 230,* 1179-1181.

5. Greenamyre J.T., Penny J.B., Young A.B., D'Amato C.J., Hicks S.P., Shoulson I.: Alterations in L-glutamate binding in Alzheimer's and Huntington's disease. *Scien*ce, 1985, 227, 1496-1499.

6. James T.C., Kanungo M.S.: Alterations in atropine sites of the brain of rats as a function of age. *Biochem. Biophys. Res. Commun., 1976, 72,* 170-175.

7. McGeer E.G.: Neurotransmitter systems in aging and senile dementia. *Prog. Neuro-Psychopharmacol., 1981, 5,* 435-445.

8. Morin A.M., Westerlain C.G.: Aging and rat brain muscarinic receptors as measured by quinuclidinyl benzilate binding. *Neurochem. Res.*, 1980, *5*, 301-308.

9. Munson P.J., Rodbard D.: Ligands: A versatile computerized approach for characterization of ligand-binding systems. *Annal. Biochem.*, 1980, *107*, 220-239.

10. Nordberg A., Wahlstrom G.: Cholinergic receptors and ageing. *Abstr. Eight Int. Congr. Pharmacol.*, 1981, 827.

11. Nordberg A., Windblad B.: Cholinergic receptors in human hippocampus: Regional distribution and variance with age. *Life Sci.*, 1981, *29*, 1937-1944.

12. Perry T.L., Gibson P.H., Blessed G., Perry R.H., Tomlinson B.E.: Neurotransmitter abnormalities in senile dementia. *J. Neurol. Sci.*, 1977, *34*, 247-265.

13. Reisine T.D., Pedigo N.W., Meiners C., Igbal K., Yamamura H.I.: Alzheimer's disease: Studies on neurochemical alterations in the brain. *In:* Ageing of the Brain and Dementia, Amaducc L., Davidson A.H., Antuono P., Eds., *Raven Press*, New York, 1980, 147-150.

14. Roth G.S., Hess G.D.: Changes in the mechanisms of hormone and neurotransmitter action during aging: Current status of the role of receptor and post-receptor alterations. A review. *Mech. Aging and Develop.*, 1982, *20*, 175-194.

15. Schwartz R., Meldrum B.: Excitatory amino acid antagonists provide a therapeutic approach to neurological disorders. *Lancet*, 1985, *2*, 140-143.

Cerebral Glucose Consumption
Effect of Ginkgo Biloba Extract

J. R. Rapin, M. Le Poncin-Lafitte

I.N.R.P.V.C., Hôpital Bicêtre. 78, Rue du Général Leclerc
F 94275 Le Kremlin Bicêtre

Summary

Deoxyglucose is transported under the same conditions as glucose from blood to cerebral tissue. After phosphorylation, 6-deoxyglucose-phosphate, which can be neither metabolized nor eliminated, accumulates in the cells. This accumulation is correlated with glucose consumption.

These two parameters, transfer rate of deoxyglucose and glucose consumption in the brain, were measured by means of quantitative autoradiography in two experimental cerebrovascular pathology models: normobaric hypoxia and carotid clamping in rats.

Normobaric hypoxia induces a decrease in both transfer rate and glucose consumption. Ligation of the carotid artery diminishes glucose consumption much more than the transfer rate.

After preventive administration of Ginkgo biloba extract, glucose consumption was partially reestablished in both experimental models.

Roy and Sherrington[8] proposed the hypothesis of local regulation of blood circulation related to cerebral metabolism. This coupling between flow and cerebral metabolism has since been confirmed numerous times, both in animals and in man. In rats, the flow is correlated with oxygen consumption and glucose consumption during different conditions such as hypothermia, hyperthermia, anesthesia, or immobilization stress, or under treatment with barbiturates, psychostimulants, and convulsants[3]. Local consumption of glucose may be used as a method for exploration of cerebral metabolism, since there is a stoichiometric relationship between mean oxygen consumption and consumption of glucose[9].

The ratio of oxygen consumption to glucose consumption, which is equal to 5.5 in man and 5.7 in rats, remains unchanged in most pathological conditions, as long as the ketone bodies only partially supplant the glucose and the anaerobic route of glucose degradation does not become preponderant[7]. Local consumption of glucose

Rökan (Ginkgo Biloba). Recent Results in Pharmacology and Clinic
Edited by E.W. Fünfgeld
© Springer-Verlag Berlin Heidelberg New York 1988, pp. 109-116

is measured in the awake animal by using the technique of Sokoloff(4) with the use of autoradiographic methods and dissection of the brain after administration of deoxyglucose. Deoxyglucose is transported under the same conditions as glucose from the blood toward the glial and neuronal tissue. Like glucose, it is then phosphorylated under the influence of hexokinase. Synthesized 6-deoxyglucose-phosphate, which cannot be metabolized or eliminated, accumulates in the cells. The level of 6-deoxyglucose-phosphate accumulated is representative of cellular activity, and from this result, it is possible to calculate local glucose consumption if the blood kinetics of deoxyglucose excretion and the glycemia value are known (*Figure 1*).

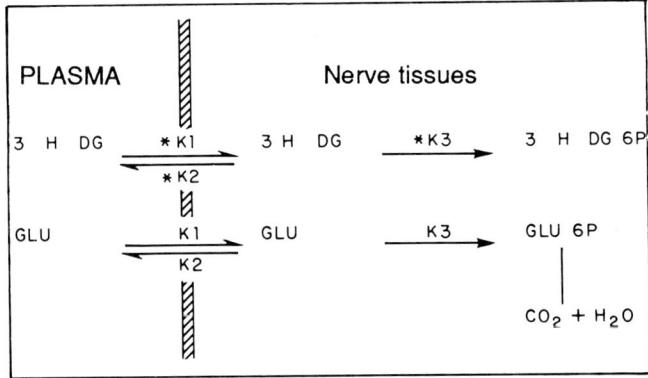

Figure 1. Representative model of cerebral glucose consumption (GLU). The tagged deoxyglucose (DG) injected intravenously enters into competition with the circulating glucose in order to cross the blood-brain barrier. Once in the glial or neuronal tissues, the deoxyglucose and glucose are phosphorylated into the 6-phosphate derivative under the influence of hexokinase (according to Sokoloff).

After intravenous administration of tagged deoxyglucose, cerebral radioactivity is essentially representative in the first three minutes of the passage of the deoxyglucose; then, as time passes, 6-deoxyglucose-phosphate accumulates, whereas the concentration of deoxyglucose diminishes(5). Two parameters therefore seem to be valuable: the rate of passage through the blood-brain barrier, measured in the short time which follows administration of the substance, and the quantity of phosphorylated derivatives accumulated (*Figure 2*).

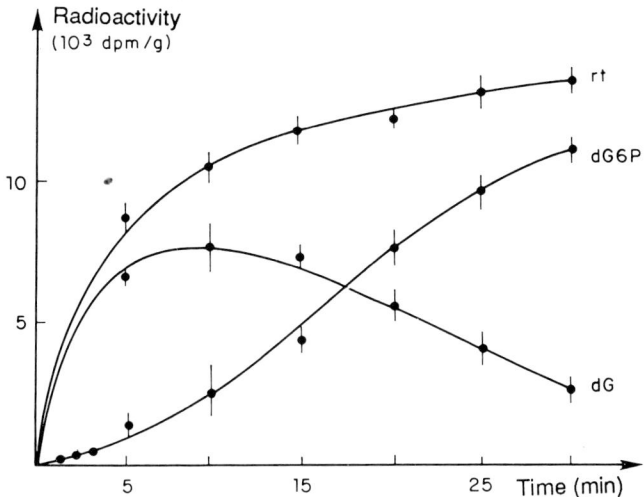

Figure 2. Fixation and cerebral conversion of deoxyglucose three hours after i.v. administration of 10 μCi/kg of tagged ose (dG = deoxyglucose, dG6P = 6P deoxyglucose, and RT = total radioactivity).

Physiologically, these two parameters are totally connected. Inversely, in pathological conditions, particularly hypoxic, a disagreement appears with relative diminution in the phosphorylation of glucose despite significant intake. It is therefore worthwhile to study these two parameters in various pathological conditions and to foresee the administration of substances reputed to be active in the treatment of cerebrovascular disorders. This is the case with Ginkgo biloba extract (EGb 761, Rökan®, Intersan), which has been shown to be active in ischemic accidents, both experimentally[1, 6] and clinically[10].

Experimental models

Two experimental models were selected for studying uptake and consumption of glucose.

In the normobaric hypoxia model, Long Evans rats weighing 300 g (four months old) were placed either in normoxia or in hypoxia in an enclosure for two hours. Hypoxia was obtained by forced ventilation with a gas mixture of 12% oxygen and 88% nitrogen. By means of a chronic venous catheter, 50 Ci 3H deoxyglucose were administered, and the rats were sacrificed either three minutes later or 30 minutes later. The arterial blood was sampled through a chronic arterial catheter 1, 2, 5, 10, 20, and 30 minutes after administration of the deoxyglucose.

In the carotid clamping model(2), since dual ligature of the primary carotids caused 100% mortality in Long Evans rats, a delay of 72 hours was allowed between the first and second ligature made under chloral anesthesia (360 mg/kg). Under these conditions, 40% of the animals survived, and the study of glucose consumption was made three hours after the second ligature under the same conditions as in the first model.

After sacrifice of the rats, the brain was rapidly separated and frozen in liquid nitrogen. Thirty sections were made by freezing microtome and freeze-dried for three hours at −30°. These sections were then placed in contact with a radioactive film for ten days (Ultrofilm LKB). After development, the autoradiographs were quantified from the values obtained with a standard deposited on the same film. For uptake, the results were expressed as percentage of quantity injected per gram of tissue, and for glucose consumption, the results were reported in mole/mn/100 g of tissue, taking into consideration the plasmatic kinetics of the radioactivity and of the glycemia according to the formula suggested by Sokoloff(9).

The animals in the treated groups received 100 mg/kg of a suspension of Ginkgo biloba extract orally in water at the rate of 0.5 mL/100 g for five days.

Results

Normobaric hypoxia (Table 1)

Low-amplitude hypoxia causes a diminution in uptake and consumption of glucose, a result which corresponds to a diminution in spontaneous activity of the animals.

Higher-amplitude hypoxia produces an increase in deoxyglucose uptake, and, depending upon the magnitude of the hypoxia, an increase and then a diminution in glucose consumption. This last observation is found when anaerobiosis is significant and the accumulation of lactates diminishes cellular activity.

Treatment with Ginkgo biloba extract, in animals placed in hypoxia, brings about an increase in deoxyglucose uptake and in glucose consumption (*Figure 3*).

This action demonstrates the protective effect of Ginkgo biloba extract against cellular hypoxia in the most vulnerable cerebral structures such as the hippocampus, the striate bodies, and the frontal cortex. In the other structures, the effect is not significant, but the protective tendency is similar.

Table 1

Effect of hypoxia on local glucose uptake and use in the Long Evans rat

Structures	Uptake: % of dose injected/g		Utilization µmoles/100 g/min	
	Normoxia	Hypoxia	Normoxia	Hypoxia
Frontal cortex	0.64 ± 0.05	*0.51 ± 0.04	85 ± 6	*67 ± 5
Parietal cortex	0.81 ± 0.08	0.68 ± 0.04	101 ± 8	88 ± 9
Occipital cortex	0.87 ± 0.07	*0.67 ± 0.05	106 ± 7	*86 ± 4
Hippocamopus	0.53 ± 0.04	*0.41 ± 0.03	73 ± 5	*59 ± 4
Caudate nuclei	0.68 ± 0.03	*0.52 ± 0.04	85 ± 6	*65 ± 4
Inferior colliculus	0.97 ± 0.07	*0.78 ± 0.05	126 ± 5	*98 ± 7
Superior colliculus	0.68 ± 0.07	*0.52 ± 0.03	84 ± 7	*64 ± 6
Thalamus	0.67 ± 0.07	0.54 ± 0.04	83 ± 7	68 ± 7
Geniculate corpus	0.84 ± 0.08	*0.62 ± 0.05	102 ± 8	*82 ± 6

Each value is the mean ± standard deviation from the mean obtained from five to seven rats. The significant differences, * $p \leq 0.05$ were obtained by analysis of variance with multiple comparisons.

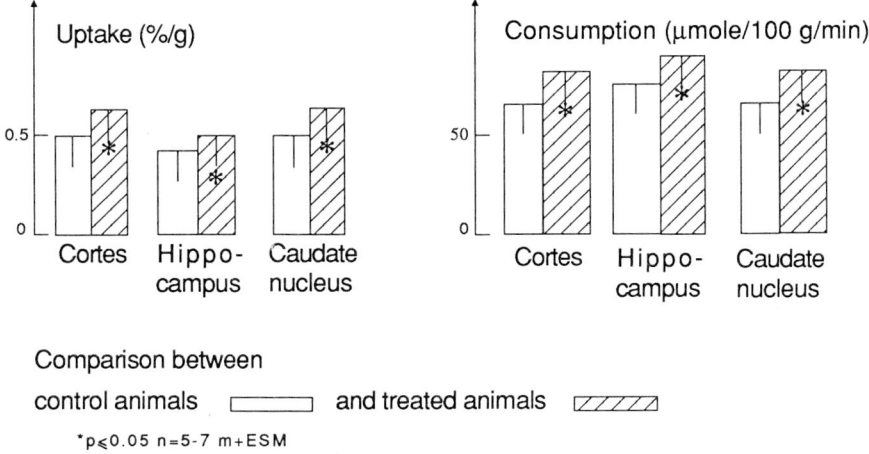

Figure 3. Effect of Ginkgo biloba extract administered preventively for five days at the rate of 100 mg/kg p.o., on glucose uptake and consumption in the frontal cortex, the hippocampus, and the caudate nuclei of rats with both carotids ligatured.

Carotid Clamping (Table 2)

A 72-hour lapse between ligatures permits partial substitution of the vertebroba-silar axis; blood flow and consequently deoxyglucose and glucose intake are therefore low (between 40 and 60% of the normal value depending upon the cerebral structures). Glucose consumption is relatively less significant than deoxyglucose uptake, which allows the supposition that the cells are no longer capable of phosphorylating the glucose, probably because of the preponderance of degradation by anaerobic route. Stimulation of hexokinase, or partial inhibition of the enzymatic activity as a result of cellular hyperacidity may be responsible for the decrease in glucose consumption. Preventive administration of Ginkgo biloba extract (*Figure 4*) does not significantly modify deoxyglucose uptake, but increases glucose consumption. This result shows that the effects of Ginkgo biloba extract on blood circulation are minor, and that the extraction of glucose, approximately 100% under these conditions, cannot be increased.

Inversely, the antihypoxic protective effect already observed is found again at the cellular level with partial reestablishment of glucose consumption.

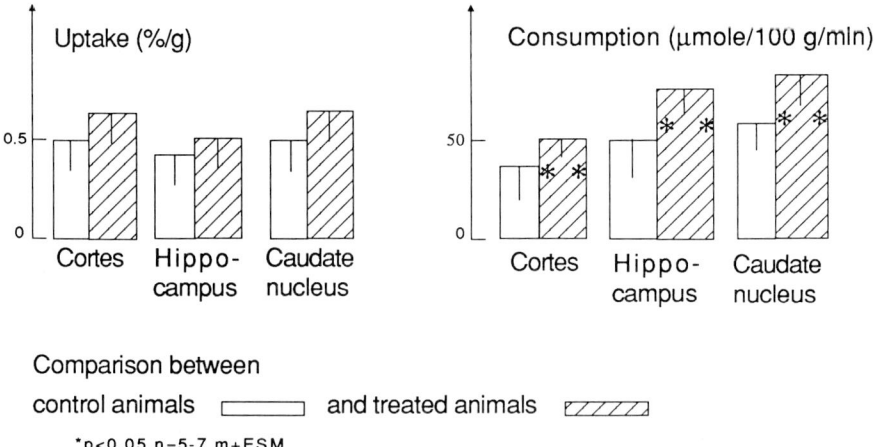

Figure 4. Effect of Ginkgo biloba extract administered preventively for five days at the rate of 100 mg/kg p.o., on glucose uptake and consumption in the frontal cortex, the hippocampus, and the caudate nuclei of animals maintained in normobaric hypoxia (O$_2$: 12%, N$_2$: 88%).

Table 2

Study of glucose uptake and local usage in the Long Evans Rat after double ligation of the common carotids separated by a time interval of 72 hours. The results correspond to the hemisphere normally irrigated last by the ligated carotid, three hours before sacrifice of the animals

Structures	Uptake: % of dose injected/g		Utilization μmoles/100 g/mn	
	Controls	Ligated carotids	Controls	Ligated carotids
Frontal cortex	0.65 ± 0.05	**0.48 ± 0.04	85 ± 6	**36 ± 4
Parietal cortex	0.81 ± 0.08	**0.53 ± 0.04	101 ± 8	**47 ± 4
Occipital cortex	0.87 ± 0.07	**0.58 ± 0.04	106 ± 7	**43 ± 5
Hippocampus	0.53 ± 0.04	**0.48 ± 0.03	73 ± 5	**48 ± 4
Caudate nuclei	0.68 ± 0.07	**0.49 ± 0.04	85 ± 6	**54 ± 5
Inferior colliculus	0.97 ± 0.07	**0.68 ± 0.03	126 ± 5	**62 ± 4
Superior colliculus	0.68 ± 0.07	*0.52 ± 0.03	84 ± 7	*41 ± 5
Thalamus	0.67 ± 0.07	0.58 ± 0.04	83 ± 7	**47 ± 4
Geniculate corpus	0.84 ± 0.08	0.66 ± 0.05	102 ± 8	**57 ± 6

Each value is the mean ± standard deviation from the mean obtained from five to seven rats. The significant differences, ** ≤ p 0.01, * p ≤ 0.05, were obtained by analysis of variance with multiple comparisons.

Conclusions

Two models of cerebrovascular pathology are suggested for study of glucose uptake and consumption. Normobaric hypoxia of low amplitude provokes a decrease in both parameters, as observed in cerebral aging in absence of any ischemic process. Ginkgo biloba extract, administered preventively in hypoxic atmosphere, brings about an increase in glucose uptake and consumption. Bicarotid clamping with a lapse of 72 hours is a substitution model combining ischemic phenomena. Although reduced as a function of blood intake, the extraction of glucose remains relatively low, probably because of a decrease in cellular metabolism. Ginkgo biloba extract administered preventively was shown to be active on this latter point, partially reestablishing glucose consumption.

References

1. Larsen R.G., Dupeyron J.P., Boulu R.G.: Modèle d'ischémie cérébrale expérimentale par microsphères chez le rat. Etude de l'effet de deux extraits de Ginkgo biloba et du naftidrofuryl. *Thérapie*, 1978, *83*, 651-660.

2. Le Poncin Lafitte M., Lespinasse P.: Mise en évidence d'une suppléance vertébro-basilaire lors d'accidents carotidiens. *J. Pharmacol.* (Paris), 1983, *14*, 99-102.

4. Sokoloff L., Reivich M., Kennedy C., Des Rosiers M.H., Patlak C.S., Pettigrew K.D., Sakurada O., Shinoara M.: The ^{14}C deoxyglycose method for measurement of local cerebral glucose utilization: theory, procedure and normal values in the conscious and anesthetized albino rat. *J. Neurochem.*, 1977, *28*, 897-916.

5. Rapin J.R., Duterte D., Le Poncin Lafitte M.: Modèles d'études des désordres cérébrovasculaires à l'aide de déoxyglucose 3H. *Radioaktive Isotope in Klinik und Forschung.*, 1980, *14*, 269-276.

6. Rapin J.R., Le Poncin Lafitte M.: Modèle expérimental d'ischémie cérébrale. Action préventive de l'extrait de Ginkgo biloba. *Semaine des hôpitaux*, 1979, *55*, 2047-2050.

7. Rapoport S.I., Ohata M., London E.D.: Cerebral blood flow and glucose utilization following opening of the blood-brain barrier and during maturation of the rat brain. *Fed. Proc.*, 1981, *40*, 2322-2325.

8. Roy C.B., Sherrington C.S.: On the regulation of the blood supply of the brain. *J. Physiol.* (London), 1980, *11*, 85-108.

9. Sokoloff L.: Relationships among local functional activity, energy metabolism and blood flow in the central nervous system. *Fed. Proc.*, 1981, *40*, 2311-2316.

10. Tea S., Celsis P., Clanet M., Marc Vergnes J.P.: Effets cliniques, hémodynamiques et métaboliques de l'extrait de Ginkgo biloba en pathologie vasculaire cérébrale. *Gazette Médicale de France*, 1979, *86*, 4149-4152.

Effect of Ginkgo Biloba Extract on the Blood-Brain Barrier

P.E. Chabrier, P. Roubert

Centre de recherche I.H.B.-I.P.S.E.N., 72, avenue des Tropiques
F 91940 Les Ulis

Summary

The different methods used to explore the blood-brain barrier (made up of cerebral capillary vessels), and notably, at molecular level, isolated microvessel preparations, have greatly improved our knowledge in this particular field. Some of these methods could be used to evaluate the protective effects of therapeutic substances, such as Ginkgo biloba extract, on the blood-brain barrier.

Subject to the same risk factors, cerebral macrocirculation and microcirculation jointly suffer the trials of aging. Although accidents which may affect the major vessels (thromboses, stenoses) can precipitate the evaluation of capillary insufficiency, both systems undergo parallel alterations with age. Also, we cannot imagine studying cerebral aging and the disorders associated with it without considering the role of the microcirculation, and first of all the evolution of the cerebral capillary.

The cerebral capillary, or cerebral microvessel, is not only the junction between the arterial and venous systems, transporting substances necessary for brain life (glucose, oxygen), it protects and regulates it by means of a unique structure constituting what is called the blood-brain barrier (BBB).

Blood-brain barrier

It has been a century since Ehrlich (1885) (6) observed that certain dyes injected systemically colored all of the organs, including the dura mater which covers the brain and the spinal medulla, but did not impregnate the cerebral tissue and the spinal medulla. Approximately 30 years later, Goldman, (9) through a dual experiment with injection of Trypan blue intravenously and intracerebroventricularly, demonstrated the existence of a barrier to diffusion between the blood and the brain, which was called the blood-brain barrier (BBB). It was first believed that this was constituted of

Rökan (Ginkgo Biloba). **Recent Results in Pharmacology and Clinic**
Edited by E.W. Fünfgeld
© Springer-Verlag Berlin Heidelberg New York 1988, pp. 117-125

the combination of cerebral microvessels with astrocytes in contact with them. At the present time, it is agreed that it is located in the endothelial cells of the capillaries. It is distinguished from the hemocerebrospinal barrier located in the capillaries perfusing the choroid plexus and the analogous periventricular formations which occupy only 1/5000th of the capillary exchange area.

The capillaries in the brain have a very different structure from those in other areas of the body (5, 15) (*Figure 1*). The cerebral endothelial cells are closely joined, connected to each other by tight junctions, forming an uninterrupted covering without gaps. They contain very few pinocytosis vesiculae, but are rich in mitochondria, indicating major energy requirements. The wall of the microvessels presents major electrical resistance, which is characteristic of an endothelium with low ionic permeability. There is also a functional polarity of the capillary: certain enzymes have a selective location on the luminal or abluminal face of the vessel. For example, 5'-nucleotidase is situated exclusively on the abluminal surface, whereas γ-glutamyl transpeptidase and alkaline phosphatase are found on both faces of the endothelium.

The cerebral capillary is closely surrounded by astrocytic processes connected by a continuous and uniform basal membrane. These astrocytes, by active transport of substances from the capillary to the neuron, and through their capacity for swelling regulating extracellular volume, represent an indispensable intermediary for nutrition of the nerve cells. In fact, they play the role of active extracellular space and regulate ion and fluid movements between the capillary and the neuron. In addition, the differentiation of the endothelial cells seems to be under their dominance.

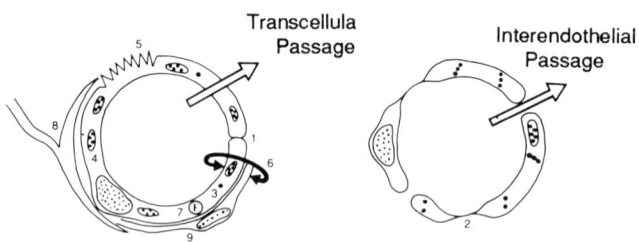

Figure 1: Diagram of a cerebral capillary illustrating transcellular and interendothelial passages. 1) closed junction; 2) opening; 3) small number of pinocytosis vesiculae; 4) numerous mitochondria; 5) increased electrical resistance of the walls; 6) polarity of structure and function; 7) specific enzymes; 8) astrocytic process; 9) pericyte.

Functions of the blood-brain barrier

Because of this special structure, substances found in the blood must traverse the cells of the endothelium in order to reach the cerebral extracellular space. Only fat-soluble substances which are capable of dissolving in the lipoprotein plasmic membrane, as well as cells profiting from an active mechanism of transport, easily penetrate the brain. More or less rapid passive diffusion depends on the more or less marked lipophilic character of substances crossing the endothelium. Thus the immediate anesthetic effect of the most fat-soluble barbiturates such as pentobarbital is explained. Water-soluble, ions, substances bound to proteins, do not cross the blood-brain barrier by this mechanism. In this case, the capillary ensures a genuine brain-protective role with respect to substances, an excess concentration of which would alter the neuronal functions, like the acetylcholine and catecholamine neurotransmitters, the circulating concentrations of which can undergo major variations.

Substances which are not fat-soluble but necessary to brain life nevertheless reach the nerve tissue by means of active and selective transport systems. This is the case with glucose, amino acids, precursors of nucleic acids, choline, and sodium-potassium exchanges. The BBB is also a metabolic barrier. The presence of l-dopa decarboxylase and monoamine oxidase enzymes has been demonstrated. Here again, this enzymatic team is a defense means for the brain with respect to potentially toxic substances.

Intrinsic innervation – biological receptors

Numerous studies suggest direct control of capillary functions by the nerve structures.(12) There is intrinsic innervation of the cerebral capillaries through the adrenergic endings and the serotoninergic and perhaps cholinergic projections. Regulation of cerebral blood circulation is certainly not the sole physiological action of innervation. Control of permeability of the BBB may also be considered. Different types of receptors have been demonstrated in the cerebral microvessels by means of binding techniques.(16) The existence of β_2 and α_1 adrenergic receptors in the capillary endothelium is not in question; this is in a ratio very favorable to the β receptors, unlike the nerve tissue. It seems that the adrenergic system may play a very subtle vasoregulating role in cerebral microvascularization. The results obtained concerning the muscarinic cholinergic receptors are contested, since the small quantities measured could originate from contamination by nerve elements from the microvessel preparations. There is no doubt with respect to the H_1 receptors. Serotoin and dopamine receptors are also found in lesser quantities. The existence of peptidergic receptors has been demonstrated for insulin and angiotensin II.(18) Very probably other peptide receptors are yet to be revealed.

Methods for investigation of the blood-brain barrier

In man, the use of nontraumatic methods such as the classical cerebral scintigraphy
or tomodensitometric examination assist the clinician in detecting possible changes
in the BBB. The pharmacologist, by radioisotopic tagging methods, obtains valuable
information on the transport of substances and on permeability of the BBB *in vivo* in
normal or pathological animals. At the molecular level, studies can be done on isolated
cerebral microvessels and on cultures of cerebral endothelial cells.

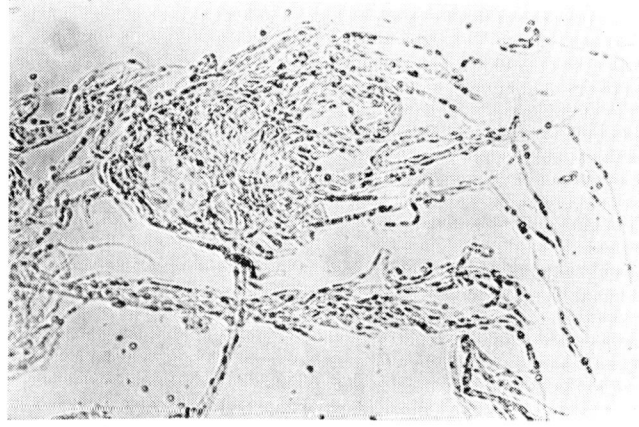

*Figure 2: Fresh purified preparation of microvessels x 160 (Kodak Tri X pan,
1000-1600 ASA film).*

In our laboratory, a pure and metabolically active preparation of cerebral microvessels is obtained after elimination of the meninges and of the medullary substance
by homogenization of the gray matter, screening, differential centrifugations, flo-
tations, and adsorption on glass balls.(17) The homogeneity and purity of the
preparation are verified by microscopic examination (*Figure 2*) and by measuring the
enzymatic activities localized specifically on the capillary, such as γ-glutamyl
transpeptidase and alkaline phosphatase. Enrichment in enzymatic activity by 25 to
30 times in comparison with the homogenate of gray matter is the mark of a good
preparation. This method has the advantage. among others, of being applicable to
various animal species (rat, gerbil) capable of suplying pathological models. The
cerebral microvessels preparation thus represents a well-defined pharmacological and
biochemical entity. Although such a preparation is not appropriate for studies of BBB
permeability, it is an in vitro system usable for very delicate biochemical and
morphological work: metabolism studies (for example, that of arachidonic acid),
characterization of biological receptors, enzymology, ultrastructural examination by
electron microscope.

Pathology

Numerous physiopathological conditions can affect the structural or metabolic integrity of the cerebral microvessels.

Aging

The cerebral capillaries are clearly sensitive to aging. From the morphological standpoint, thickenings of the capillary wall, diminutions in the number of endothelial cells as well as in the number of mitochondria have been observed in the elderly subject.(10) These modifications are parallel to those in adrenergic functions: increases in concentration of noradrenalin and of β-adrenergic receptors have been found. (7, 13) Such changes can have major repercussions on permeability of the BBB, on neuronal functions, and on regulation of the cerebral microcirculation in elderly persons.

In Alzheimer's Disease

Degenerative ultrastructural changes and significant increases in the volume of the capillaries of the cerebral cortex have been reported. (3) Hypotheses relating the formation of senile plaques and degeneration of the cerebral capillary have been advanced.(21) In all cases, changes in the structure and properties of the BBB, particularly in its permeability, seem to be well established in this disease.

In Hypertension

Structural and functional lesions of the microvessels are apparent. In particular, an elevation in blood pressure, acute or chronic, brings about hyperpermeability of the BBB through rupture of the endothelium and formation of edema.(1, 11)

Diabetes

This affects the capillary. In animals rendered hyperglycemic, the intravenous injection of radio-tagged albumin demonstrates ruptures in the BBB. At the same time a larger number of pinocytosis vesicuale are observed.(19)

In these last two conditions, the number of β-adrenergic receptors is diminished. (12)

Cerebral Ischemia – Effect of EGb

We know that cerebral ischemia brings about major biochemical changes: metabolic disturbances, disturbances in the concentration of neurotransmitters, of lipids, and of protein synthesis.(4) In particular, in the course of the ischemic phase, unsaturated fatty acids, and first of all arachidonic acid, are released in massive quantities. In the post-ischemic period, these substances are converted into endoperoxides, thromboxanes, prostacyclin, prostaglandins, and leukotrienes, which are responsible for changes provoking ruptures in the BBB and bringing about disturbances in recirculation. Even prostacyclin, whose beneficial effects on blood circulation are well known, modifies vasomotoricity in the ischemic zone, provoking a state of vasodilatation ranging up to vasoparalysis which is damaging for the BBB. An obvious therapeutic approach to ischemia is to prevent the formation of these substances. Also, we investigated whether EGb could exert an effect on the production of arachidonic acid metabolites in the cerebral capillaries.

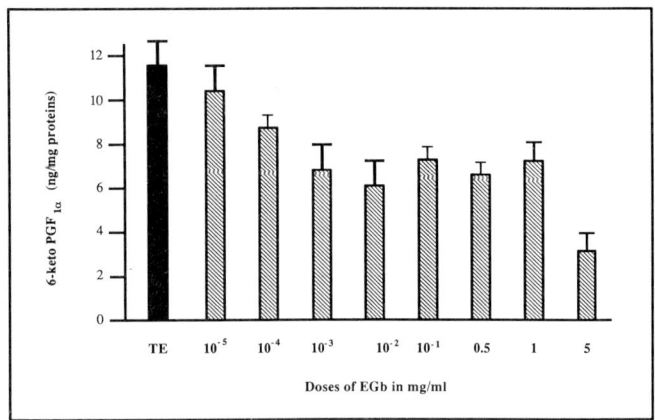

Figure 3: Effect of Ginkgo biloba extract on production of 6-keto PGF$_{1\alpha}$ on a homogenate of beef microvessels.

Although their role is still not well known, several studies have supplied proof of the synthesis of prostaglandins by the cerebral microvessels of various animal species.(20, 22) By far the most substantial synthesis is that of prostacyclin (PGI$_2$), measured by its stable metabolite 6-keto PGF$_{1\alpha}$. (8, 14)

At low doses, EGb decreases the production of 6-keto PGF$_{1\alpha}$ in a cerebral microvessel preparation from beef (*Figure 3*). This inhibiting or regulating effect, however, reaches a plateau (maximum effect), since at very high doses the formation of 6-keto PGF$_{1\alpha}$ is not inhibited as it may be with indomethacin or acetylsalicyclic acid.

This effect does not seem to be limited to the synthesis of PGI_2, it applies for PGE_2. Under these conditions, EGb seems capable of decreasing the metabolism of arachidonic acid. EGb could thus ensure a true protective role toward the BBB, added to its vasoregulating effect.(2)

Conclusion

The blood-brain barrier constitutes a homeostasis mechanism. Its function is to ensure the nutrition and protection of the most remarkable biological structure in the body: the human brain. In numerous pathological conditions, the BBB becomes deficient, it can no longer play its role, and severe disorders follow. Certain of these, we believe, may be avoided or corrected by the appropriate therapy, the purpose of which would be to preserve the structure and the properties of the cerebral capillary. Clinical investigators, pharmacologists, chemists, and biochemists now have the opportunity to approach these problems according to their own particular approach to the entire organism, at the cellular or molecular level.

One hundred years after Ehrlich's discovery, the advances made in knowledge of the BBB, and more particularly in methods for exploring it, are opening perspectives for research and exciting potentials for therapeutic application, notably by making it possible to test the effect of certain drugs.

At low doses, Ginkgo biloba extract (EGb 761, Rökan®, Intersan) seems to exert on the cerebral microvessels of beef a protective effect which is all the more interesting because it is in addition to its vasoregulating effect.

References

1. Adachi M., Rosenblum W.I., Feigin I.: Hypertensive disease and cerebral edema. *J. Neurol. Neurosurg. Psychiat.*, 1966, *29*, 451-455

2. Auguet M., Delaflotte D., Hellegouarch A., Clostre F.: Bases pharmacologiques de l'impact vasculaire de l'extrait de Ginkgo biloba. *Presse Méd.*, 1986, *15*, 1524-1528.

3. Bell M.A., Ball M.J.: Morphometric comparison of hippocampal microvasculature in ageing and demented people: diameters and densities. *Acta Neuropathol.*, 1981, *53*, 299-318.

4. Boulu R.G.: Conséquences biochimiques de l'ischémie cérébrale. *Act. Pharm. Biol. Clin.*, 1983, *2*, 35-54.

5. Cornford E.M.: The blood brain barrier, a dynamic regulatory interface. *Molecular Physiology*, 1985, *7*, 219-260.

6. Ehrlich, P.: Das Sauerstoff-Bedürfnis des Organismus: eine farbenanalytische Studie. Berlin, *Hirschward, 1885*.

7. Embree L.J.G., Kakson D.W., Ordway F., Roubein I.F.: Aging effect on the noradrenaline content of rat brain microvessels. *Soc. Neuroscience*, 1960, *6*, 282.

8. Goehlert U.G., Ying Kin N.M.K., Wolfe L.S.: Biosynthesis of prostacyclin in rat cerebral microvessels and the choroid plexus. *J. Neurochem.*, 1981, *36*, 1192-1201.

9. Goldmann E.E.: Vitalfärbung am Zentralnervensystem. Berlin, *Eimer*, 1913.

10. Hunziker O., Abdel'as S., Schlulz V.: The aging human cerebral cortex: a stereological characterization of changes in the capillary rat. *J. Gerontology*, 1979, *34*, 345-350.

11. Johansson B., Li C.L., Olsson Y., Klatzo I.: The effect of acute arterial hypertension on the blood brain barrier to protein tracers. *Acta Neuropath.*, 1970, *16*, 117-127.

12. Kobayashi H., Magnoni M.S., Govoni S., Izumi F., Wada A., Trabucchi M.: Neuronal control of brain microvessel function. *Experientia*, 1985, *4*, 427-558.

13. Kobayashi H., Maoret T., Spano P.F., Trabucchi M.: Effect of age on beta-adrenergic receptors on cerebral microvessels. *Brain Research*, 1982, *244*, 374-377.

14. Maurer P., Moskovitz M.A., Levine L., Melamed E.: The synthesis of prostaglandins by bovine cerebral microvessels. *Prostaglandins and Medicine*, 1980, *4*, 153-161.

15. Partridge W.M.: Brain Metabolism: A perspective from the blood-brain Barrier. *Physiological Reviews*, 1983, *63*, 1481-1535.

16. Peroutka S.J., Moskowitz M.A., Reinhard J.F., Snyder S.H.: Neurotransmitter receptor binding in bovine cerebral microvessels. *Science*, 1980, *208*, 610-612.

17. Roubert P.: Biosynthèse de dérivés de l'acide arachidonique dans les capillaires sanguins de cerveau de boeuf. Thèse de Docteur en Pharmacie (1986). Université Paris-Sud, Chatenay-Malabry.

18. Speth R.C., Harik S.I.: Angiotensin II receptor binding sites in brain microvessels. *Pro. Natl. Acad. Sci. U.S.A.*, 1985, *82*, 6340-6343.

19. Stauber W.T., Ong S.H., McCuskey R.S.: Selective extravascular escape of albumin into the cerebral cortex of the diuretic rat. *Diabetes*, 1981, *30*, 500-503.

20. White R.P., Ainsworth A.M.: Cerebrovascular actions of prostaglandins. *Pharmac. Ther.*, 1982, *18*, 313-331.

21. Wisniewski H.M., Koslowski P.B.: Evidence for blood brain barrier changes in senile dementia of the Alzheimer type (SDAT). *Ann. N.Y. Acad. Sci.*, 1982, *396*, 119-129.

22. Wolfe L.S.: Eicosanoids, prostaglandins, thromboxanes, leukotrienes and other derivatives of C-20 unsaturated fatty acids. *J. Neurochem.*, 1982, *38*, 1-19.

Protective Effects of Ginkgo Biloba Extract on Early Rupture of the Blood-Brain Barrier in Rats

C. Grosdemouge, M. Le Poncin-Lafitte, J.R. Rapin

Groupe de Neurophysiologie Cerebrovasculaire, C.H.U. St. Antoine
F 75012 Paris

Summary

During the hours immediately after a hypertensive flare-up or cerebral ischemia induced by intracarotid administration of microspheres, rupture of the blood-brain barrier is observed for molecules of low molecular weight, such as angiotensin, whereas albumin or large proteins are not extravasated and edema is negligible. In hypertensive animals Ginkgo biloba extract diminishes the cerebral uptake of angiotensin, and this effect is proportional to the dose of extract used (50-100 mg/kg). An identical effect is observed in animals with unilateral cerebral embolism, and the explanation of this mechanism is probably related to the membrane-stabilizing effect of Ginkgo biloba.

Abrupt rupture of the blood-brain barrier (BBB) may be induced by a very significant elevation in blood pressure (5, 7) or by administration of a substance which provokes osmotic shock.(6, 13) In these cases, the passage of proteins, demonstrated by the use of Evans blue or of iodoalbumin, is immediate, and cerebral edema develops at the time the blood-brain barrier is ruptured. Inversely, in precoma periods in encephalopathies, the BBB is not breached, whereas the passage of polypeptides of low molecular weight is greatly increased. (1, 3)

In a unilateral ischemia model, cerebral edema appears slowly, not until six hours after administration of the embolizing agent, whereas the hemodynamic and metabolic changes are immediate.(8, 9) It is therefore important to study the transfer of a small molecule such as polypeptide, angiotensin, in the first pre-edematous period of the ischemia. In this study, we are reporting the results concerning the transfer of this polypeptide at the time of a moderate hypertension not causing rupture of the BBB.

In these models Ginkgo biloba extract EGb761 (EGb) was tested because of its anti-ischemic activity observed in cerebral microembolism(10, 11) and its stabilizing effect on the membrane.(4)

Rökan (Ginkgo Biloba). Recent Results in Pharmacology and Clinic
Edited by E.W. Fünfgeld
© Springer-Verlag Berlin Heidelberg New York 1988, pp. 126-132

Material and Methods

The experiments were made on male Sprague-Dawley rats (Lessieux) with a mean weight of 250 ± 10 g. Three groups of rats were formed at random from the colony: a control group receiving 9 g/L NaCl orally (0.4mL) for seven days, two treated groups receiving orally for seven days either 50 or 100 mg/kg EGb. Uptake of angiotensin II by the brain was measured.

At the time of a hypertensive flare-up

The control animals or those treated with Ginkgo biloba were kept under chloral anesthesia (360 mg/kg) and were infused through the jugular vein for four hours (flow: 1.5 mL/hour) with:
– either 9 g/L physiological saline solution;
– or 7.5 ng•kg-1•min-1 angiotensin II.
At the end of four hours, the animals whose pressure had been measured without bleeding received i.v. a tracer dose of angiotensin II tagged with iodine 125. Three minutes after this administration, the animals were sacrificed by decapitation. A fraction of blood was removed for determination of the circulating angiotensin II by radioimmunological assay. The brain was rapidly removed, and the radioactivity present in the cerebral tissues was determined by means of a counter (Packard instruments), the window of which was regulated on the photoelectric peak of the iodine 125.

The percentage of water in the brain was determined by the difference between the weight at the time of removal and that after drying in the oven.

At the time of cerebral ischemia

On the seventh day of treatment, the rats were anesthetized with chloral and the external and internal carotids were removed.

2,000 microspheres tagged with strontium 85 with a diameter of 50 microns were injected within 30 seconds into the internal carotid flow through the external carotid. At the end of administration, the external carotid was ligated and under these conditions the internal carotid flow was almost unchanged. Immediately after ischemia, an infusion (NaCl g/L, 1.5 mL/hour) was placed in the jugular vein of the animals for four hours.

At the end of the infusion, the animals received intravenously a tracer dose of angiotensin II tagged with iodine 125. Three minutes after the injection, the animals were sacrificed by decapitation. The brain was separated into the two hemispheres along the interhemispheic line and the radioactivities of iodine 125 and of strontium

85 were counted in two different windows and corrected with reinjections. On the basis of the strontium 85 counting result, the number of embolizing microspheres was calculated, and it was found to be equal in all cases to 420 ± 30 in the embolized hemisphere and 35 ± 5 in the other hemisphere. In both hemispheres, the edema was measured by determination of the percentage of water (dry weight and moist weight).

Results

Figure 1 shows the effects of Ginkgo biloba on the quantity of angiotensin taken up by the brain in three minutes. The results are expressed as percentage of the quantity of angiotensin administered. The systolic pressure, measured just before sacrifice of the animals, was equal to $11 \text{ mmHg} \pm 1$. The relatively low value of the blood pressure is explained by the fact that the animals were kept under anesthesia during the sodium chloride infusion. The treatment with EGb brought about a decrease in hemoence-phalic permeability with respect to the angiotensin II, without modifying the circulating concentrations of radioactive angiotensin and cold angiotensin. Finally, there was a dose-effect relationship of EGb in this model of permeability of the BBB to polypeptides.

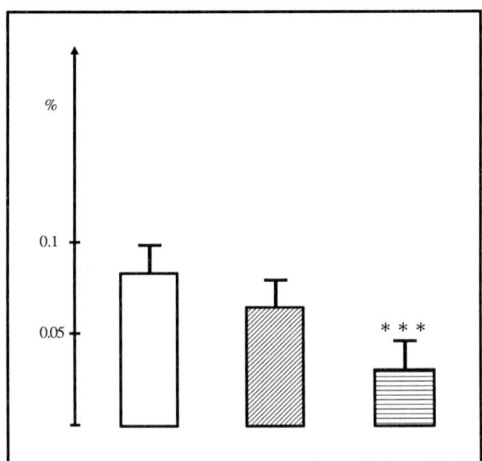

*Figure 1: Study of cerebral uptake of angiotensin II in normotensive animals pretreated with Ginkgo biloba extract (EGb). The results are expressed as percentage of the dose of angiotensin administered: n=10, m ± MSE. ☐ = normotensive control animals; ⁄⁄⁄⁄ = normotensive animals treated with 50 mg/kg EGb p.o.; ▤ = normotensive animals treated with 100 mg/kg EGb; P ≤ 0.005, ***P ≤ 0.0005: comparison between control animals and treated animals.*

In hypertensive animals

The administration of angiotensin II by infusion for four hours increased systolic blood pressure to 140 mmHg in the anesthetized animal. Parallel to this increase in blood pressure, the quantity of nonradioactive angiotensin was increased by 300%, which had the effect of diminishing the circulating specific radioactivity at the time of administration of the tracer dose of radioactive angiotensin, with the circulating radioactivity not varying. In the brain (*Figure 2*) a very significant increase of fixed angiotensin was observed, without taking into account the decrease in specific radioactivity of the blood. In fact, it is difficult to take this specific radioactivity into consideration, since two substances are involved (angiotensin II or iodoangiotensin II), for which the transfer constant in the brain is different. Nevertheless, the competition between radioactive and nonradioactive molecules produces an error by default in the quantity of angiotensin fixed by the brain. Furthermore, no edema corresponding to rupture of the BBB was observed, and the percentage of water in the brain was equal to $76.6 \pm 0.2\%$ in all cases. Preventive treatment with EGb (100 mg/kg) suppresses the elevation in angiotensin II uptake by the cerebral tissue, and a dose-effect relationship was observed in all of the normotensive animals.

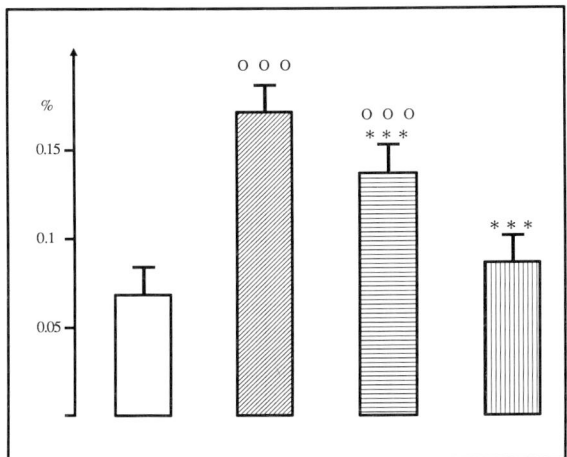

Figure 2: Study of uptake of angiotensin II in hypertensive animals pretreated with Ginkgo biloba extract (EGb). The results are expressed as percentage of the dose of angiotensin administered: $n = 10$, $m \pm MSE$. ☐ = normotensive control animals; ▨ = hypertensive control animals; ▤ = hypertensive animals treated with 50 mg/kg EGb; ▥ = hypertensive animals treated with 100 mg/kg EGb; ***$P \leq 0.0005$: comparison between hypertensive control animals and hypertensive treated animals; $^{ooo}P \leq 0.0005$: comparison between normotensive control animals and hypertensive animals.

In ischemic animals

The intracarotid injection of 2000 microspheres causes embolization in the ipsilateral hemisphere, whereas the number of embolisms found in the contralateral
hemisphere was small. Four hours after this embolism, cerebral edema had not yet
developed (76.8 ± 0.3 on the contralateral side and 77.2 ± 0.3 on the ipsilateral side),
and cerebral blood flow was much decreased on the embolized side alone.

These effects did not modify the circulating angiotensin, but brought about a
variation in fixation of angiotensin at the cerebral level (*Figure 3*). The increase in
fixation of angiotensin was significant both on the embolized and nonembolized
sides; however, the increase was greatest on the embolized side. Treatment with EGb
decreased the quantity of angiotensin fixed in both hemispheres, and a dose-effect
relationship was also reported.

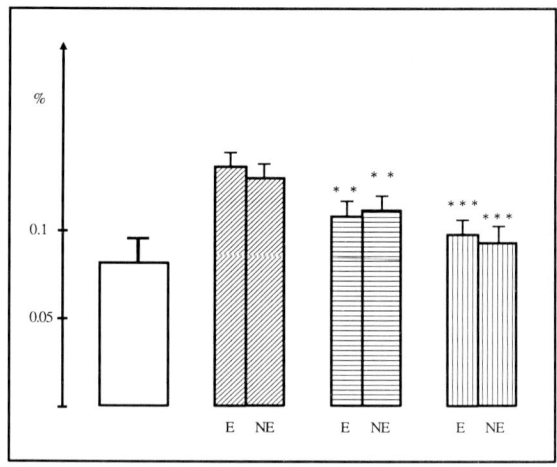

*Figure 3: Study of cerebral uptake of angiotensin II in ischemic animals pretreated
with Ginkgo biloba extract (EGb). E = embolized hemisphere; NE =nonembolized
hemisphere; n = 10, m ± MSE.*☐*= control animals;*▨*= ischemic control animals;*
▤*= control animals treated with 50 mg/kg EGb;*▥*= control animals treated with
100 mg/kg EGb; ***P ≤ 0.0005, **P ≤ 0.01: comparison between ischemic animals
and treated ischemic animals. The results are expressed as percent of the quantity of
angiotensin administered.*

Discussion

Rupture of the BBB may be limited to certain molecules whose molecular weight
is low or moderate. Angiotensin II may be considered as one of these molecules.

Outside of a physiological passage at the level of the central organs for regulation of thirst, where the barrier phenomenon is very particluar,(14) angiotensin practically never ruptures the blood-brain barrier. Its "brain uptake index", determined by simultaneous administration of tagged angiotensin and of a diffusible indicator (tritium-labeled water) was equal to 5 to 6%,(14) a very low value if we compare it with that of lipophilic or diffusible substances.

The hypertensive flare-up induced under our experimental conditions did not provoke rupture of the barrier, which we verified by administration of Evans blue, and which was confirmed by the nonappearance of edema. Furthermore, this hypertensive flare-up was too minor to modify cerebral blood flow,(15) this being kept constant by means of the self-regulation mechanism.(2) The increase in quantity of angiotensin fixed therefore corresponds well to a modification in permeability of the BBB at the time of a hypertensive flare-up.

At the time of a quantitative ischemia, the facts observed are rather similar as to the increase in fixation of angiotensin, despite a significant decrease in cerebral circulation on the embolized side.(12) After embolization, the decrease in flow observed in the entire hemisphere corresponds to the resulting local diminutions in flow in ischemic areas and the local increases in the areas of reactive hyperemia. The edema and rupture of the BBB did not appear until six hours after the embolization, whereas permeability has already been modified for the angiotensin, on both the embolized and nonembolized sides, without our being able to explain this last phenomenon. These results are similar to those observed at the time of precomatose periods when permeability is greatly increased for substances such as angiotensin or insulin and not modified for albumin and large proteins.(3) It is possible that this may be a consistent factor in all encephalopathies regardless of their origin, and that it corresponds to a modification in ionic movements perhaps in liaison with an alteration in the energetic mechanisms.

EGb may be considered as a membrane stabilizer, and its preventive action against extension of the edema has already been reported.(11) EGb is capable of diminishing the permeability of the BBB toward angiotensin, both in control animals and in the animals in both pathological models. It is possible that the membrane-stabilizing effect may be the primary mechanism explaining the decrease in traumatic and ischemic edemas observed after administration of Ginkgo biloba extract.

References

1. Bloch P., Delorme M.L., Rapin J.R., Granger A., Boschat M., Opolon P.: Reversible modifications of neurotransmitters of the brain in experimental acute hepatic coma. *Surg. Gynecol. Obstet.*, 1978, *146*, 551-558.

2. Boisvert D.P., Jones J.V., Harper A.M.: Cerebral blood flow autoregulation to acutely increasing blood pressure during sympathetic stimulation. *Acta Neurol. Scand.*, 1977, *56*, 46-47.

3. Crinquette J.F., Faguer P., Delorme M.L., Boschat M., Rapin J.R., Opalon P.: Modifications précoces de la perméabilité de la barrière hématoméningée après anastomose portocave (APC) et ischémie hépatique (IH) chez le rat. *Gastroenterol. Clin. Biol.*, 1979, *3*, 94-96.

4. Etienne A., Baranes J., Hecquet F., Hellegouarch A., Clostre F.: Effet stabilisateur de membrane d'un extrait de Ginkgo biloba. *Planta Medica.*, 1980, *39*, 237.

5. Haggendal E., Johanson B.: Pathophysiological aspects of the blood brain barrier change in acute arterial hypertension. *Eur. Neurol.*, 1971, *72*, 24-28.

6. Hardebo J.E., Nilsson B.: Hemodynamic changes in brain caused by local infusion of hyperosomolar solutions, in particular relations to blood-brain barrier opening. *Brain. Res.*, 1980, *181*, 49-59.

7. Johansson B.B., Martinsson L.: The blood-brain barrier in adrenaline-induced hypertension. Circadian variations and modification by beta-adrenoreceptor antagonists. *Acta Neurol. Scand.*, 1980, *62*, 96-102.

8. Kogure K., Busto R., Scheinberg P., Reinmuth O.M.: Energy metabolites and water content in rat brain during the early stage of development of cerebral infarction. *Brain*, 1974, *97*, 103-114.

9. Lageron A., Le Poncin-Lafitte M., Rapin J.R., Saffroy M., Bulach C.: Brain rat histoenzymological changes induced by microsphere injection during ischemia. *Acta Histochem.*, 1979, *64*, 184-190.

10. Larsen R.G., Dupeyron J.P., Boulu R.G.: An experimental model of cerebral ischemia induced by microspheres in the rat. Effect of 2 Gingko biloba extracts and of naftidrofuryl. *Therapie*, 1978, *33*, 651-660.

11. Le Poncin-Lafitte M., Rapin J., Rapin J.R.: Effects of Ginkgo biloba on changes induced by quantitative cerebral microembolization in rats. *Arch. Int. Pharmacodyn. Ther.*, 1980, *243*, 236-244.

12. Rapin J.R., Grosdemouge C., Le Poncin-Lafitte M.: Pathophysiol. Pharmacother. of cerebrovascular disorders. Betz., Grote Eds. *Verlag Gerhard Witestrock.*, 1980, 163-166.

13. Rapoport S.I., Hori M., Klatzi I.: Testing of a hypothesis for osmotic opening of the blood-brain-barrier. *Am. J. Physiol.*, 1972, *223*, 323-331.

14. Simpson J.B., Routtenberg A.: Subfornical organ: site of drinking elicitation by angiotensin. *Science.*, 1973, *181*, 1772-1775.

15. Symon L., Held K., Dorsch N.W.C.: A study of regional autoregulation in the cerebral circulation to increased perfusion pressur in Normocapnia and Hypercapnia. *Stroke.*, 1973, *4*, 139-147.

Mechanisms of Effect of Ginkgo Biloba Extract on Experimental Cerebral Edema

A. Etienne, F. Hecquet, F. Clostre

Centre de recherche I.H.B.–I.P.S.E.N., 72, avenue des Tropiques
F 91940 Les Ulis

Summary

Oedema is one of the major complication of cerebral ischaemia being at the same time a consequence and an aggravating factor. Its first phase is intracellular and cytotoxic, with breakdown of ionic pumps through loss of energy, resulting in a whole sequence of ionic pertubations characterized by loss of intracellular K^+ and accumulation of water and Na^+, Cl^-, and Ca^{2+} ions in the cells of the ischaemic zone.

The second phase, termed vasogenic, applies to the accumulation of lactates, inorganic phosphates and free polyunsaturated fatty acids and in particular, arachidonic acid. This last compound is responsible for the production of membrane "aggressors", amongst which free radicals play an important role.

Ginkgo biloba extract limits the formation of cerebral oedema and suppresses its neurological consequences, whether the oedema is of cytotoxic (triethyltin) or vasogenic (unilateral traumatic oedema) origin. Several membrane mechanisms could be implicated in the protective action manifested by Ginkgo biloba extract against cerebral oedema.

Any damage to the circulatory integrity of a tissue induces functional changes in the cellular and subcellular membranes (in particular, the mitochondrial), sources of ionic and metabolic disturbances which generate tissue edema.

In the brain, edema constitutes a major complication of ischemia, of which it is both a result and an aggravation factor. Cerebral edema takes place in two stages:(9) the first is intracellular and early, directly porportional to the magnitude of the energy deficit; it is qualified as cytotoxic. The second, extracellular and more subtle, can have dramatic consequences in the so-called "shadowy" area (perifocal to the ischemic zone) where edema added to the energy deficit which is present there can cause a tissue to pass from the reversible functional stage to that of severe metabolic alteration resulting in irreversible necrosis.

Cerebral edema represents a major step in the evolution of cerebral ischemia. Its mechanisms of installation are hemodynamic, ionic, and metabolic (*Figure 1*).

Rökan (Ginkgo Biloba). Recent Results in Pharmacology and Clinic
Edited by E.W. Fünfgeld
© Springer-Verlag Berlin Heidelberg New York 1988, pp. 133-142

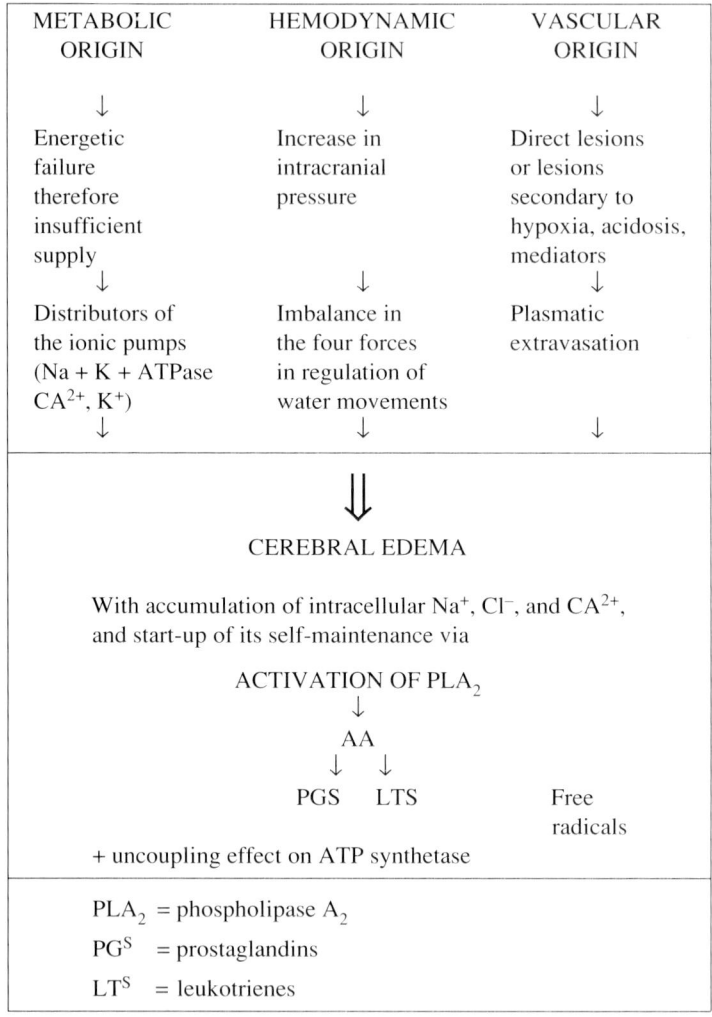

Figure 1: The two stages of cerebral edema.

Principal mechanisms of ischemic cerebral edema

Ischemic edema appears as a biphasic and even triphasic event, if there are added to it disturbances of the blood-brain barrier, which are much later.

The initial phase is a direct and immediate consequence of failure of energy supply. This deficit is indicated by a breakdown of the ionic pumps: extracellular Na^+ massively invades the intracellular medium; intracellular K^+ then escapes toward the extracellular space. This potassium movement sets off entrance of Cl^- into the intracellular medium by a mechanism of passive diffusion related to the concentration of extracellular K^+ and is accompanied by the intake of an osmotic equivalent of water.(18) It also induces intake of Ca^{2+} from a certain threshold of mebranal depolarization and consecutive to the potassium outflow. This intracellular invasion of Ca^{2+} in itself represents an important factor in aggravation of the ischemia which has just been added to the osmotic consequences of the edema.(24)

This ionic imbalance causes movement of water toward the cells (*Figure 2*). In a first stage, only redistribution of the tissue water is involved, but after a delay of five to six hours, start-up of the production of potent vasogenic metabolites begins self-maintenance of the tissue edema.

These second-wave factors are as numerous as they are various: lactates and their acidosic effects,(22) lysosomial proteases, cytostructural destruction factors, increase in intracellular inorganic phosphates, the source of osmotic swelling of the mitochondria;(17) polyunsaturated free fatty acids, in particular arachidonic acid, play a major role as sources of factors in the particularly fearful second attack.(5, 6, 23).

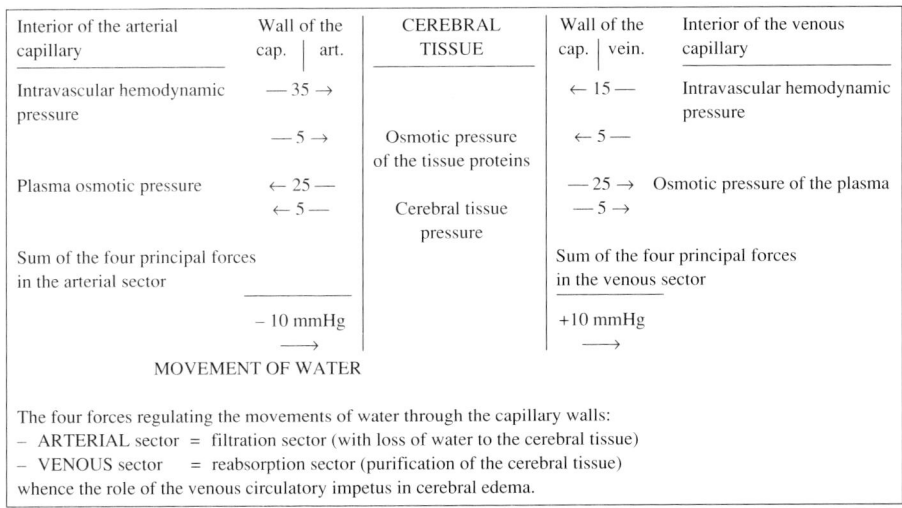

Figure 2: Forces and pressures participating in regulation of movement of water through the capillary walls.

The chain for production of these toxic metabolites may be summarized thus: Ca^{2+}, which accumulates during the initial phase of the edema, activates the A_2 phospholipases which, from membranal phospholipids, supply significant quantities of arachidonic acid. The latter plays two roles: one consists of uncoupling the respiratory chain, making the mitochondrial membranes too permeable to be selective in their exchanges, the other effect of arachidonic acid being the initiation of its succession of reactions which, through the cyclo-oxygenase pathway, would produce endoperoxides (source of production of oxygenated free radicals) or of thromboxane A_2, and by the lipoxygenase pathway, hydroperoxides, excellent sources of free radicals and of leukotrienes (LTC_4 and LTD_4), potent inductors of plasmatic extravasation through capillary hyperpermeability.(27)

Blood-brain barrier (BBB) disorders are more belated, but will be produced earlier when the ischemia is lasting. The destruction of the capillary structure of the BBB is reflected by loss of plasma proteins and water to the adjacent cerebral tissue, causing exaggeration of the vasogenic phase of the cerebral edema.(1)

Ginkgo biloba extract in experimental cerebral edema

Whatever the origin of the cerebral tissue damage (ischemic, hypoxic, traumatic, or toxic), the edema phase is an inevitable stage in its evolution. Thus, in most of the experimental cerebral damage models currently used, whether they are obtained by ligation, by hypoxia, or by embolization, measurement of the various parameters of the evolution of the phenomenon makes it possible to objectively assay the efficacy of a therapy.

There are, however, more specific models for the creation of experimental edema. They have the advantage of better discerning the evolution of the phenomenon and of better locating the mechanisms which set it off. This is the case with unilateral traumatic edema through removal of the dura mater in rabbits,(2) but it is mainly the case in edema induced by triethyletain (TET), which provokes selective edema of the central nervous system through still incompletely elucidated mechanisms, certain of which – inhibition of $Na^+K^+ATPase$ and uncoupling of oxidative phosphorylations – are identical or similar to those which are encountered in human physiopathology. Also, the value of this model is that it is possible to combine determination of intracerebral ionic disturbances with behavioral observations (neurological index). (3)

Ginkgo biloba extract reduces the edema phase in the course of unilateral cerebral embolization in the rat with microspheres calibrated and tagged with Sr 85.(19) It also combats the appearance of cerebral edema and ionic disturbances – accumulation of intracellular Na^+ and loss of K^+ – in the ischemic hemisphere after unilateral ligation in the gerbil.(25) Outside of these observations, the effects of Ginkgo biloba extract have been studied in models of unilateraltraumatic edema in the rabbit and of triethletain-induced edema in the rat.

Unilateral traumatic edema in the rabbit(4)

Unilateral stripping of the dura mater in the rabbit is followed by the appearance of edema in the cerebral hemisphere corresponding to the injury. The most distinct consequences from the installation of edema are profound disturbances in cortical electrogenesis characterized by degradation of the physiological arousal rhythms (θ and β waves), an increase in slow waves (α), and mainly by the appearance of δ waves, signs of cerebral distress and of deterioration in cerebral function at this level.

In untreated control rabbits, the ($\theta + \beta/\alpha + \delta$) ratio is decreased after traumatic edema mainly because of the strong increase in δ waves and a joint diminution in θ and β waves. Ginkgo biloba extract, administered as curative treatment 18 hours before the injury, at doses of 12.5, and 50 mg/kg orally, erases the disturbances in cortical electrogenesis without modifying the physiological θ waves, but strongly decreasing the number of pathological δ waves, a sign not of an effect on normal cortical electrogenesis, but of a direct effect on the cerebral edema, source of the electrical disturbances recorded (*Table 1*).

Triethyletain-induced (TET) edema in the rat (3, 15)

Cerebral edema is induced in Sprague-Dawley rats by ingestion for two weeks of an aqueous solution of TET (0.002%) supplied as the only drink. The neurological deficit consecutive to the installation of the edema is evaluated by determination of the ultimate angle of a grilled inclined plane compatible with movement of the animal and the index of walking. The following scoring is used for this latter: 10 = normal gait, 8 = gait on the tips of the paws, 2 = muscular hypertonic gait with paws spread, 0 = semilateral decubitus.

The neurological index is evaluated on the tenth and 15th days of treatment. After the last observation, the animals are sacrificed, the percentage of edema is evaluated by the water content by weighing the brain before and after drying, and the content of Na^+ and K^+ by flame photometry.

The results obtained by Borzeix(4) with Ginkgo biloba extract are summarized in *Table 2*. At doses of 10, 30, and 90 mg/kg (oral route, treatment for 15 days), the Ginkgo biloba extract totally annulled the neurological disturbances induced by the TET. These results were confirmed by regulation of the water and cerebral electrolytes content, which were returned to normal by 30 and 90 mg/kg Ginkgo biloba extract.

Thus in these two experimental edema models, but particularly in the TET model, Ginkgo biloba extract opposes the development of edema and of the ionic disturbances which accompany it, and above all annuls the functional consequences of the latter.(21)

Table 1

Unilateral traumatic edema in the rabbit.
Effects of ginkgo biloba extract on evolution of the $\theta + \beta/\delta + \alpha$ ratio
(according to Borzeix(4))

Evaluation elements	Hours after treatment	Controls n = 10	Ginkgo biloba extract (mg/kg[1], p.o.)		
			12,5 (n = 10)	*25 (n = 10)*	*50 (n = 10)*
Reference value		$51 \pm 4,6$	$43 \pm 5,2$	$44 \pm 3,9$	$38 \pm 2,8$
Differences in comparison with the reference value	1	$-3 \pm 3,0$	$-1 \pm 3,8$	$+3 \pm 3,3$	$+7 \pm 3,8*$
	2	$-4 \pm 3,1$	$-1 \pm 3,1$	$+2 \pm 4,4$	$+5 \pm 3,9$
	3	$-1 \pm 2,8$	$+3 \pm 4,3$	$-1 \pm 3,8$	$+8 \pm 3,5*$
	4	$-6 \pm 3,1$	$+2 \pm 4,9$	$0 \pm 3,3$	$+12 \pm 5,6*$
	5	$-2 \pm 3,1$	$+3 \pm 4,4$	$+1 \pm 3,7$	$+10 \pm 3,4*$
	6	$-4 \pm 3,6$	$+4 \pm 3,8$	$-1 \pm 3,3$	$+12 \pm 4,9*$

*$p \leq 0.05$ (t = test).

Table 2

Triethyletain-induced (TET) edema in the rat.
Effects of treatment with ginkgo biloba extract (EGb) on intracerebral
content of water and electrolytes, and on the neurological index

Series	Daily dose in mg/kg (p.o)	n	Cerebral concentration			Neurological index		Gait index (inclined plane)	
			%	mmol/kg dry weight					
			H_2O	Na^+	K^+	*D 10*	*D 15*	*D10*	*D15*
Controls	–	15	$78,3 \pm 0,10$	$201 \pm 1,8$	$382 \pm 7,7$	10	10	90	90
Intoxicated with TET	–	15	$80,5 \pm 0,17$ (*)	$290 \pm 5,3$ (*)	$373 \pm 8,2$	4,1(*)	0(*)	30(*)	0(*)
Treated with EGb	10	15	$79,7 \pm 0,18*$	$249 \pm 6,0*$	$372 \pm 4,9$	9,7*	9,7*	90*	90*
EGb	30	15	$78,6 \pm 0,14*$	$209 \pm 3,5*$	$377 \pm 6,7*$	10*	10*	90*	90*
EGb	90	15	$78,4 \pm 0,07*$	$202 \pm 2,4*$	$390 \pm 4,3$	10*	10*	90*	90*

D 10, D 15 = on the 15th day of treatment; (*) = $P \leq 0.001$ in comparison with controls; * = $P \leq 0.001$ in comparison with rats intoxicated with TET.

Mechanisms of effects of Ginkgo Biloba extract on cerebral edema

First of all we must stress the fact that the hemodynamic and vascular components of Ginkgo biloba extract, guarantees of the maintenance of an effective tissue perfusion flow(10) and of less deficit in the energy supply,(7, 8) but also the revealed antagonism by the Ginkgo biloba extract to experimental capillary hyperpermeabilities to histamine and bradykinin (in the rabbit), to dextran and galactosamine (in the rat),(20) would be sufficient in themselves to explain the protection exerted by this product against cererbal edema and its neurological consequences.

But it is in the membranes that most of the edematogenic factors are located which intervene, let us remember, in two successive stages of membranal attack. The first phase of disturbance, direct consequence of the deficit in energy supply, is essentially ionic and can be summarized as paralysis of $Na^+K^+ATpase$, with a loss of potassium and an influx of intracellular calcium. In the second phase, the membranal phopholipids produce a group of metabolites aggresive toward the membranal structures (arachidonic acid, leukotrienes, oxygenated free radicals) and thus support the edema, particularly by increasing the magnitude through vasogenic mechanisms. At these levels we find the "keys" to the membranal mechanisms of Ginkgo biloba extract which explain the protection which it exerts on cerebral edema. In fact, the latter decreases the osmotic fragility of the erythrocytic membranes placed under debilitating conditions, *in vitro* and *ex vivo*.(13) It stabilizes the lysosomial membranes(26) and exerts an antiproteasic component.(20) Ginkgo biloba extract inhibits uncoupling of oxidative phosphorylations at the mitochondrial level,(16) manifests scavenging effects on oxygenated free radicals,(11) inhibitors of peroxidation of membranal phospholipids (demonstrated on homogenates of brains of rats and mice through inhibition of the formation of malonaldehyde) and antagonists of adriamycin-induced inflammatory edema (*in vivo*), an inflammatory reaction due to membranal lipoperoxidation.(12, 14)

In conclusion, the protection which Ginkgo biloba extract gives against cerebral edema, whether this is of cytotoxic type (triethyletain-induced edema) or vasogenic (unilateral traumatic edema) is manifested both in regard to the ionic disturbances and the neurological deficit which is its direct consequence. These antiedematous effects of Ginkgo biloba extract are the indirect result of vascular impacts (maintenance of effective tissue perfusion flow) and metabolic impacts, but may be explained mainly by the network of direct actions which Ginkgo biloba extract exerts in the cellular membranes and certain subcellular fractions.

References

1. Baron J.C.: Phénomènes physiopathologiques au cours de l'ischémie focale aiguë du cerveau. *Revue Méd.*, 1983, *38*, 1853-1863.

2. Borzeix M.G., Labos M., Cahn J.: A propos d'un modèle expérimental d'œdème cérébral pour l'étude des substances agissant sur le débit sanguin et/ou le métabolisme cérébral. *Agressologie*, 1972, *13*, 257-260.

3. Borzeix M.G., Weber S., Akimjak J.P.: Cerebral edema induced by triethyltin (TET) in the rabbit and in the rat. *In:* Proc. of the 7th International Congress of Pharmacology, Satellite Symposium of Reims, 1978.

4. Borzeix M.G.: Effect of Ginkgo biloba Extract on 2 types of cerebral edema. *In:* Effects of Ginkgo biloba Extract on Organic Cerebral Impairment, Agnoli A., Rapin J.R., Scapagnini V., Weitbrecht W.V., Eda, *John Libbey*, London, 1985, 51-56.

5. Braquet P., De Feudis F.V., Deby C., Braquet M.: Involvement of oxygen free radicals in biologic and pathologic processes. *In:* Cerebral Ischaemia, Bes A., Braquet P., Paoletti R., Siesjö B.K., Eds., *Excerpta Medica*, Amsterdam, 1984, 265-283.

6. Braquet P., Braquet M., Deby C.: Oxidative damages induced by cerebral ischemia: protective role of some radical scavengers and related drugs. *J. Cerebral Blood Flow and Metabolism*, 1983, *3*, supl. 1, 564-565.

7. Chatterjee S.S., Gabard B.: Protective effect of an extract of Ginkgo biloba and other hydroxyl radical scavengers against hypoxia. *Eighth International Congress of Pharmacology*, 1981, Tokyo, Abstract 866.

8. Chatterjee S.S.,: Effects of Ginkgo biloba Extract on metabolic processes. *In:* Effects of Ginkgo biloba Extract on Organic Cerebral Impairment, Agnoli A., Rapin J.R., Scapagnini V., Weitbrecht W.V., Eds., *John Libbey*, London, 1985, 5-15.

9. Cohadon F.: Physiopathologie de l'œdème cérébral ischémique. *Circulation et Métabolisme du Cerveau*, 1983, *1*, 45-54.

10. DeFeudis F.V., Auguet M., Delaflotte S., Hellegouarch A., Baranes J., Chapelat M., Braquet M., Etienne A., Drieu K., Clostre F., Braquet P.: Some *in vitro* and *in vivo* actions of an extract of Ginkgo biloba (GbE 761). *In:* Effects of Ginkgo biloba extract on Organic Cerebral Impairment, Agnoli A., Rapin J.R., Scapagnini V., Weitbrecht W.V., Eds. *John Libbey*, London, 1985, 17-29.

11. Doly M., Braquet P., Droy M.T., Bonhomme B., Vennat J.C.: Effets des radicaux libres oxygénés sur l'activité électrophysiologique de la rétine isolée de rat. *J. Fr. Ophtalmol.*, 1985, *8*.

12. Etienne A., Baranes J., Hecquet F., Hellegouarch A., Clostre F.: Effet stabilisateur de membrane d'un extrait de Ginkgo biloba. *Planta Medica*, 1980, *39*, 327.

13. Etienne A., Chapelat M., Braquet M., Clostre F., Drieu K., DeFeudis F.V., Braquet P.: *In vivo* studies of free radical scavenging activity; relation to cerebral ischaemia. *In:* Cerebral Ischaemia, Bes A., Braquet P., Paoletti R., Siesjö B.K., Eds. *Excerpta medica*, Amsterdam, 1984, 379-384.

14. Etienne, A., Hacquet F., Clostre F., DeFeudis F.V.: Comparaison des effets d'un extrait de Ginkgo biloba et de la chlorpromazine sur la fragilité osmotique *in vitro* d'érythrocytes de rat. *J. Pharmacol.*, 1982, *13*, 291-298.

15. Gabard B., Chatterjee S.S.: Cerebral edema induced by triethyltin in the rat: Effects of an extract of Ginkgo biloba. *Naunym Schmiedeberg's Arch. Pharmacol.*, 311, (suppl.) R 68.

16. Karchel I., Zagermann P., Krieglstein J.: Effect of an Extract of Ginkgo biloba on rat brain energy metabolism in hypoxia, *Naunym Schmiedeberg's Arch. Pharmacol.*, 1984, *327*, 31-35.

17. Kariman K.: Mecanisms of cell damage in brain ischemia: a hypothesis. *Life Sciences*, 1985, *37*, 71-73.

18. Kimelberg H.K.: Glial enzymes and ion transport in brain swelling. *In:* seminar in neurological surgery. In: Neural trauma, Pepp A.J., Bourke R.S., Melson L.R., Kimelbert M.K., Eds., *Raven Press*, 137-155.

19. Le Poncin Lafitte M., Rapin J.R.: Effects of Ginkgo biloba on changes induced by quantitative cerebral micro-embolization in rats. *Arch. Int. Pharmacodyn.*, 1980, *243*, 236-244.

20. Marcy R.: Dossier d'AMM Tanakan, Rapport d'expertise pharmacologique, 1980.

21. Otani M., Chatterjee S.S., Gabard B., Kreutzberg G.W.: Effect of an extract of Ginkgo biloba on triethyltin-induced cerebral edema. *Acta Neuropathol.*, 1986, *69*, 54-65.

22. Overgaard, J.: Cerebral blood flow brain edema. *Circulation et Métabolisme du cerveau*, 1984, *2*, 11-22.

23. Pickard J.D., Walker V.: Current concepts of the role of prostaglandins and other eicosanoïds in acute cerebrovascular disease. *In:* Lers vol., 2 Mackenzie E.T. ed., *Raven Press*, New York, 191-218.

24. Siesjö B.K.: Cell damage in the brain: A speculative synthesis. *J. Cerebral Blood Flow and Metabolism*, 1981, *1*,155-185.

25. Spinnewyn B., Blavet N., Clostre F.: Effets du Ginkgo biloba sur l'ischémie cérébrale expérimentale chez la gerbille. *Presse Méd.*, 1986, *15*, 1511-1515.

26. Van Caneghen P.: Influence of some hydrosoluble substances with vitamin P activity on the fragility of lysosomes *in vitro*. *Biochem. Pharm.*, 1972, *21*, 1543-1548.

27. Williams T.J., Jose P.J., Wedmore C.V., Peck M.J., Forrest M.J.: Mechanisme underlying inflammatory œdoma: The importance of synergism prostaglandins, leukotrienes and complement derived peptides. *In:* Advances in Prostaglandin, Thromboxane, and Leukotriene Research, vol. 11, Samuelsson B., Paoletti R., Ramwell P. Eds., *Raven Press,* New York, 33-37.

Effects of Ginkgo Biloba Extract on a Cerebral Ischemia Model in Gerbils

B. Spinnewyn, N. Blavet, F. Clostre

Centre de recherche I.H.B.-I.P.S.E.N., 72, avenue des Tropiques
F 91940 Les Ulis

Summary

Certain anatomical characteristics peculiar to the gerbil make it the animal model best adapted to experimental pathology studies of acute ischaemia.

In this animal species, devoid of any substitute vertebro-basilar vascular tissue, unilateral ligature of the carotid artery produces a cerebral ischaemia with neurological signs (well quantifiable), metabolic perturbations (especially mitochondrial) and cerebral oedema development closely resembling the symptoms revealed by physiopathology in human clinical studies.

Using this model and under the experimental conditions described, clear-cut, highly significant results were obtained with Ginkgo biloba, whether by oral or intravenous administration.

These results were normalization of mitochondrial respiration, diminution of cerebral oedema, correction of the accompanying ionic pertubarations, and practically total functional restoration revealed by a normal neurological index in the gerbils treated with Ginkgo biloba extract.

In man, cerebral ischemia, whatever its origin – thrombosis, spasm, hypotension or elevation of intracranial pressure – engenders a sequence of complex vascular and metabolic events which is difficult to reproduce in its entirety in laboratory animals.

There are numerous experimental models. Many have value, all have limitations. The hypoxia models are often easy to realize. Some are crude, others more sophisticated, but all of them have the disadvantage of causing a generalized state of hypoxia, not specific for the cerebral sphere. Experimental ischemia models can be obtained by ligation or by microembolization. Fieschi and Lenzi(4) counted more than 25 different ones, usually achieved in rats, cats, dogs, monkeys, and gerbils.

But the anatomical differences which distinguish the rat, cat, and dog from man are numerous; in dogs, for example, the cerebral vascular supply is assured almost totally by the vertebral network. In this case, it is understood that extrapolation from animals to man is very hazardous.

Rökan (Ginkgo Biloba). Recent Results in Pharmacology and Clinic
Edited by E.W. Fünfgeld
© Springer-Verlag Berlin Heidelberg New York 1988, pp. 143-152

The advantage of the gerbil is that in 40 to 60% of cases it presents an abnormality in the circulus arteriosus, preventing any communication between the carotid and vertebral systems.(8, 12) This lack of vertebrobasilar substitution makes it possible to obtain ischemia localized in the ipsilateral hemisphere in gerbils by simple ligation of one of the common carotids.(3)

Gerbils are small, black rodents – found in Africa and Asia – in size intermediate between mice and hamsters. We have worked with the Mongolian gerbil (*Meriones unguiculatus* Taminoto K, 1943). In adulthood a male weighs between 80 and 90 grams and the female between 70 and 80 grams. Since 1954, strains indtroduced initially in Japan have been developed in the United States, and for the past several years, in Europe.(15)

Gerbils possess physiological and morphological qualitities as well as dietary habits which allow them to adapt to often difficult climatic conditions. But the most remarkable – and the most surprising – are certain organized characteristics of their group behavior.(17)

Thus, the value of the gerbil as a model for experimental ischemia is dual: histopathological, biochemical, and electrophysiological studies have shown that the disturbances observed during ischemia in the gerbil were close to those described in human pharmacology; furthermore, this is an animal strain with rich behavioral characteristcs which are not – unlike the rat, dog, and cat – limited in the expression of their potentialities by the constraint of the breeding or laboratory environment.(16)

The experiment was carried out on gerbils having undergone unilateral ligation of the carotid, causing cerebral ischemia revealed by neurological signs quantifiable according to the scale defined by C.P. MacGraw,(13) by mitochondrial biochemical disturbances identified by determination of a respiratory index or respiratory control ratio(1) and by the installation of cerebral edema verified objectively by an increase in the weight of the ischemic hemisphere and by loss of potasssium and accumulation of sodium at this level.

The combination of these three groups of parameters in the same experiment has the advantage of making it possible to correlate the different types of disturbances in the installation and evolution of cerebral ischemia in the gerbil, but also, and mainly, of being able to dissociate the effects of products with specific impact (vascular or metabolic) from those which present a broader spectrum of action.

Material and Methods

The experiment involved 180 gerbils weighing 50 grams to 80 grams, divided into nine groups of 20 animals.

Induction of the ischemia

After prior selection made 15 days before the beginning of the experiment (ten-second clamping of the left carotid, selection of the animals presenting with ptosis of the left eye), the gerbils were divided at random into nine groups, and, under ketamine anesthesia (80 mg/kg i.p.), their right carotids were carefully occluded (preserving the adjacent nerve fibers). The control animals underwent the same operation, but without occlusion of the carotid ("sham-operated").

Determination of the neurological index (stroke index)

After two hours and every hour until six hours after the ischemia, the gerbils were placed individually in an enclosure (48 x 38 x 19 cm) for analysis of their behavior for three minutes according to the scale of C.P. MacGraw (13) (*Table 1*).

Table 1

MacGraw Scale. The sum of the coefficients constitutes the neurological index.

Criteria	Coefficient
– piloerection – tremor	1
– loss of balance	1
– slowness of movements	1
– palpebral ptosis	2
– epilepsy	2
– inclination of the head	3
– eye fixedly open	3
– splayed contalateral rear paw	3
– circular rotation	3
– convulsions	3
– coma	6
– death	34

Quantification of the cerebral edema

Immediately after the behavioral observation, the gerbils were decapitated and the brain was rapidly divided into three portions: the right and left occipital areas were weighed, then dried for determination of the cerebral edema and electrolytes; the right fronto-parietal zone was used for determination of mitochondrial respiration.

The water content was calculated by the following equation:(7)

$$\text{Water content } (\%) = \frac{\text{fresh weight} - \text{dry weight}}{\text{fresh weight}} \times 100.$$

Then the occipital zones were taken up with 3 mL of a 3N nitric acid solution, and the sodium and potassium concentrations were determined by flame photometry and expressed as mEq/kg dry weight according to the equation:

$$C \text{ mEq/kg} = \frac{3}{1000} \times \frac{1}{\text{dry weight}} \times 1000.$$

Measurement of the coefficient of mitochondrial respiration (respiratory control ratio)

The mitochondria in the right frontal parietal zone were isolated according to the method of D. Holtzman et al., (6) modified by J.P. Nowicki et al.(14)

Mitochondrial respiration was studied in the temperature-controlled cell of a Gilson oxygraph.(14) The RCR, indicator of mitochondrial respiratory efficacy, is represented by the ratio of stage 3 oxygen consumption (pyruvate + malate in the incubation medium with ADP) to stage 4 oxygen consumption (pyruvate + malate in the incubation medium without ADP).(1)

Treatments

In the course of this experiment, three products were tested as preventive treatment seven days before the ischemia:
– vincamine, 10 mg/kg i.p.
– nicergoline, 10 mg/kg p.o.
– Ginkgo biloba extract (EGb 761, Rökan®, Intersan), 10 mg/kg i.p. and 50 mg/kg p.o.

Expression of the results

All of the experimental data were processed by the analysis of variance test. The findings illustrated with an asterisk represent the magnitude of the ischemia or the differences in comparison with the ischemic controls, those represented by a black triangle, the differences in comparison with the "sham-opreated" controls, in order to evaluate a possible return to normal.

Results

Cerebral edema and Na⁺ and K⁺ concentrations

The cerebral edema in the ischemic hemisphere was partially decreased by all three products, but correction of the ionic disturbances consecutive to the ischemia (loss of K^+ and accumulation of Na^+ in the ischemic hemisphere) was more distinct after treatment with Ginkgo biloba extract or with vincamine than with nicergoline (*Table 2*).

Index of mitochondrial respiration

Cerebral ischemia in gerbilis is reflected at the mitochondrial level by severe inhibition of the rate of ATP synthesis combined with uncoupling of the mitochondrial function (stage 3 0_2 consumption ist decreased, but that of stage 4 is increased) which causes breakdown of the RCR. Nicergoline, vincamine, and Ginkgo biloba extract (in increasing order of efficacy) limit the decrease in the RCR in a statistically significant manner. This shows that these products permit the mitochondria in the ischemic hemisphere to recover a major part of their functional respiratory activity, that is, ensure adequate ATP synthesis for the maintenance of an effective cellular energy store (*Figure 1*).

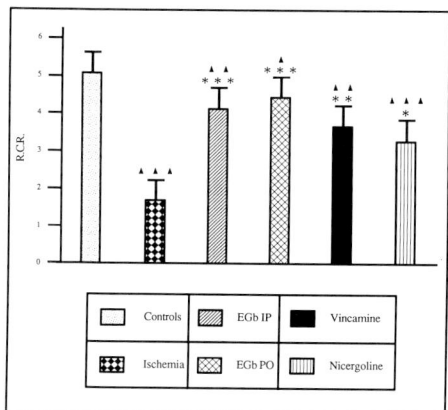

Figure 1: Mitochondrial respiration index (RCR) six hours after cerebral ischemia in the gerbil.

* or ▲, ** or ▲▲, and *** or ▲▲▲ signify respectively P < 0.05, P < 0.01, and P < 0.01 for the analysis of variance test.
*: comparisons with ischemic controls.
▲: comparisons with sham controls.

Table 2

Cerebral edema and concentration in Na^+ and K^+ in the ischemic hemisphere six hours after ligation of the right carotid in gerbils

Treatment	Water content[1]		Sodium levels (mEq/kg dry weight)		Potassium levels (mEq/kg dry weight)	
	Right hemisphere	Left hemisphere	Right hemisphere	Left hemisphere	Right hemisphere	Left hemisphere
Controls	78.3 0.06	78.2 0.07	203.9 7.19	210.9 6.26	480.4 0.21	475.7 0.22
Untreated ischemic gerbils	79.7 0.60 ♦♦♦	78.3 0.08 ***	317.8 3.08 ♦♦♦	206.6 8.66 ***	430.2 2.26 ♦♦	466.2 1.24
EGb 10mg/kg IP	79.0 0.32 ♦	78.2 0.06 *	282.4 2.21 ♦♦	220.6 5.66 *	428.9 1.45 ♦♦	475.9 0.32 *
EGb 50 mg/kg PO	79.1 0.25 ♦♦	78.4 0.20 *	287.1 2.34 ♦♦♦	219.1 5.37 **	447.6 2.11	477.8 0.80
Vincamine 10 mg/kg IP	79.3 0.32 ♦♦	78.5 0.11 *	296.9 2.33 ♦♦♦	224.7 4.35 **	434.2 1.40 ♦	480.1 0.35 *
Nicergoline 10 mg/kg PO	79.2 0.32 ♦	78.1 0.9 **	350.3 2.65 ♦♦♦	240.3 6.10 ***	395.6 1.92 ♦♦♦	478.6 0.45 ***

* or ♦, ** or ♦♦, and *** or ♦♦♦ signify respectively P < 0.05, P < 0.01, and P < 0.001 by analysis of variance test.

*: Right hemisphere/left hemisphere comparisons.

♦: Treated right hemisphere/nonligated control right hemisphere comparisons (recovery) or ischemic right hemisphere/nonischemic right hemisphere comparisons.

(1) Water content = $\dfrac{\text{fresh weight} - \text{dry weight}}{\text{fresh weight}} \times 100$

of the occipital zones (left) of the healthy hemisphere and of the ischemic hemisphere (right).

Neurological index (or stroke index)

Cerebral ischemia brings the neurological index to the mean score of 9.2 after six hours of ischemia. Nicergoline diminishes it slightly, but not in a statistically significant manner. Vincamine and particularly Ginkgo biloba extract (for the latter, regardless of route of administration) very distinctly improve the stroke index after ischemia. With respect to the groups treated with Ginkgo biloba extract, their stroke index was not statistically different from that of the nonischemic group, which proves almost total functional restoration in the ischemic gerbils treated with this product (*Figure 2*).

Discussion

In the gerbil deprived of vertebrobasilar vascular substitution, unilateral ligation of the carotid causes a cerebral accident, with well-quantifiable neurological signs, major biochemical disturbances, in particular mitochondrial, and the development of cerebral edema developing within several days toward necrosis and cell death. The mitochondria which, through oxidative phosphorylation reactions, ensure the cellular energy requirements, are the sites most sensitive to ischemic and/or hypoxic effects. Mitochondrial changes, both ultrastructural and biochemical, are the first signs of ischemia. They are reflected very early by disengagement of oxidative phosphorylations, which signifies that a much greater quantity of oxygen is found necessary for the same ATP production.

After six hours of ischemia, there was found in the ischemic hemisphere:

– a breakdown in mitochondrial respiratoy efficacy revealed by a decrease of more than 50% in the RCR:

– the installation of cerebral edema with increased Na^+ concentration and a decrease in that of K^+ in the ischemic hemisphere;

– a behavioral index (stroke index) which attains code 9, a sign of profound neurological disturbances.

In this cerebral ischemia model, by unilateral ligation of the carotid in gerbils, the effects of nicergoline were moderate, both on the ionic and mitochondrial disturbances and on the neurological index (in this last case, they were not statistically significant). Vincamine (10 mg/kg i.p.) influences all of the disturbances in a statistically significant manner: mitochondrial RCR, cerebral edema, and disturbances in the Na^+ and K^+ exchanges, neurological index. These results confirm the value attributed to this product by B. Gotti et al.,(5) who states that vincamine is one of the substances capable of significantly reducing the extent of the necrotic area after a focal cerebral edema.

But the most distinct and the most significant results were recorded with EGb, whether this was administered i.p. or p.o. There was observed:
– distinct recovery of the mitochondrial RCR,
– a decrease in the cerebral edema and significant correction of the ionic disturbances which accompany it,
– functional restoration, revealed by total recovery of a normal neurological index.

These experimental findings confirm those which have already been recorded and published in the metabolic field (9, 11) and in the neurological field.(10)

They confirm that the triple vascular, metabolic, and neurological impact of EGb explains its efficacy in this cerebral ischemia model.(2)

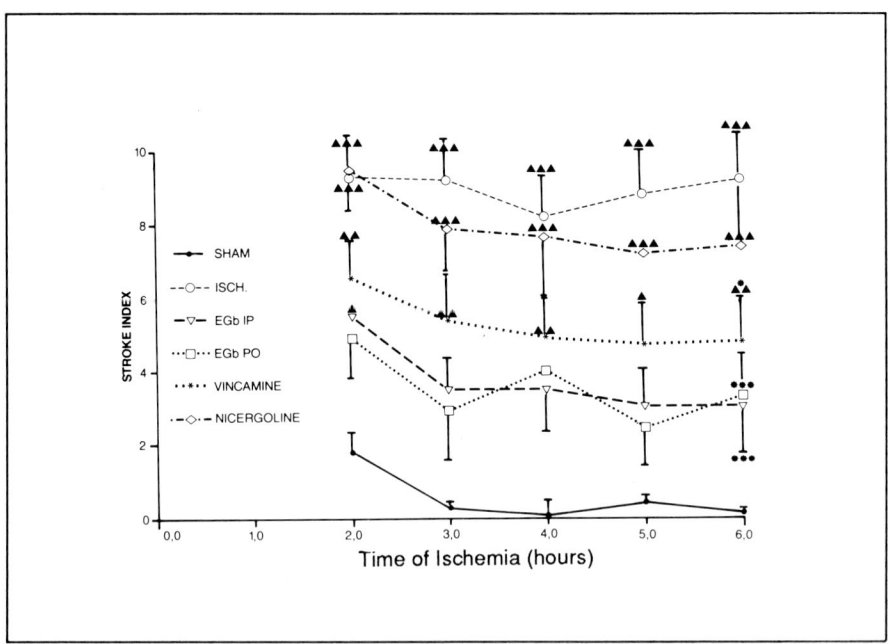

Figure 2: Neurological index (stroke index) in the course of cerebral ischemia in gerbils.

* or ▲, ** or ▲▲, and *** or ▲▲▲ signify respectively P < 0.05, P < 0.01, and P < 0.01 for the analysis of variance test.
*: comparisons with ischemic controls.
▲: comparisons with sham controls.

Conclusion

The value of the cerebral ischemia model in gerbils is that it faithfully mimics the sequences of the disturbances of human cerebral ischemia. The prime mover for all cellular disorders is damage to the membranal integrity of the vascular cells (edema and ionic disturbances), of the mitochondria (uncoupling of oxidative phosphorylations), or the neurons (functional and neurological disorders). Under our experimental conditions, Ginkgo biloba extract was shown to be the most effective of the products tested in the treatment of the metabolic and neurological disorders induced in gerbils by cerebral ischemia.

References

1. Chance B., Williams G.R.: The respiratory chain and oxydative phosphorylation. *Nature,* 1955, *175,* 1120-1121.

2. Chatterjee S.S.: Effects of Ginkgo biloba Extract on cerebral metabolic processes. *In:* Effects of Ginkgo biloba on organic cerebral impairment, Agnoli A., Rapin J.R., Scapagnini V., Weitbrecht W.V. Eds., *John Libbey,* London, 1985, 5-15.

3. Delbarre B., Delbarre G.: La gerbille comme modèle d'ischémie cérébrale. *J. Int. Médecine,* 1984, *9,* Suppl. n° 50, 11-14.

4. Fieschi C., Lenzi G.L.: Experimental models of focal cerebral ischemia. *In:* Cerebral Ischemia, Bes A., Braquet P., Paoletti R., Siesjö B.K. Eds., *Excerpta Medica,* 1984, 57-62.

5. Gotti B., Mackenzie E.T., Nowicki J.P., Young A.R.: Pharmacothérapie de l'ischémie cérébrale focale. *Actua Clin. Ther.* 1983, *10,* 114-124.

6. Holtzman D., Lewinston N., Herman N.M., Desantel M., Brewer E., Robin E.: Effects of osmolar changes on isolated mitochondria of brain and liver. *J. Neurochem.,* 1978, *30,* 1409-1419.

7. Ito U.: Brain edema during ischemia and after restoration of blood flow. Measurement of water, sodium, potassium content and plasma protein permeability. *Stroke,* 1979, *10,* 542-547.

8. Kahn K.: The natural course of experimental cerebral infarction in the Gerbil. *Neurology,* 1972, *22,* 510-515.

9. Karcher L., Zagermann P., Krieglstein J.: Effect of an extract of Ginkgo biloba on rat brain energy metabolism in hypoxia. *Naunyn–Schmiedeberg's Arch. Pharamacol.*, 1984, *327*, 31-35.

10. Larssen R.G., Dupeyron J.P., Boulu R.G.: Modèle d'ischémie cérébrale expérimentale par microsphères chez le rat. Etude de l'effet de deux extraits de Ginkgo biloba et du naftidrofuryl. *Thérapie*, 1978, *33*, 651-660.

11. Le Poncin Lafitte M., Martin P., Lespinasse P., Rapin J.R.: Ischémie cérébrale après ligature non simultanée des artères carotides chez le rat: effet de l'extrait de Ginkgo biloba. *Sem. Hôp. Paris*, 1982, *58*, 403-406.

12. Levines S., Payan H.: Effects of ischemia and other procedures on the brain and retina of the gerbil (Meriones unguiculatus). *Exp. Neurol.*, 1966, *16*, 255-262.

13. MacGraw C.P.: Experimental cerebral infarction. Effects of pentobarbital in mongolian gerbils. *Arch. Neurol.*, 1977, *34*, 334-336.

14. Nowicki J.P., MacKenzie E.T., Spinnewyn B.: Effects of agents used in the pharmacotherapy of cerebrocvascular disease on the oxygen consumption of isolated cerebral mitochondria. *J. Cerebral Blood Flow Metabolism*, 1982, *2*, 33-40.

15. Petter F.: La diversité des Gerbillidés. *In:* Rodents in desert environment, Junk W. Ed., *The Hague*, 1975, 47-52.

16. Petter F.: Les principales particularités du comportement des rongeurs de la famille des gerbillidés. *Sci. Tech. Anim. Lab.*, 1984, *9*, 229-231.

17. Tanimoto K.: Ecological studies on plague-carrying in Manchuria Dobutsugaku Zasski. *Zool. Mag. Tokyo*, 1943, *55*, 111-127.

Effects of Ginkgo Biloba Extract on Two Models of Experimental Myocardial Ischemia

J.M. Guillon[1], L. Rochette[2], J. Baranès[1]

(1) Centre de recherche I.H.B.-I.P.S.E.N., 72, avenue des Tropiques.
    F 9140 Les Ulis
(2) Laboratoire de Pharmacodynamie et Physiologie pharmaceutique,
    Faculté de Médecine et Pharmacie. 7, boulevard Jeanne d'Arc.
    F 21033 Dijon Cedex

Summary

Ginkgo biloba extract, a free radical scavenger containing kaempferol and quercetine esters, which are potent radical scavengers, was studied on various models of cardiac ischaemia, both in vitro *and* in vivo.

On the two in vitro *models of ischemia-reperfusion described (rat and guinea-pig hearts) Ginkgo biloba extract was without effect on cardiac functional parameters. However, it induced a significant decrease in the intensity of ventricular fibrillation during the reperfusion stage.*

On normal or hypertrophied heart in vivo, *Ginkgo biloba extract provided effective protection against the electrocardiographic disorders induced by ischaemia.*

On the different models of global or localized ischaemia (followed or not by reperfusion), a decrease of arrhythmia without change in cardiovascular parameters was regularly noted.

Cardiovascular diseases, and particularly myocardial ischemia, carry a very high mortality rate. The therapeutic approach to acute myocardial ischemia may be in two ways: by analysis of the functional disturbances and by analysis of metabolic disorders consecutive to the ischemia.

Under normal conditions, there is a balance between oxygen intake and requirements of the myocardium for oxygen by self-regulation (adjusted or refined by the autonomic system). Ischemia is the rupture of this equilibrium, either through diminution of supplies without increase in requirements (Prinzmetal's spastic angina), or through increased requirements without a concomitant increase in supply (effort angina). We shall devote ourselves here to the functional aspect of the first, by studying various models of coronary occlusion.

Rökan (Ginkgo Biloba). Recent Results in Pharmacology and Clinic
Edited by E.W. Fünfgeld
© Springer-Verlag Berlin Heidelberg New York 1988, pp. 153-161

Physiopathology

The quantitative and qualitative use of oxygen by the myocardium is therefore the keystone of the ischemic condition.

Although the toxicity of dioxygen has long been known, its role and that of its radical derivatives (superoxide O_2^- anion radical, OH hydroxyl radical) in the genesis of functional and metabolic disorders of cardiac ischemia are difficult to discern.

In the course of long-lasting ischemia, the electrical and contractile abnormalities observed are the result of depletion of the energy reserves (ATP), of the influx of calcium into the cell, of alternations in the sarcolemma, and of microvascular damages.

ATP depletion has two major consequences: dissociation of intramitochondrial transport from the electrons releasing the Q_{10} coenzyme (ubisemiquinone) and superoxide free radicals(5) for the one part, an increase in xanthine concentration(3) for the other part. In the course of ischemia, there is conversion of xanthine-dehydrogenase into xanthine-oxidase. Xanthine-oxidase combined with xanthine and hypoxanthine constitutes a system capable of producing superoxide radicals and hydrogen peroxide. The latter, via a Fenton-type reaction or a Haber-Weiss-type reaction catalyzed by ferrous ions, is itself the source of hydroxyl radicals, the strong oxidizing property of which makes it a very dangerous cytotoxic agent.(2)

Calcium desequestration permits activation of phospholipase, which stimulates the metabolism of arachidonic acid, certain intermediates of which produce free radicals.(8)

In the case of reperfusion after ischemia, reoxygenation causes a veritable explosion in production of free radical derivatives of dioxygen.(4) These, very reactive, attack practically all substrates (sugars, proteins, lipids). The concomitant release of cytosolic and mitochondrial enzymes, good markers for the damage suffered by the myocardium, is much greater in case of reperfusion.

A pharmacological approach through the use of free radical "scavengers" such as Ginkgo biloba extract (EGb 761, Rökan®, Intersan) allows us at least to confirm, if not to understand, certain of these hypotheses.

Glossary

ATP:	adenosine triphosphate
EGb:	Ginkgo biloba extract
VES:	ventricular extrasystole
VT:	ventricular tachycardia
VF:	ventricular fibrillation
AII:	angiotensin II

Methodology

The "oxy-radical scavenger" and antilipoperoxidative capacities of EGb led us to test it on various cardiac ischemia models: one model, *in vitro*, of ischemia-reperfusion in rats; one model, *in vitro*, of total ischemia-reperfusion in guinea pigs; one model of localized ischemia, without reperfusion, *in vivo*, in anesthetized rats.

In vitro models

The effects of EGb on the heart perfused through the left atrium (working heart) subjected to ischemia followed by reperfusion, have been studied in two different species, the rat and the guinea pig.

The hearts were removed and immediately placed in perfusion fluid (modified Krebs-Henseleit) at 0°C. They were then mounted on an apparatus derived from that described by Neely et al.(6) The hearts were initially perfused by the retrograde aortic route (Langendorff) under pressure of 80 cm of water. After a 15-minute stabilization period, ventricular work was created by opening of the canalization connecting the left auricle to the auricular chamber. The precharge was 10 cm of water and the postcharge was 80 cm of water.

In the rat heart, localized ischemia was obtained by occlusion of the left coronary artery according to the technique of Selye et al.(7) after 30 minutes of perfusion. The ischemia was maintained for ten minutes, then relieved. The perfusion was studied then for ten minutes.

In the guinea pig heart, which presents development of its collateral network such that ligation of the coronary artery does not cause ischemia, *overall* ischemia was obtained by the zero-flow-method,(4) depriving the heart of any nutritive fluid and of oxygen for ten minutes. Reperfusion was also studied for ten minutes.

In both models, EGb was added to the perfusion fluid (at concentrations of 1 mg/L for rats, and 10 mg/L for guinea pigs), 15 minutes before precipitation of the ischemia, then maintained until the end of the experiment.

In vivo models

Localized myocardial ischemia was obtained by ligation of the left coronary artery of the rat anesthetized with a nembutal-urethane mixture. After placement on artificial ventilation (1.5 mL/100 g), catheterization of the carotid artery, and realization of a chest flail at the level of the fourth space, the heart was exteriorized by simple pressure on the sternum of the animal fixed in dorsal decubitus. The ligation strand was passed around the left coronary artery, then the heart was replaced. The ligation was not done until 15 minutes afterward in order to allow a sufficiently long stabilization period.

Any animal presenting with dysrhythmia or blood pressure below 70 mmHg during this period was eliminated from the study. The ligature was kept tightened for 30 minutes, and recording of the EKG on the D II Lead allowed quantification of the rhythm disorders engendered by the localized ischemia: ventricular extrasystoles (VES), ventricular tachycardia (VT), ventricular fibrillations (VF). The rat was selected as the experimental animal, since it presents the peculiarity of having spontaneously reversible episodes of fibrillation during ischemia.(1, 7)

EGb was used in its lyophilized injectable form and was administered at the dose of 50 mg/kg in perfusion into the jugular vein for 45 minutes (15 minutes of stabilization + 30 minutes of ischemia). The volume injected, in order to avoid any danger of volemic expansion, was 0.02 mL/minute.

Ginkgo biloba extract and ischemia of the hypertrophied heart

Ventricular hypertrophy is a predisposing factor for myocardial infarction. The heart, a major consumer of oxygen, sensitive to toxic derivatives of dioxygen, would be more vulnerable to their attack when it is hypertrophic. In fact, a hypertrophic heart consumes more oxygen than a normal heart. Cardiac hypertrophy is created by infusion of angiotensin II (AII) (8 nmoles/hour) for 14 days by means of Alzet osmotic minipumps. Hypertension (HT), through an adaptive reaction of the heart, causes cardiac hypertrophy. But angiotensin II probably has other direct effects on the development of this hypertrophy.

At the end of 14 days of infusion, the animals were submitted to ischemia induced by ligation. Treatment with EGb at the dose of 50 mg/kg p.o. each day, began six days before implantation of the minipumps and continued for the 14 days of infusion. The animals were divided into four groups. AII + saline, AII + EGb, EGb, saline. They were kept in individual cages and received water and standardized nourishment *ad libitum*.

Results

In vitro models

Effect of EGb on coronary, aortic, and cardiac flows during ischemia and reperfusion.

In the rat heart, coronary ligation causes a reduction of approximately 50% in coronary flow. Reperfusion, performed following removal of the ligation, does not allow coronary flow to recover its initial value (9.7 ± 2.3 mL/minute with reperfusion against 18.4 ± 0.6 mL/minute before ligation). Under the effect of EGb (1 mg/L), changes in the various flows during the pre-ischemic, ischemic, and reperfusion phases are not observed with the series of control hearts.

In the guinea pig heart, EGb (10 mg/L) has no effect on the pre-ischemic value of coronary flow, but does permit attaining and even exceeding it significantly upon reperfusion ($127 \pm 6.8\%$ against $99 \pm 2.4\%$ for the control series; $P > 0.01$).

The aortic pre-ischemic flow is not modified under the influence of EGb. During reperfusion, EGb exerts a depressant effect on aortic flow ($89 \pm 2.7\%$ against $98 \pm 1.4\%$ for the control series; $P < 0.01$). EGb therefore has no influence on cardiac flow (sum of the aortic and coronary flows).

Action of EGb on evolution of heart rate and aortic pressure

In the rat heart, perfusion of EGb causes no significant modification in heart during the pre-ischemic or reperfusion phases. During ischemia, aortic pressure expressed as percent of initial value is equal to $62.4 \pm 5.5.\%$ in the control series. Under influence of EGb, a tendency was noted to an increase in this percentage. However, the variation was not statistically significant.

In the guinea pig heart, no influence of EGb was noted on heart rate during the pre-ischemic and reperfusion phases. EGb slightly increased the heart rate under global ischemia, but this was not significant. EGb permitted total recovery of aortic pressure after ten minutes of reperfusion, whereas the controls only partially recovered the pre-ischemic aortic pressure (103% EGb series against 86% controls series).

Effects of EGb on ischemia and reperfusion arrhythmias

Under the influence of EGb, a significant reduction was observed ($P < 0.05$) in the duration of ventricular fibrillations during the reperfusion phase (425.9 ± 42.7 seconds for the controls; 252.3 ± 66.8 for the EGb-treated animals). The duration of the post-ischemic ventricular tachycardia was increased significantly.

In vivo models

The number of VES, the VT time (in seconds), the fibrillation time during the 30 minutes of ischemia were compared by the F test of analysis of variance, according to a group-block scheme. The total numbers of disorders registered were compared, as well as their respective evolutions every five minutes after ligation.

The results were expressed by $P < 0.001***, P < 0.01**, P < 0.05$. EGb used in i.v. perfusion at the rate of 50 mg/kg caused a significant reduction in the total number of VES (EGb: 152.4 ± 22.0; saline: 307.6 ± 56.9; $P < 0.001$), as well as in the number of VES during the five-to-ten-minute and ten-to-15 minute periods after ligation, which are the periods richest in disturbances (five to ten minutes: EGb 23.7 ± 10.9; saline: 70.1 ± 12.3; $P < 0.05$; ten to 15 minutes: EGb 96.8 ± 15.7; saline: 140.4 ± 33.9; $P < 0.05$) (*Figure 1*).

The total time for VT(s) is also significantly lowered (EGb: 29.6 ± 13.4; saline: 59.0 ± 21.2: P < 0.001). Also, the VT time during the ten-to-15-minute period after ligation is less in the treated series in comparison with the physiological controls (EGb: 11.1 ± 4.7; saline: 40.8 ± 12.9; P < 0.001) (*Figure 2*). Wistar rats present little fibrillation, and EGb has no effect on these disturbances. Whatever the period or the disorders considered (VT or VES), the values recorded in the treated animals were always less than those of the controls, but without the differences (except for those previously cited) being statistically significant.

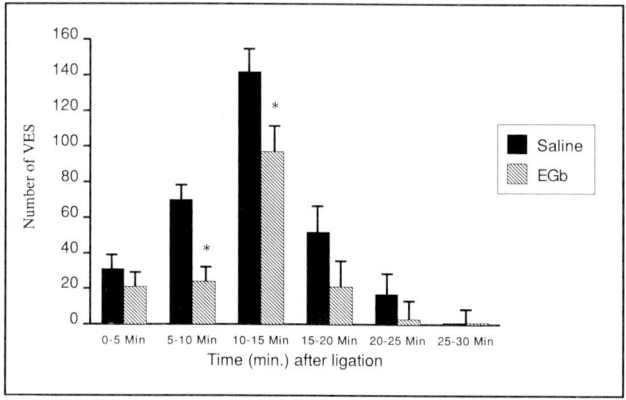

Figure 1: Evolution of the number of ventricular extrasystoles in the course of ligation. Effect of EGb in perfusion (50 mg/kg).

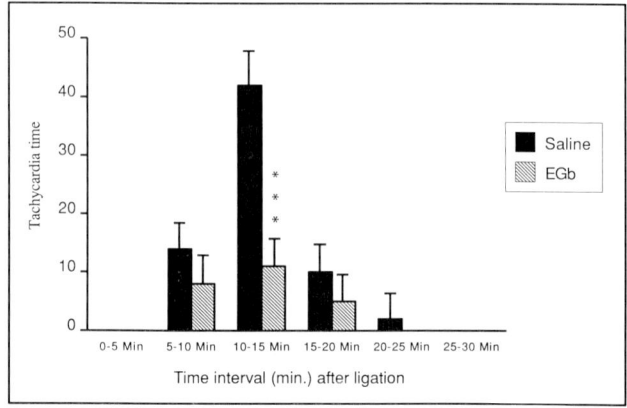

Figure 2: Evolution of ventricular tachycardia time during ligation. Effect of EGb in perfusion (50 mg/kg).

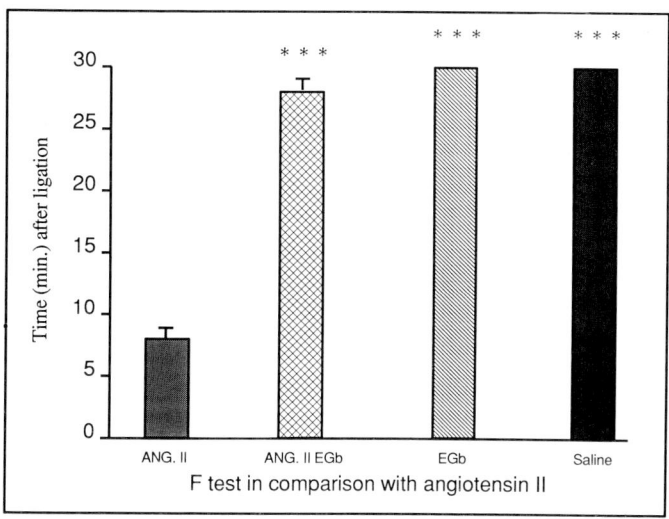

Figure 3: Time before occurence of death. Effects of angiotensin and EGb.

In the ischemic heart

Cardiac hypertrophy is measured by the ratio

$$\frac{\text{weight of both ventricles}}{\text{animal weight}} \times 100$$

The action of AII is very significant, and EGb does not combat this hypertrophy.

Ligation of the left coronary artery caused the death of rats in the AII group 8.2 ± 0.7 minutes after ligation, whereas only one animal in the AII + EGb group died (mean for Group 2: 20.2 ± 1.8 minutes). Total VF time was much less in the animals in Group AII + EGb than in Group AII (AII group 1325.6 ± 45.5; AII + EGb group 162.0 ± 18.7; $P < 0.001$***) (*Figures 3 and 4*). The hypertrophied heart was therefore protected very effectively from fibrillation by EGb, but the values for other disturbances were not returned to normal. EGb p.o. has no antiarrhythmic action on the normal heart subjected to localized ischemia.

EGb alone has no effect at this level on the normal heart. However, the animals in the AII + EGb group presented with numerous disorders (particularly VF and VT) in comparison with the physiological controls. There was therefore "replacement" of severe disorders (VF, irreversible or not) by these less serious disturbances (VT and VES).

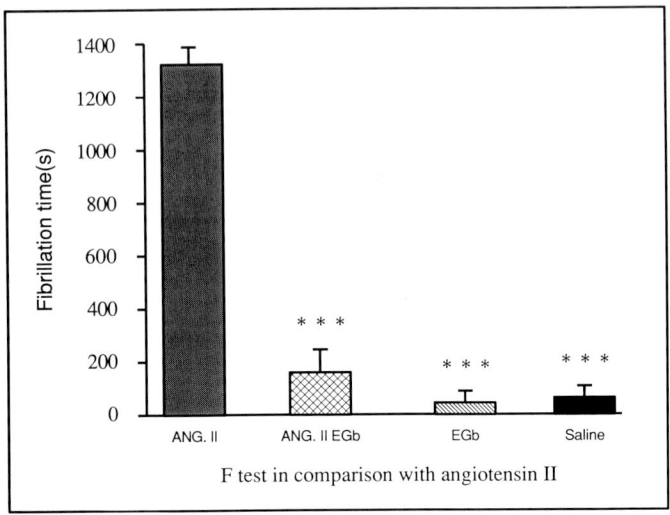

Figure 4: Measurement of total fibrillation time. Effects of angiotensin and of EGb.

Discussion and Conclusion

EGb causes no changes in the evolution of cardiac functional parameters (*in vitro*). However, in rat heart *in vitro* a significant reduction is observed in the intensity of ventricular fibrillations. *In vivo*, EGb supplies very significant protection with respect to the functional disturbances engendered by ischemia (normal heart), mainly during the critical periods five to ten and ten to 15 minutes after ligation: a reduction in the total number of VES and in the total VT time, reduction in the number of VES during these two periods, reduction in the VT time in the course of the ten-to-15-minute period. EGb spectacularly protects the heart rendered hypertrophic by angiotensin II from fibrillations, whether irreversible or not, but without returning the other parameters to normal.

In view of the potent free-radical-"scavenging" effect and the antilipoperoxidative properties of EGb (probably due to the coumaric esters of kaempferol and of quercetine which it contains, see the article by C. Deby et al. *Presse Méd. 15*, 1986, pages 1468-1474), this physiological approach to left ventricular hypertrophy and ischemia causes us to believe that the role of free radicals is preponderant in myocardial ischemia. Their implication in the genesis of left ventricular hypertrophy seems to be much more moderate.

References

1. Clark C., Foreman M.I., Kane K.A., McDonald F., Paratt J.R.: Coronary artery ligation in anaesthetized rats as a method for the production of experimental dysrhytmias and for the determination of infarct size. *J. Pharmacol. Methods,* 1980, *3*, 357-368.

2. Halliwel B., Gutterridge J.M.C.: Oxygen toxicity, oxygen radicals, transition metal and disease. *Biochem. J.,* 1984, *219*, 1-14.

3. Jennings R.B., Reimer K.A.: Lethal myocardical ischaemia injury. *Am. J. Pathol.,* 1981, *102*, 241-255.

4. Manning A.S., Hearse D.J.: Reperfusion-induced arrythmias: mechanisms and prevention. *J. Mol. Cell. Cardiol.,* 1984, *16*, 497-518.

5. Nayler W.G., Poole-Wilson P.A., Williams A.: Hypoxia and Calcium. *J. Mol. Cell. Cardiol.,* 1979, *11*, 683-706.

6. Neely J.R., Libermeister M., Battersby E.J., Morgan H.E.: Effect of pressure development on oxygen consumption by isolated rat heart. *Am. J. Physiol.,* 1967, *212*, 804-814.

7. Selye H., Bajusz E., Graslo S., Mendell P.: Simple techniques for the surgical occlusion of coronary vessels in the rat. *Angiology,* 1960, *11*, 398-407.

8. Vandervusse I., Reneman R.S.: Pharmacological intervention in acute myocardial ischaemia and reperfusion. *TIPS* 1985, *6*, 76-79.

Effect of Ginkgo Biloba Extract on Arteriolar Spasm in Rabbits

S. Reuse-Blom[1], K. Drieu[2]

(1) Laboratoire de Physiologie. Faculté des Sciences psychologiques et pédagogiques.
  Université libre de Bruxelles, 2 rue Evers. 1000 Bruxelles. Belgique.
(2) Centre de recherche I.H.B.-I.P.S.E.N., 17, avenue Descartes, F 92350 Le Plessis-Robinson

Summary

Injectable Ginkgo biloba extract, administered intravenously to rabbits, suppressed the vasospasm induced by the topical application of autologous serum on the brain surface.

This effect was dose-dependent with respect to normalization of the arterial diameter and duration of spasm. In animals previously treated with oral Ginkgo biloba extract, the almost complete disappearance of spasm was observed at intervals of time similar to those observed after intravenous injection of the extract.

The etiology of cerebral vasospasm can be diverse, and its mechanisms are still poorly elucidated. Numerous animal models have been suggested. Primates have an anatomy similar to that of man, but they constitute models which are costly and difficult to handle. Methods using smaller mammals must take into consideration the particular anatomy of each species when angiographic measurements or measurements of circulation after occlusion of a vessel are to be made.(4)

Experimental procedures

Direct observation of vessels on the brain surface makes possible vizualization of the precapillary arterioles under the microscope, but has the disadvantage of suppressing intracranial pressure. Isometric or isotonic measurements of muscle tension of the vessel walls can be made on isolated arteries, but this involves *in vitro* measurements not taking into consideration the neuronal regulation of the vessels.

Spasm may be produced by injuring a vessel by intracisternal injection of blood, of heparin, or of blood originating from patients suffering with subarachnoidal hemorrhage. In these cases, the spasm may be evaluated by angiographic measure-

Rökan (Ginkgo Biloba). Recent Results in Pharmacology and Clinic
Edited by E.W. Fünfgeld
© Springer-Verlag Berlin Heidelberg New York 1988, pp. 162-168

ments of circulation, which uses complex material and indicates only total or regional circulation and not local circulation, which is the most important for the neurological implications.

Open-skull experiments use the topical application of nonphysiological spasmogenic substances such as barium sulfate, for example, or physiological spasmogenic substances such as serotonin or autologous serum. Whole blood cannot be used, since direct observation of the vessels at the surface of the skull could then scarcely be effected.

Up to the present, only the efficacy of certain calcium antagonists could be demonstrated experimentally by the diminution in contraction (induced by serotonin and noradrenalin) of the cerebral vessels of animals with vasospasm induced by intracisternal injection of blood.(2, 10)

Ginkgo biloba extract , EGb 761, has long been known as a vasoactive substance, particularly in the cerebral area. The chemical complexity of the extract explains the multiplicity of its effects:(6) flavonoid glycosides have an antiradical and/or antilipoperoxidizing effect, responsible for the protective action of the extract toward the cellular membranes.(7) The effects of EGb on capillary hyperpermeability, on protection of the blood-brain barrier, and its antiedematous effect, in particular in the brain,(5, 8) are certainly significantly related to this membranal action. Terpenes, other constituents of EGb, possess potent antagonistic activity to PAF-acether (Platelet Activating Factor) which seems to be implicated in numerous pathological situations. Finally, in isolated organs, interactions of Ginkgo biloba extract with the neuromediators(1) have been demonstrated.

It appeared worthwhile to test its action on precapillary arteriolar spasm *in vivo*. A first experiment was carried out by administering Ginkgo biloba extract intravenously after production of the spasm.(9) In a second experiment, the spasm was provoked in animals pretreated with EGb administered preventively p.o.

Material and Methods

We developed a model which reproduces the vascular spasm observed after leptomeningeal hemorrhages. Also, the observation being done at the level of the precapillary arterioles, the reactivity of the vessels was studied at the actual level of the neuronal implications due to ischemia.

Observation of the piamatral circulation shows that the arterioles plunge into the cerebral mass (the vessels seem to end with a small enlargement in their diameter) and we are able reasonably to suppose that the variations in diameter observed on the surface are reflected in the deep layers.

Rabbits of both sexes and weighing approximately 2.5 kg are anesthetized with Nembutal; the effect of Nembutal on the cerebral circulation, being manifested both in the controls and in the treated animals, may be disregarded in the interpretation of the results. A tracheal cannula permits the animal to breathe spontaneously throughout the duration of the experiment. An opening is made in the skull by trepan, making it possible to lay bare an area of approximately $2\,cm^2$ in the temporal cortex.

The dura mater is carefully resected and the edges folded back over the circumference of the bony opening in order to avoid, insofar as possible, infiltrations of blood over the area. Artificial cerebrospinal fluid at $38°$ C dropwise keeps the preparation moist.

A cold light is conducted by optic fibers in order to light the preparation which is placed under a Nikon SMZ 10 microscope equipped with 4X lens and two 20-power eyepieces. A Panasonic video camera is used to continously record the images on a magnetoscope.

The analysis is done by measuring the diameters of several vessels at the same level on the screen of a television monitor from minute to minute on the tape and still-frames.

Replacement of the artificial cerebrospinal fluid with an autologous serum induces a spasm of the arterioles within several minutes. This spasm lasts as long as the serum is present and may be suppressed by washing the preparation with artificial cerebrospinal fluid. However, if the spasm is allowed to endure for a sufficiently long time, edema appears, and visual observation of the preparation shows very clearly the increase in volume of the brain. The experiment being carried out on an open skull, intracranial pressure cannot be measured.

No modification in the caliber of the veins or veinules was observed.

In the first experiment, Ginkgo biloba extract in injectable form (IPS 200) was administered i.v. when the vessels had reached their minimal diameter. Increasing doses were used: 2, 5, 7, 10, 15, 20, and 25 mg/kg to groups of two, two, two, five, five, three, and four rabbits respectively.

In the second experiment, three rabbits received 60 mg/kg Ginkgo biloba extract orally for eight, nine, and ten days before test day. Recording of the images and measurement of the caliber of the vessels made it possible to calculate the percentage of decrease in comparison to normal (baseline) after installation of the spasm, and the increase in diameter after treatment in comparison with the spasmed vessels.

The difference in diameter, expressed as percentage in comparison with the baseline diameter ($\Delta\,\%$) indicates the effect of the treatment. Reactivity of the vessels is a function of their diameter. We present all of of the results for both groups of vessels: 15 to $50\,\mu$ and 50 to $125\,\mu$ in diameter.

Table 1

Control animal: effect of repeated application (6) of serum after lavage of the brain surface with artificial cerebrospinal fluid. Δ% = percent decrease in comparison with the initial diameter.

Artery, 15 to 50 μ in diameter			Artery, 50 to 125 μ in diameter		
n Vessels	Δ %	Time	n Vessels	Δ %	Time
8	– 37.90	30'	8	– 38.75	30'
8	– 48.58	60'	8	– 44.16	60'
8	–28.42	90'	8	– 28.52	90'
8	– 46.52	120'	8	–34.60	120'
8	– 37.16	160'	8	– 35.88	160'
8	– 36.20	210'	8	– 15.81	210'

Results

Intravenous administration

Table 1 demonstrates the perfect reproducibility of realization of the spasm in a control animal: after return to the baseline diameter by washing with artificial cerebrospinal fluid, application of the serum caused the spasm to reappear.

Table 2

Effect of increasing doses of Ginkgo biloba extract injected i.v. five minutes after realization of the spasm. Δ% = percent of residual difference in diameter of the vessels in comparison with the initial diameter at the indicated time.

Intravenous		Artery, 15 to 50 μ in diameter			Artery, 50 to 125 μ in diameter		
doses	n Rabbits	n Vessels	Δ%	Time	n Vessels	Δ%	Time
2 mg/kg	2	12	– 22.35	25'00	06	– 07.95	22'30
5 mg/kg	2	10	– 06.40	23'30	09	– 09.05	24'00
7 mg/kg	2	09	– 04.30	09'00	09	– 01.66	09'30
10 mg/kg	5	23	+ 00.40	17'30	29	– 03.50	16'30
15 mg/kg	5	26	+ 01.70	10'30	29	– 01.75	10'30
20 mg/kg	3	12	– 03.60	08'15	16	– 03.05	05'00
25 mg/kg	4	18	+ 07.10	07'00	16	+ 01.80	10'00

Table 2 gives the results obtained with EGb administered intravenously five minutes after the appearance of spasm. The Δ % represents the difference in diameter in comparison to the baseline, which is obtained after the time when maximal recuperation is attained. A dose-effect relationship of EGb is observed; the diameter of the arterioles returns to normal at the dose of 10 mg/kg; the time for return to the initial diameter is reduced when the dose is increased.

Prolonged observation of several animals for a period of 3 1/2 hours with repeated application of the autologous serum every 30 minutes (seven times) showed that the effect of a single injection of EGb (15 mg/kg) continues throughout this entire duration and that the spasm engendered by the serum clears up within the same period (on the order of 11 to 15 minutes).

Oral administration

Table 3 indicates the results obtained. No difference was observed as a function of the duration of the prior treatment. The oral dose of 60 mg/kg administered for eight, nine, or ten days does not modify the induction of the spasm by the autologous serum. But after a delay of five to seven minutes (even briefer than that observed after acute treatment i.v.), a return of the spasmed arteries almost to the initial diameter is noted.

It should be noted that the intensity of the spasm (Δ 1%) in these pretreated animals is on the same order as that observed in 23 untreated rabbits in identical experiments:
– 57.9% for arteries 15 to 50 μ in diameter;
– 44.4% in arteries 50 to 125 μ (average for 23 animals).

Table 3

Effect of Ginkgo biloba extract administered preventively p.o. (60 mg/kg). n = number of calibrated vessels; Δ 1% = percentage of decrease in comparison with the initial diameter after application of serum; Δ 2% = percentage of decrease in comparison with the initial diameter after the lapse of time t necessary for relief of the spasm.

Duration of treatment	Artery, 15 to 50 μ in diameter				Artery, 50 to 125 μ in diameter			
60 mg/kg	n	Δ 1%	Δ 2%	t	n	Δ 1%	Δ 2%	t
8 days	9	– 60.9	– 5.25	6'	23	– 43.9	– 2.9	5'30
9 days	12	– 57.4	– 8.8	6'45	12	– 40.8	– 15	7'30
10 days	5	– 34.2	+ 1.3	5'	11	– 24	– 5.5	5'

Effects of pretreatment with antiplatelet serum

In order to attempt to understand the mechanism underlining the action of the autologous serum, we pretreated three animals with antiplatelet serum 24 hours before the experiment. In these rabbits thus "deplatelated", the application of serum provokes the appearance of spasm as in normal rabbits; but this spasm gradually disappears of itself, and the diameter of the vessels returns to a value approximately 15% less than that of the initial value within an average time of 15 minutes. This lag time is essentially the same as that brought about by active doses of EGb, and the profiles of both recording curves for two hours with several successive applications of serum are essentially identical.

Discussion

For the pharmacologist, the experimental model used demonstrates the activity of Ginkgo biloba extract, which combats arteriolar spasm induced by the application of autologous serum to the cerebral cortex of the rabbit. This effect is observed after both curative intravenous treatment and preventive oral treatment, and it is interesting to compare it with the antiedematous activity of Ginkgo biloba extract.(3)

For the physiologist, the use of Ginkgo biloba extract, as well as that of other parmacologically active substances, can assist in elucidating the mechanism of effect of the serum: our previous studies have already emphasized that the topical application of serotonin has less effect and particularly a less reproducible effect than does the serum. Ginkgo biloba extract is not a cerebral vasodilator: after injection into animals without spasm, only insignificant changes are noted in the diameter of the vessels.

The similarity in evolution of the spasm in "deplatelated" animals in comparison with that of animals treated with EGb may suggest the implication of an effect on the platelets, when we remember the anti-PAF activity of a constituent of Ginkgo biloba extract.

Later experiments will allow us to study the hypothesis of the participation of platelets in the maintenance of spasm and also to investigate what would be the active fraction of the serum.

Thanks: We express our recognition for Dr. B. Vargaftig (Institut Pasteur) who kindly supplied the antiplatelet serum, and we thank M. Prévot for his technical assistance.

References

1. Auguet M., Hellegouarch A., Delaflotte S., Baranès J., DeFeudis F., Clostre F., Braquet P., Drieu K.: Effects of Ginkgo biloba extract on rabbit isolated blood vessels. *In:* Cerebral ischemia, Bes A., Braquet P., Paoletti R., Siesjö B.K., Eds., *Elsevier,* Amsterdam, 1984, 347-354.

2. Bevan J.A., Bevan R.D., Frazee J.: Experimental chronic vasospasm in the monkey: protection by diltiazem. *J. Cerebral Blood flow and Metabolism,* 1985, *5,* suppl. 1, S. 429.

3. Borzeix M.G.: Effects of Ginkgo biloba extract on two types of cerebral edema. *In:* Effects of Ginkgo biloba extract on organic cerebral impairment, Agnoli A., Rapin J.R., Scapagnini V., Weitbrecht W.V., *Eds. John Libbey,* London, 1985, 51-56.

4. Boullin D.J.: Cerebral Vasospasm. *Wiley,* New York, 1980.

5. Cahn J.: Effects of Ginkgo biloba extract (GbE) on the acuse phase of cerebral ischemia due to embolisms. *In*: Effects of Ginkgo biloba extract on organic cerebral impairment, Agnoli A., Rapin J.R., Scapagnini V., Weitbrecht W.V., *Eds. John Libbey,* London, 1985, 43-49.

6. Drieu K.: Multiplicity of effects of Ginkgo biloba extract: current status and new trends. *In*: Effects of Ginkgo biloba extract on organic cerebral impairment, Agnoli A., Rapin J.R., Scapagnini V., Weitbrecht W.V., *Eds. John Libbey,* London, 1985, 63-68.

7. Etienne A., Chapelat M., Braquet M., Clostre F., Drieu K., De Feudis F.V., Braquet P.: *In vivo* studies of free radical scavenging activity; relation to cerebral ischemia. *In:* Cerebral ischemia, Bes A., Braquet P., Paoletti R., Siesjö B.K., Eds., *Elsevier,* Amsterdam, 1984, 379-384.

8. Le Poncin-Lafitte M., Rapin J., Rapin J.R.: Effects of Ginkgo biloba on changes induced by quantitative cerebral microemolization in rats. *Arch. Int. Pharmacodyn.,* 1980, *243,* 236-244.

9. Reuse-Blom S., Drieu K.: Effet de l'extrait de Ginkgo biloba sur le spasme artériolaire chez le lapin. *J. Cerebral Blood Flow and Metabolism,* sous presse.

10. Sahlin Ch., Owman Ch., Chang J.Y., Delgado T., Svengaard N.A.: Experimental subarachnoïd hemorrhage in monkeys markedly increases the contractile response of intracranial arteries to norepinephrine and serotonine: effects of the calcium antagonist, nimodipine. *J. Cerebral Blood Flow and Metabolism,* 1980, *5,* suppl. 1, S. 427.

The Pharmacological Bases for the Vascular Impact of Ginkgo Biloba Extract

M. Auguet, S. Delaflotte, A. Hellegouarch, F. Clostre

Centre de recherche I.H.B.-I.P.S.E.N., 72, avenue des Tropiques
F 91940 Les Ulis

Summary

The preferential tissue irrigatory effect of Ginkgo biloba extract in ischaemic areas is largely explained by the direct impact of this product on both arteries and veins.

The adrenergic vasoregulatory system and the vascular endothelium are the preferential targets for arterial impact. Ginkgo biloba extract reinforces the physiological vasoregulation of the sympathetic nervous system directly, by acting on neuromediator release, and indirectly, by inhibiting their extraneuronal degradation by catechol-orthomethyltransferase (C.O.M.T.).

In the arterial endothelium Ginkgo biloba extract stimulates the release of endogenous relaxing factors, such as endothelium-derived relaxing factor (EDRF) and prostacyclin.

The action of Ginkgo biloba extract on the venous system has been shown to have a venoconstrictor component that maintains the degree of parietal tonus essential to the dynamic clearing of toxic metabolites accumulated during tissue ischemia.

The originality of the vascular impact mechanisms of Ginkgo biloba extract is due to the fact that the product can at the same time combat the phenomena resulting from vascular spasm and with the same efficiency restore circulation in areas subject to vasomotor paralysis.

The tissue-irrigating effects of Ginkgo biloba extract (EGb 761, Rökan®, Intersan) have been demonstrated in man at both the cerebral and peripheral levels. In animals, EGb revealed protective effects with respect to hemodynamic, metabolic, ionic, and functional disturbances observed in different models of cerebral ischemia obtained by ligation(32) or by experimental microembolizations.(23, 25)

These effects of EGb are partially explained by hemorheological impact, demonstrated *in vitro* and *in vivo*, in platelet hyperagregability and experimental thromboses of the cortical vessels,(8) as well as in risks of osmotic debilitation of the erythrocytic membranes.(15) But they are explained mainly by an arterial and venous

Rökan (Ginkgo Biloba). Recent Results in Pharmacology and Clinic
Edited by E.W. Fünfgeld
© Springer-Verlag Berlin Heidelberg New York 1988, pp. 169-179

impact, the mechanisms of which we have studied in the vessels (thoracic aorta and vena cava of the rabbit), isolated in order to better focalize the direct or indirect interactions of EGb on the various types of receptors and endogenous substances which participate in the regulation of vasomotoricity.

Action of Ginkgo Biloba extract on the isolated rabbit aorta

Fragments of thoric aorta sliced spirally were taken from New Zealand rabbits and suspended vertically under 2 g tension in cells containing Krebs Henseleit glucose solution maintained at 37°C and traversed by a current of carbogen. The endothelium of certain preparations was scraped off by a mechanical instrument in order to dissociate the role of the receptors and/or mediators of the endothelial layer in the vasomotor mechanisms of EGb.

The contractions were recorded by means of isometric sensors connected to a polygraph. The effects of EGb were studied at three levels of the arterial parietal structure: the intima, the media, and the adventitia.

Glossary

α:	α-adrenergic receptor
AA:	arachidonic acid
AC:	adenylcyclase
ACh:	acetylcholine
AD:	adrenalin
5'-AMP:	5-adenosine monophosphate
cAMP:	cyclic adenosine monophosphate
ATP:	adenosine triphosphoric acid
β:	β-adrenergic receptor
COMT:	catechol-O-methyltransferase
EDRF:	endothelium-derived relaxing factor
EGb:	Ginkgo biloba extract
GC:	guanylcyclase
5'-GMP:	5'-guanosine monophosphate
c-GMP:	cyclic guanosine monophosphate
M:	muscarinic receptor
MAO:	monoaminoxidase
NA:	noradrenalin
PDE:	phosphodiesterase
PGI_2:	prostacycline

The *intima* is formed of the endothelium, a monocellular layer playing an important role in control of homeostasis and of vascular tonus.(18) Furchgott and Zawadzki(17) demonstrated *in vitro* that acetylcholine induced relaxation of the thoracic aorta of the rabbit only when the endothelium was intact. The vasodilatation induced by acetylcholine takes place through stimulation of the muscarinic receptors situated in the endothelial layer which causes release of prostacycline,(16) but mainly that of a substance inducing relaxation of the artery through stimulation of the guanylcyclase in the smooth muscle cells.(18, 29) This product, the endothelium-dependent relaxing factor or EDRF, which could be a metabolite of arachidonic acid, is inactivable by certain antioxidants and/or scavengers of free radicals.(12)

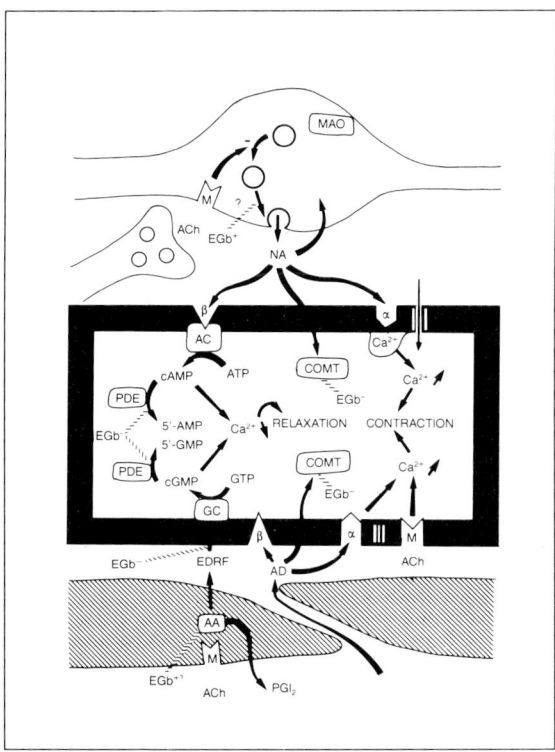

Figure 1: Diagram of possible sites of action of Ginkgo biloba extract in comparison with those of acethylcholine and of the catecholaminergic mediators (AD, NA) in the adrenergic nerve fibers and the smooth muscle and endothelial cells of the isolated rabbit aorta. + = stimulation; – = inhibition; ? = unknown mechanism

At concentrations on the order of 10 to 200 mcg/mL, EGb stimulates the release of prostacycline by the arterial endothelium(10, 20) *in vitro*. At comparable concentrations, it also provokes relaxation of the isolated rabbit aorta, which, like that provoked by carbachol (cholinergic agonist), depends on the integrity of the vascular endothelium, which includes the release of EDRF (*Figure 1*). Relaxation is not, however, modified by atropine. Thus, the release of EDRF by EGb is independent of stimulation of the muscarinic cholinergic receptors of the endothelium (*Figure 2*).(11, 13) Incubated at higher concentration (300 mcg/mL), EGb inhibits the relaxation induced by carbachol in the isolated rabbit aorta, and this effect can be attributed to the free radical scavenging properties of EGb. Rutin, a flavonol glycoside contained in EGb, induces neither release nor inhibition of EDRF (*Figure 2*).

The *media,* the intermediate layer, is rich in myocytes, contractile elements of the artery, whose level of excitation regulates the caliber of the arterial wall. It is at the level of the myocytic membranes that we find most of the specific receptors of the neurotransmitters which participate in regulation of arterial and arteriolar vasomotricity. Here also is located, in part, the extraneuronal metabolism of the catecholamines, the degradation of which at this level is assured by COMT.(28) EGb (100 mcg/mL) brings about potentiation of the contraction induced by noradrenalin,(2) which could be explained partially by inhibition of COMT. There is then observed, at high concentrations (CE_{50} ≈ 1.0 mg/mL), a true contracturant effect of EGb on the isolated rabbit aorta. This effect, partially antagonized by phentolamine (α-blocker), could partially be due to direct (or indirect) stimulation of the adrenergic receptors.(1)

At high concentration, EGb can also provoke relaxation of an isolated rabbit aorta the tonus of which has previously been increased by a contracting agent (*Figure 2*),(11) this type of relaxation being comparable to that of a spasmolytic inhibitor of phosphodiesterase such as papaverine.(3) Inhibition of enzymatic systems like COMT and/or phosphodiesterases have been described for certain flavonoids.(7, 30)

The adventitia is rich in adrenergic nerve endings. The fact that the contraction of an isolated rabbit aorta induced by Ginkgo biloba extract is inhibited by prior reserpinization of the animals (the reserpine provokes exhaustion of the stocks of endogenous catecholamines) and is diminished by inhibitors of neuronal recapture of catecholamines, such as cocaine and desipramine, tend to prove that Ginkgo biloba extract is capable of stimulating, at this level, the release of endogenous catecholamines.(1)

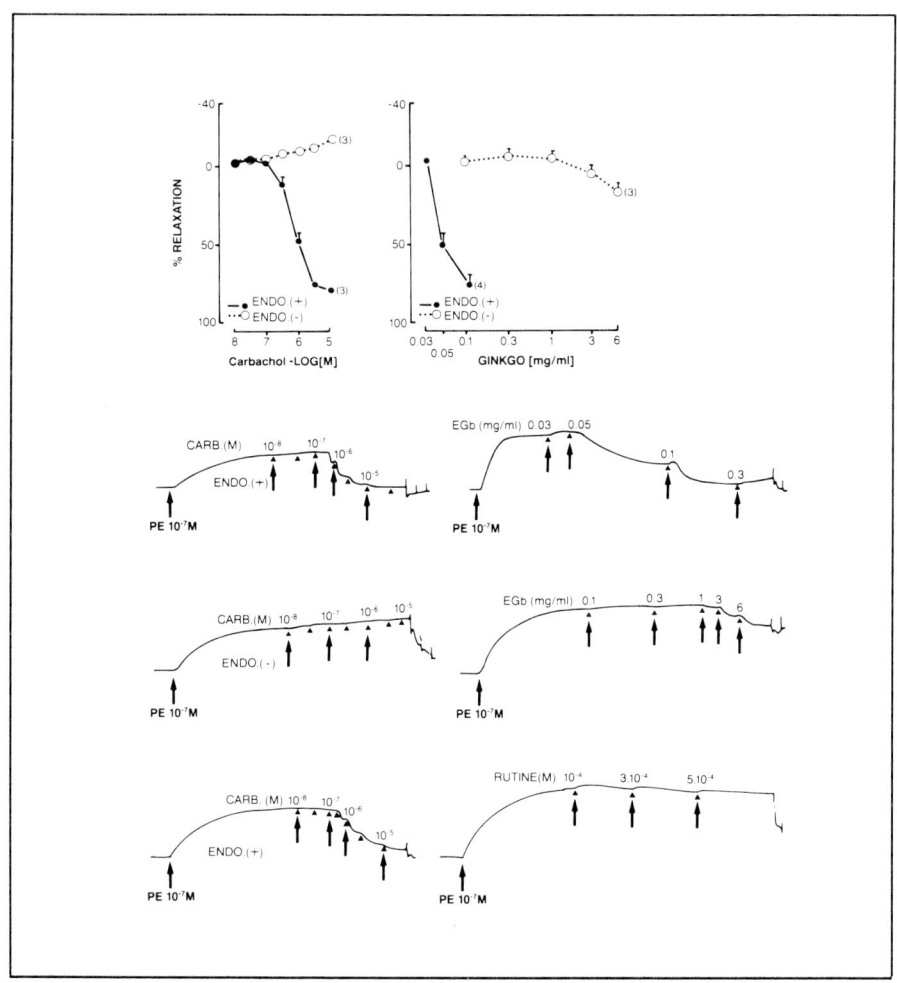

Figure 2: Upper portion: effects of carbachol (left) and EGb (right) on isolated rabbit aortas precontracted by phenylephrine (PE 10^{-7}M), with intact endothelium (• = endo +) or endothelium not intact (○: endo −). Mean ≡ MSE (n).

Lower part: Tracings representative of the action of carbachol (CARB) (at left) on the isolated rabbit aorta, with intact endothelium (ENDO +) or endothelium not intact (ENDO −); it is noted (at right) that EGb at the lowest concentrations tested relaxed only the artery with intact endothelium, whereas rutin had no effect. The arrows indicate the moment the different products were introduced.

Action of Ginkgo biloba extract on the isolated rabbit vena cava

At low concentration ($CE_{50} \approx 86$ mcg/mL) in comparison with the rabbit aorta, EGb provokes contraction of the isolated rabbit vena cava. This contraction is reduced by half an irreversible α-blocker such as phenoxybenzamine and is therefore only partially dependent on the catecholaminergic system (*Figure 3*).(4) The difference in sensitivity observed between the aorta and the vena cava could be explained by variations in the mode of innervation(21) or in the specificity of the endothelial function(33) between the two types of vessels, but they show that the venous tonic effect of EGb occurs through mechanisms certain of which still remain to be discovered.

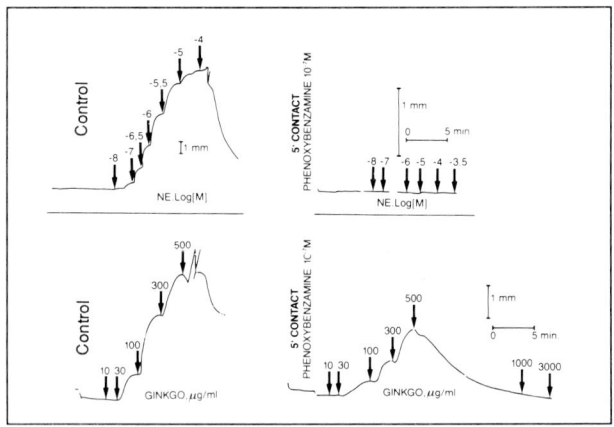

Figure 3: Effects of phenoxybenzamine on contraction induced by noradrenalin (NA) (top) and Ginkgo biloba extract on the isolated rabbit vena cava (reproduced from reference 4).

Discussion

The experimental approach to proof of the effects of a drug in a vascular area is generally realized by *in vivo* methods, with determination of perfusion pressures, of global or regional circulations, or even of circulation rate. These methods make it possible to quantify the effect, but not to explain its mechanisms. For this, only isolated preparations of an artery, a vein, and even today of microvessels(11) permit this type of analysis.(19)

The isolated vessel techniques in themselves can be supplemented by specific neurochemical or immunocytochemical determinations at the level of the mediators and/or of their vascular metabolites and would thus permit passing from the cellular level to the molecular level.

Extrapolation of the results obtained in an isolated vessel to those found in man may appear to some to be hazardous and speculative. It is still, however, the only way to explain the specific components of a global hemodynamic effect and may be accepted provided several elements are taken into consideration. Thus the types and population of vascular receptors, as well as the endothelial response, vary according to the animal species, age, type and caliber of the vessels, and the pathological condition of the latter.(6, 26) The action and metabolism of a neutrotransmitter, at the level of a vessel, depends on the type and density of innervation which is specific to it.(28)

The studies made on the isolated rabbit thoracic aorta revealed that the mechanisms of vascular action of EGb at the arterial level are exerted on two major targets. These are the endothelial cells at the level of which EGb stimulates the release of the endogenous vascular-releasing factors, EDRF and prostacycline. However, a biphasic effect is found, since EGb is also capable of inhibiting the synthesis of prostacycline in a preparation of cerebral microvessels(9) and of opposing, at stronger concentration, EDRF-dependent relaxation due to carbachol. The second target is represented by the smooth muscle layer in which EGb restores effective vascular tonus by maintenance of α-adrenergic constrictive vasoregulation and β-adrenergic relaxant vasoregulation. EGb prolongs the vasoregulating effects of catecholamines by inhibition of their extraneuronal degradation by COMT. To this is added inhibition of phosphodiesterases which reinforces the cAMP-dependent relaxant component. This maintenance of sympathetic vasoregulation is supplemented, in the adventitia, by stimulation of catecholamine release from the postsynaptic sympathetic endings. The relative importance of these effects depends on the concentration of EGb, on incubation time, and on prior tonus of the vessel.

The vascular impact of EGb is characterized by a balance between the arterial and venous tonic effects, capable of restarting circulation in a territory in a state of vasomotor paralysis, and relaxant effects, allowing it to battle effectively against vascular spasms. These experimental facts permit us to better understand that *in vivo* the effects of EGb are more distinct on an ischemic vascular area than on a normally irrigated area.

Finally, it is worthwhile to note that a major portion of the vascular effects of EGb is related to the adrenergic system. However, it must be remembered that the latter plays a dual capital role in the regulation of cerebral circulation.(31) It plays a role of natural vasoregulation through the distribution of its α and β receptors intervening respectively in contraction or dilatation of the cerebral vessels as a function of need or of the physiopathological situations.(14) It also plays a trophic and protective role, as shown by the studies of Mueller,(27) for example: unilateral sympathetic denervation in the rat very distinctly increases the probability of hemorrhagic and ischemic vascular accidents on the sympathectomized side. It also plays a part in the maintenance of the quality of the exchanges in the cerebral capillaries and therefore in the good functioning of the blood-brain barrier.(9)

Conclusion

Hypoxia of an ischemic cerebral tissular area precipitates arteriolar vasodilatation, increased capillary permeability, and venous atony leading rapidly to paralysis of the exchanges and to severe disturbances in the neurogenic vasoregulating systems (particularly adrenergic), which can no longer ensure their controlling role.

If vasodilatation is considered as a phenomenon of compensation for a deficit in energy supplies to the ischemic area, the therapist might be tempted to prescribe essentially vasodilatating substances in the treatment of circulatory cerebral insufficiency. It is known today that this can be the opposite of what is desirable. In fact, by dilating the healthy areas preferentially to the detriment of the ischemic areas (this is the risk of cerebral vascular "flight" described by Lassen(24)), they provoke hemodeflection capable of aggravating even more the blood diversion capable of activating even more the effects of the ischemia. Furthermore, since the hypoxia, itself causing vasodilatation, could range as far as vasoparalysis, why wish to add to it an additional pharmacological vasodilatation?(22) In order to effectively combat the circulatory and microcirculatory disturbances in an ischemic area, today it appears increasingly evident that a single vasomotor component is inadequate.(5)

Ginkgo biloba extract, as shown by the studies made on isolated vessels, reveals vasoregulating properties, certain of which occur through the maintenance of catecholaminergic vasomotor regulation, and others through activation of endothelial functions. All of the mechanisms of the vascular effects of EGb are not yet explained. The studies currently conducted on preparations of cerebral microvessels will supply new indications on the basis of pharmacological impacts of EGb at this level.

We could thus observe that the effects of EGb in cerebral ischemia, both experimental and clinical, are explained by a triple vascular, rheological, and metabolic impact; that these vascular effects implicate arterial, capillary, and venous vasoregulating properties; and finally, that at the arterial level, its mechanisms involve the endothelium, the smooth muscle layer, and the adventitia at the same time.

References

1. Auguet M., DeFeudis F.V., Clostre F., Deghenghi R.: Effects of an extract of Ginkgo biloba on rabbit isolated aport. *Gen. Pharmac.*, 1982, *13*, 225-230.

2. Auguet M., DeFeudis F.V., Clostre F., Deghenghi R.: Effects of Ginkgo biloba on arterial smooth muscle responses to vasoactive stimuli. *Gen. Pharmac.*, 1982, *13*, 169-171.

3. Auguet M., Clostre F.: Effects of an extract of Ginkgo biloba and diverse substances on the phasic and tonic components of the contraction of an isolated rabbit aorta. *Gen. Pharmac.*, 1983, *14*, 277-280.

4. Auguet M., Hellegouarch A., Delaflotte S., Baranes J., DeFeudis F.V., Clostre F., Braquet P., Drieu K.: Effects of Ginkgo biloba extract on rabbit blood vessels. *In:* Cerebral ischemia, Bes A., Braquet P. Paoletti R., Siesjö B.K., Eds. *Elsevier,* Amsterdam, 1984, 347-354.

5. Baron J.: Phénomènes physiolpathologiques au cours de l'ischémie focale aiguë du cerveau. *Revue de Médecine,* 1983, *38,* 1853-1863.

6. Bevan J.A.: Autonomic pharmacologist's guide to the cerebral circulation. *TIPS,* 1984, 234-236.

7. Borchardt R.T., Huber J.A.: Catechol O-Methyltransferase-5 structure – activity relationships for inhibition by flavonoids. *J. Med. Chem.*, 1975, *18*, 120-122.

8. Borzeix M.G., Labos M., Hartl C.: Recherches sur l'action anti-agrégante de l'extrait de Ginkgo biloba. Activité au niveau des artères et des veines de la pie-mère chez le lapin. *Sem. Hôpitaux,* 1980, *56,* 383-398.

9. Chabrier P.E., Roubert P.: Capillaires cérébraux barrière hémato-encéphalique et effet de l'extrait de Ginkgo biloba. *Presse Méd.* 1986, *15*, 1498-1501.

10. Chatterjee S.S.: Effects of Ginkgo biloba extract on cerebral metabolic processes. *In:* Effects of Ginkgo biloba extract on organic cerebral impairment, Agnoli A., Rapin J.R., Scapagnini V. Weitbrecht W.V. eds, *John Libbey,* London, 1985, 5-15.

11. DeFeudis F.V., Auguet M., Delaflotte S., Hellegouarch A., Baranes J., Chapelat M., Braquet M., Etienne A., Drieu K., Clostre F., and Braquet P.: Some in vitro and in vivo actions of an extract of Ginkgo biloba (GBE U761). *In:* Effects of Ginkgo biloba extract on organic cerebral impairment, Agnoli A., Rapin J.R., Scapagnini V. Weitbrecht W.V. eds, *John Libbey,* London, 1985, 17-29.

12. DeFeudis F.V.: Mechanism of endothelium-dependent vasorelaxation. *Medical Hypotheses,* 1985, *17,* 363-374.

13. Delaflotte S., Auguet M., DeFeudis F.V., Baranes J., Clostre F., Drieu K., Braquet P.: Endothelium-dependent relaxations of rabbit isolated aorta produced by carbachol and by Ginkgo biloba extract. *Biomed. Biochim. Acta,* 1984, *43,* 5212-5216.

14. Edvisson L.: Vascular autonomic nerves and corresponding receptor in brain vessels. *Path. Biol.,* 1982, *30,* 261-268.

15. Etienne A., Hecquet F., Clostre F., DeFeudis F.V.: Comparaison des effets d'un extrait de Ginkgo biloba et de la chlorpromazine sur la fragilité osmotique, in vitro, d'érythrocytes de rat. *J. Pharmacol.* (Paris), 1982, *13,* 291-298.

16. Forsterman V., Neufang B.: The endothelium-dependent vasodilator effect of acetylcholine: characterization of the endothelial relaxing factor with inhibitors of arachidonic acid metabolism. *Eur. J. Pharmacol.,* 1984, *103,* 65-70.

17. Furchgott R.F., Zawadzki J.V.: The obligatory role of endothelial cells in the relaxation of arterial smooth muscle by acetyl-choline. *Nature,* 1980, *288,* 373-376.

18. Furchgott R.F.: The role of endothelium in the responses of vascular smooth muscle to drugs. *Ann. Rev. Pharmacol. Toxicol.,* 1984, *24,* 175-197.

19. Harik S.I.: Neurotransmitter receptors in cerebral microvessels. *In:* Neurotransmitters and the cerebral circulation. MacKenzie E.T., Seylaz J., Bes A. eds, *Raven Press.* New York, 1984, 1-9.

20. Herman A.G., Beetens J.R.: Effects of vasoactive substances on prostacycline synthesis. XV Bad Herrenalber angiologisches Gespräch 1983, 22-23 April, 83-87.

21. Keatinge W.R., Clare Harman M.: Local mechanisms controlling blood vessels. *Academic Press inc,* London, 1980.

22. Krahengühl B.: Vasodilatateurs dans les affections artérielles occlusives? *Med. et Hyg.,* 1982, *40,* 171-172.

23. Larsen R.G., Dupeyron J.P., Boulu R.G.: Modèle d'ischémie cérébrale expérimentale par microsphères chez le rat. Etude de l'effet de deux extraits de Ginkgo biloba et du naftidrofuryl. *Thérapie,* 1978, *33,* 651-660.

24. Lassen N.A.: The luxury-perfusion syndrome and its possible relation to acute metabolic acidosis localised within the brain. *Lancet,* 1966, *2,* 1113-1115.

25. Le Poncin-Lafitte M., Rapin J., Rapin J.R.: Effect of Ginkgo biloba on changes induced by quantitative cerebral micro-embolization in rats. *Arch. Int. Pharmacodyn.,* 1980, *243,* 236-244.

26. Morishita H.: Distribution and characterization of the adrenoceptors in dog coronary arteries. *Arch. Int. Pharmacodyn.,* 1979, *239,* 195-207.

27. Mueller S.M., Heistad D.D., Marcus M.L.: Effect of the sympathetic nerves on cerebral vessels during seizures. *Am. J. Physiol.*, 1979, *237*, H178-H184.

28. Osswald W., Guimaraes S.: Adrenergic mechanisms in blood vessels: morphological and pharmacological aspects. *Rev. Physiol. Biochem. Pharmacol.*, 1983, *96*, 53-122.

29. Rapoport R.M., Murad F.: Endothelium-dependent and nitro-vasodilator-induced relaxation of vascular smooth muscle: Role of cyclic GMP. *J. Cyclic Nuc. Res.*, 1983, 9, 281-296.

30. Ruckstuhl M., Beretz A., Anton R., Landry Y.: Flavonoïds are selective cyclic GMP phosphodiesterase inhibitors. *Biochem. Pharmac.*, 1979, *28*. 535-538.

31. Seylaz J.: Rôle du système nerveux autonome dans la régulation de la circulation sanguine cérébrale. *Circ. et Métabolisme du Cerveau*, 1985, *2*, 115-132.

32. Spinnewyn B., Blavet N., Clostre F.: Effets du Ginkgo biloba sur l'ischémie cérébrale expérimentale chez la gerbille. *Presse Méd.*, 1986, *15*, 1511-1515.

33. Vanhoutte P.M., Miller U.M.: Heterogeneity of endothelium-dependent responses in mammalian blood vessels. *J. Cardiovasc. Pharmacol.* 1985, *7*, S12-S23.

From the Body to the Cellular Membranes: The Different Levels of Pharmacological Action of Ginkgo Biloba Extract

F. Clostre

Centre de recherche I.H.B.-I.P.S.E.N., 72, avenue des Tropiques. F 91940 Les Ulis

Summary

The pharmacological study of Ginkgo biloba extract has required numerous experiments over several years: different pathological models of cerebral ischaemia to evaluate its effects, and experiments at both cellular and molecular levels to determine its mechanisms of action.

In experimental models of ischaemia, oedema and hypoxia, Ginkgo biloba extract reduced vascular, tissular and metabolic disturbances as well as their neurological and behavioural consequences.

The pharmacological effects of Ginkgo biloba extract concern vascular, rheological and metabolic processes. Several membrane mechanisms seem to be involved: protection of the membrane ultrastructure against free radicals, modulation of some enzymatic systems and ionic pumps.

The originality of the pharmocological properties of Ginkgo biloba extract lies in preferential focusing of its effects on ischaemic areas.

The pharmacological study of Ginkgo biloba extract (EGb 761, Rökan®, Intersan) has required many years of experiments both in the organism and in global models of ischemia, hypoxia, or experimental cerebral tissue distress, and at the cellular and membranal level in order to explain the components and to discover its mechanisms. Ginkgo biloba extract is an ensemble of several active principles, with specific pharmacological properties interfering with each other, which singularly complicates the task of pharmacologists in quest of their sites of membranal fixation and the keys to their mechanisms. In this case, the experimental approach is therefore more complex than for a single entity: discovery rather than research is involved.

Rökan (Ginkgo Biloba). Recent Results in Pharmacology and Clinic
Edited by E.W. Fünfgeld
© Springer-Verlag Berlin Heidelberg New York 1988, pp. 180-198

Ginkgo biloba extract in experimental cerebral ischemia

The brain is extremely sensitive to ischemia. Its functions and its homeostasis require large amounts of energy, of which, unlike other organs, it has little or no tissue reserves. In man, cerebral ischemia, regardless of origin, sets off a sequence of vasomotor and metabolic disturbances which are rapidly reflected in behavioral and functional disorders.

The principal objective of experimental pharmacology in this field is to create models as close as possible to human physiopathological reality and thus to make it possible to show objectively the vascular, metabolic, and functional impacts of a drug. Clinically, the evolution of a cerebral vascular accident can be evaluated on the basis of psychometric criteria which are difficult to apply in animals, even in the most evolved primates. Faced with this stumbling block, pharmacologists have resorted to hemodynamic, biochemical, behavioral, and electrical criteria which must be objective, reproducible, and quantifiable.

These models, as similar as possible to clinical reality, make it possible to explore the circulatory hemodynamics: overall regional and local flows, vascular resistance, prefusion pressures. They also study metabolic activity: extraction, uptake, and consumption of glucose and oxygen, production of ATP, filtering of metabolic debris, cerebral concentrations of various metabolites and/or neuromediators. They also evaluate the magnitude of cerebral edema and of the membranal ionic disturbances ($Na+$, K^+, Cl^-, Ca^{2+}) which accompany it, and functional recovery, through behavioral observation tests, combined or not with cortical electrogenesis recordings.

Glossary

α:	α-adrenergic receptor
AA:	arachidonic acid
ADP:	adenosine diphosphoric acid
cAMP:	cyclic adenosine monophosphate
ATP:	adenosine triphosphoric acid
CVA:	cerebral vascular accidents
β:	β-adrenergic receptor
BBB:	blood-brain barrier
COMT:	catechol-O-methyltransferase
EDRF:	endothelium-derived relaxing factor
EGb:	Ginkgo biloba extract EGb 761
LTs:	leukotrienes
O_2^-:	superoxide ion
$OH^.$:	hydroxyl radical
PDE:	phosphodiesterase
PGI_2:	prostacyclin
PGs:	prostaglandins
PLA_2:	A_2 phospholipase
TxA_2:	A_2 thromboxane

Numerous models exist, many have value, all have their limitations. The experimental ischemia models are the most numerous. They can be obtained by complete or incomplete ligation of a carotid or of various cerebral arteries. Fieschi cites more than 25 different ones, indicating the value of those obtained in gerbils.(25) Outside of ligations, certain of these were realized by experimental embolization with radio-tagged calibrated microspheres. The hypoxia models, easy to realize and frequently used for this reason in preliminary studies, however have the disadvantage of inducing generalized hypoxia, not specific for the cerebral sphere.(44) As for specific experimental models of cerebral edema (cytotoxic, induced by triethyletain, or vasogenic, due to experimental trauma), they have the advantage of outlining the parameters of evolution of the cerebral edema phase and of better locating the ionic mechanisms which are associated with it.(14)

These various experimental models of cerebral ischemia, hypoxia, and edema have made it possible to demonstrate and to quantify the efficacy of Ginkgo biloba extract with respect to vascular, metabolic, ionic, and neurological disturbances of cerebral ischemia. In a model of cerebral ischemia induced by unilateral ligation of the carotid artery in the gerbil,(44) Ginkgo biloba extract regulates mitochondrial respiration, source of ATP production, diminishes cerebral edema, corrects the ionic disturbances (K^+ and Na^+) which accompany it, and restores a normal neurological index. Unilateral cerebral embolization due to intracarotid injection of calibrated microspheres causes, in the ischemic hemisphere, circulatory disturbances (notable particularly in the hippocampus and striatum), a deviation in mitochondrial glycolysis toward the anaerobic route, and cerebral edema in the embolized hemisphere.(34, 35)

Ginkgo biloba extract normalizes the circulation in the areas most affected by the microembolization (hippocampus and striatum), diminishes the deficit in mitochondrial ATP production, and reduces the magnitude of the edema. The studies by Larsen,(33) also carried out in a cerebral ischemia model in rats by microembolization with microspheres, confirm and supplement the preceding results, revealing obvious behavioral functional recovery in rats treated with Ginkgo biloba extract. In experimental models of cerebral hypoxia, Ginkgo biloba extract lengthens survival time of mice in hypobaric hypoxia,(13) returns to normal the uptake of deoxyglucose in the brains of mice subjected to normobaric hypoxia,(40) and antagonizes the principal biochemical disorders of hypoxia in rats.(31)

Ginkgo biloba extract has been shown to be particularly effective in various experimental models of cerebral edema, regardless of their origin.(25) It neutralizes the appearance of δ waves, signs of cerebral distress consecutive to the installation of vasogenic edema of traumatic type (by unilateral stripping of the dura mater) in rabbits.(9) It is interesting to note that the recovery of normal cortical electrogenesis in animals treated with Ginkgo biloba extract is more the result of inhibition of the number of cerebral distress waves than an effect of this product on the physiological arousal waves, thus reflecting the existence for this product of an antiedematous effect and not of a psychotropic effect. Triethyletain-induced edema is a model of choice for better understanding of membranal ionic disturbances and cellular metabolic disturbances similar to those encountered in human physiopathology.(28) The studies of Borzeix et al.(7) in this field have shown that Ginkgo biloba extract opposes not only the development of the edema and its ionic disturbances, but reestablishes a normal neurological index, sign of abatement of the functional consequences of cerebral edema.

The effects of Ginkgo biloba extract on experimental cerebral ischemia models thus involve vascular, tissular, and metabolic disturbances as much as their neurological and behavioral consequences. This range of the spectrum of action suggests several different mechanisms at the tissular and cellular levels.

The vascular impacts of Ginkgo biloba extract

The mechanisms of the vasomotor effects of Ginkgo biloba extract and of the influences which it exerts on the factors that control and regulate tissue blood flow have been demonstrated by *in vitro* isolated vessel techniques.

In a vascular, cerebral, coronary, or peripheral territory, *in vivo* explorations as precise as they may be, can account only for the total circulatory phenomena. In order to separate its arterial, arteriolar, microcirculatory, venular, or venous components and to explain the mechanism or mechanisms of each of these, we must resort to isolated vessel methods, which must be supplemented by neurochemical or immunocytochemical determinations, or even by those of the rates of binding of a mediator to its specific receptors.

For the arteries, the experimental pharmacology studies conducted *in vivo* on intact animals have shown that Ginkgo biloba extract increases the perfusion rate in the various territories, regardless of their initial vascular pathological condition, observations that have been confirmed in clinical pharmacology.(1)

Studies performed by Auguet(4) on isolated rabbit aorta demonstrated that Ginkgo biloba extract plays a part in catecholaminergic vasomotor regulation: it potentiates the effects of noradrenalin on arterial tonus through a triple influence on neuronal and extraneuronal metabolism of this neurotransmitter: stimulation of its release (potentiation of the arterial effect of noradrenalin by Ginkgo biloba extract is diminished after reserpinization of the rabbits), partial inhibition of its neuronal recapture (noradrenalin-Ginkgo biloba extract interaction is diminished by other inhibitors of neuronal recapture of catecholamines), and, lastly, inhibition of its extraneuronal enzymatic degradation.(3) Furthermore, the contracturant effects of Ginkgo biloba extract are partially inhibited by phentolamine (α_1 and α_2 blocker). It is thus clear that Ginkgo biloba extract plays a part in the vasoregulating and vascular trophic role of the catecholamines, which play an essential role in the maintenance of cerebral vasomotricity (through the bias of the α-constrictor receptors and the β-dilator receptors), of the trophicity and integrity of the blood-brain barrier.(21, 37) Furthermore, like carbachol (cholinergic agonist), Ginkgo biloba extract manifests an endothelio-dependent arterial relaxant effect.(17) This effect does not operate through a cholinergic effect: atropine does not modify it.(18)

For the veins, Ginkgo biloba extract has shown *in vivo*, on the intact animal, that it was capable of maintaining venous capacitance at its normal level, regardless of the initial condition of central venous pressure (experimentally increased or decreased).

In vitro studies on the isolated vena cava have explained this venous vasoregulating effect of Ginkgo biloba extract. EGb presents venous tonic effects which are particular to it and which are only partially due to catecholaminergic mediation.(3) At higher concentration, it is capable of relieving an experimental venous spasm.(5)

These results explain how, in all of the *in vivo* experimental models, whether ischemia, hypoxia, or microembolization were involved, Ginkgo biloba extract has always ensured cleansing of metabolic wastes (lactates, CO_2) accumulated at the time of the ischemia.

Adding that Ginkgo biloba extract inhibits experimental capillary hyperpermeabilities and increases resistance of the capillaries through a direct effect on their parietal cement,(32) we understand that the term arterial, capillary, and venous vasoregulation could have been used to qualify the vascular effects of Ginkgo biloba extract. But today this term seems incomplete, since in addition to an anatomical trivasoregulation (artery, vein, and capillary), pharmacological tests at the cellular level have demonstrated that there is also trivasoregulation involving the various cellular layers of the arterial wall.

Cellular Mechanisms

Arterial wall

The importance of the integrity of the endothelium in regulating vasomotoricity and maintaining vascular homeostasis was reported by Furchgott.(27) In the media and the smooth muscle cellular membranes are found most of the receptors which are specific for the neuromediators which participate in arterial and arteriolar vasomotor regulation. Lastly, the adventitia, composed principally of collagen and elastin, is in direct contact with the postsynaptic endings which are potential releasers of of neuromediators.

Studies by Auguet(4) on the isolated rabbit aorta, with or without endothelium, have made it possible to identify a certain number of cellular mechanisms which could explain the arterial vasoregulating effects of Ginkgo biloba extract. In the endothelial cells, the vasodilatating component of Ginkgo biloba extract is explained by direct stimulation of the release of EDRF (endothelium-derived relaxing factor(s)).(18) In the smooth muscle layer, Ginkgo biloba extract potentiates the vasomotor regulation of endogenous catecholamines (α-constrictive or β-relaxant) through inhibition of their extraneuronal degradation by catechol-O-methyltransferase (COMT), as well as by partial inhibition of their neuronal recapture.(5) Also, inhibition of phosphodiesterases, thus increasing the intracellular concentration of cAMP, is added to the arterial relaxing component.(2) In the adventitia, the maintenance of sympathetic vasoregulation is supplemented by stimulation of the release of endogenous catecholamines from the sympathetic endings.(4)

In conclusion, the vasomotor effects of Ginkgo biloba extract may be expressed through a balancing effect as a function of the vascular pathological state of the ischemic area. In the vascular relaxation "plateau" we find the mechanisms: release of EDRF, inhibition of phosphodiesterases, and maintenance of the β-adrenergic effects (through indirect effects, one of which is inhibition of COMT). And in the reinforcing "plateau" of arterial and venous tonus are found the direct effects (certain of which are still unexplained), and indirect effects occuring through the maintenance of sympathetic regulation (*Table 1*).

Neuronal cells

The cellular biochemical modifications of cerebral ischemia are essentially due to a deficit in energy supply closely linked to the mitochondrial anoxia responsible for an entire chain of reactions generating membranal disturbances, as well as to an accumulation of toxic wastes due to insufficient venous cleansing.

When the cerebral circulation diminishes, aerobic glycolysis continues to function for some time, causing an accumulation of CO_2 in the ischemic tissue. Then the tissular anoxia brings about an anaerobic deviation of glycolysis with diminution in pyruvate and an obvious accumulation of the lactate which, in the total ischemia areas, is no longer evacuated. The anaerobic glycolysis uses up the tissue stocks of glucose rather quickly, then those of glycogen. The severe diminution in aerobic metabolism causes a fall in ATP production, a fall which even a massive increase in anaerobic glycolysis cannot compensate.

The scarcity of ATP causes overwhelming of Na^+K^+-ase: Na^+ penetrates massively into the cell, bringing water with it; K^+ exits from the neuronal milieu and accumulates in the extracellular space, from which it is repumped partially by the glial cells; Ca^{++} penetrates en masse into the intracellular compartment. Complex movements of water bring about massive intracellular edema. This "cytotoxic" edema, very precocious and directly proportional in magnitude to the degree of ischemia, aggravates pre-existing neuronal hypoxia.(14)

Table 1

The cellular and membranal mechanisms of the vasoregulating effects of Ginkgo biloba extract

Site of action	Upstream flow (arterioles)			Exchange area (capillaries)			Downstream flow (venous cleansing)	
Tissular pathological conditions	Arterial spasm	Arterial thrombosis	Vascular atony	Hypoxic vasoparalysis	Capillary hyperpermeability and plasmatic extravasation	Debilitation of the capillary walls	Venous relaxation and vaso-paralysis	Venular spasms
Effects found with Ginkgo biloba extract	Vasorelaxation	Diminution in platelet hyper-aggregability	Restitution of arterial tonus	Diminution in the accumulation of toxic wastes: K^+, CO_2, lactates	Antagonism of capillary hyperpermeability	Increased capillary resistance	Venous tonic effect	Antagonism of experimental venous spasms (high concentrations)
Cellular and membranal mechanisms which explain them	Release of EDRF from the endothelium; Inhibition of PDE; Potentiation of α-adrenergic effects (partially through COMT inhibition)	Release of PGI_2; Direct membranal effect	Direct effect; Potentiation of α-adrenergic effects (partially through COMT inhibition)	Consequence of a venous tonic effect; Mitochondrial metabolic restart	Direct membranal effect (ionic flow?)	Direct membranal effect	Direct effect; Indirect effect via the α-adrenergic effects	Inhibition of PDE?; Release of dilatating PGs

Metabolic and ionic disturbances are reflected by an accumulation of intracellular Ca^{2+}, overproduction of oxygenated free radicals which overwhelm the mitochondrial enzymatic systems responsible for detsroying them, and an accumulation of proteolytic enzymes, three events whose consequences are aggressive toward the integrity of the cellular membranes(10, 16, 19) (*Figure 1*).

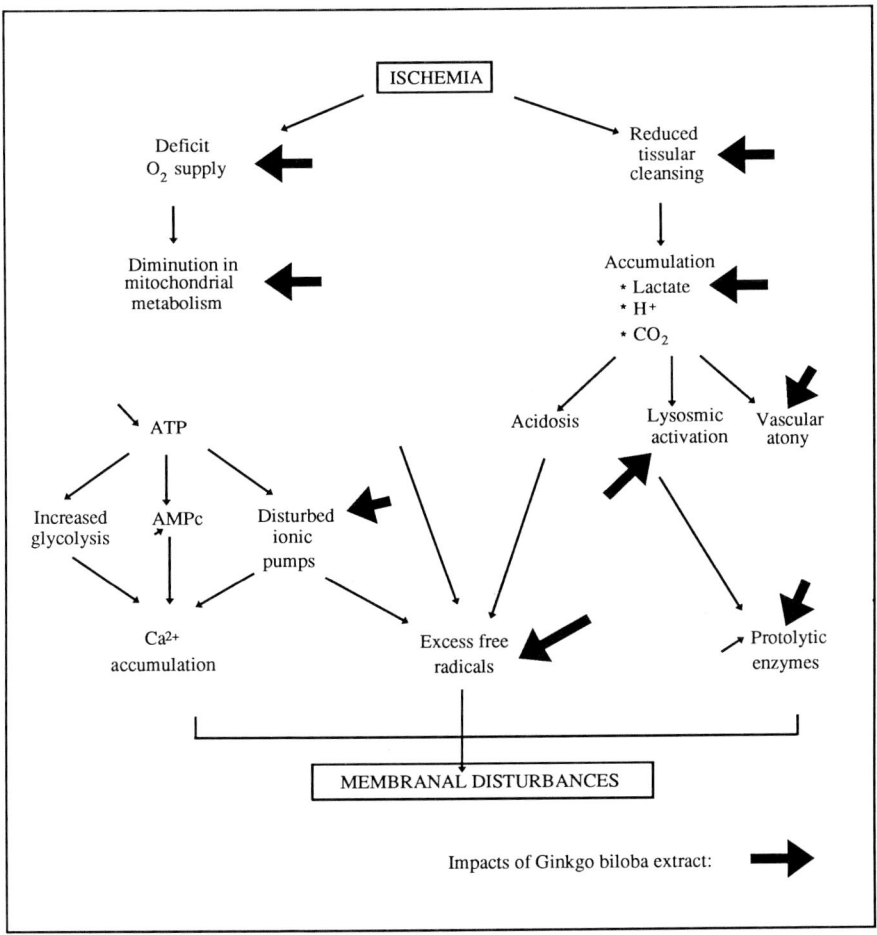

Figure 1. Sequence of cellular metabolic and ionic events in cerebral ischemia. The impacts of Ginkgo biloba extract (←).

Ginkgo biloba extract acts in most of these cellular metabolic disturbances. In fact, it increases the intake of metabolites and of O_2 through the maintenance of an effective perfusion flow, the direct consequence of the arteriolar vasoregulating effects.[4] It improves glucose and O_2 uptake, which promotes the reestablishment of mito-chondrial metabolism and restarting of aerobic glycolysis and therefore of ATP synthesis.[40] It also facilitates tissue cleansing through its tonic effects on the vein.[3] The difference between the concentrations of lactates in an ischemic he-misphere and a normal hemisphere (model of cerebral embolization by microspheres) is diminished by Ginkgo biloba extract. [40] Also there is stabilization of the lysosomial membranes, antiproteasic activity, and restoration of vascular tonus.

These protective effects on normal cellular metabolism, the mechanisms of which are membranal and molecular, explain for the most part the results recorded with Ginkgo biloba extract in various models of cerebral ischemia and hypoxia.

Platelets

The rheological effects of Ginkgo biloba extract have been studied *in vitro* and *in vivo* in platelet and erythrocytic hyperaggregability, as well as in different models of microcirculatory experimental thromboses. Ginkgo biloba extract inhibits human platelet aggregation induced by various aggregation inducers such as ADP, collagen, or thrombin. In the microcirculation in the hamster cheek, Ginkgo biloba extract slows the rate of growth of the platelet thrombi induced by micro-ionophoresis of ADP *in situ*. Finally, in experimental microthromboses induced in rabbits in the cortical artery by electrical stimulation, and in the cortical veins by intravenous injection of sodium lactate, Ginkgo biloba extract diminishes both the number of thrombi and the number of embolized vessels.[8] This demonstrates *in vivo* that Ginkgo biloba extract exerts an inhibiting action on platelet hyperaggregability, both arterial and venous, in the cerebral microcirculation.

But the rheological impact of Ginkgo biloba extract is not limited solely to platelet function; it also concerns the aggregability of the erythrocytes ("sludge"), as shown by the studies of Ernst.[22] Ginkgo biloba extract, without modifying the filterability of the erythrocytes, distinctly decreases their aggregability.

Inhibition of platelet and erythrocytic aggregability by Ginkgo biloba extract is possibly explained by a direct membranal effect,[23, 24] but also by stimulation of prostacyclin release,[13] as well as by antiradical properties in the cellular mem-branes.[16, 38]

Erythrocytic membrane

Erythrocytes are currently used for studying cellular membranal functions. Easy to obtain in men and animals, the erythrocyte is the best model for study of ionic flows for three reasons: its transport systems are now well described;(29) there is only a single intracellular compartment for the ions; finally, the intracellular and extracellular ionic concentrations can easily be determined.

In this model, it has been demonstrated that Ginkgo biloba extract increases membranal resistance of erythrocytes placed under conditions of experimental osmotic lysis *in vitro*(24) and *in vivo*(3) after single or repeated treatment of rabbits with Ginkgo biloba extract orally. It activates the intracellular exchange of Na^+ with extracellular K^+, with this occurrence being linked to activation of the sodium pump, membranal Na^+K^+ATP-ase.

This membranal protective effect, combined with improved yield from the active mechanisms of Na^+ transport, assumes a major role in the vascular and metabolic effects of Ginkgo biloba extract, explains its remarkable efficacy in cerebral edema, and allows us to foresee better membranal polarization, necessary for good functioning of all of the excitable tissues, in particular the nerve tissues.

Membranal and molecular actions of Ginkgo biloba extract

The first line of defense in the integrity of the cell and of its organites, the membrane plays an essential role in cellular life. The structure of the cellular membranes is ubiquitous through its phospholipids, and specific through the variety of its proteins capable of recognizing a signal and transmitting it either to other membranal proteins which convert it, or to the second messengers which are found within the cell.

Both fluid barriers, exchange sites, electrical structures, the site of molecular information transmissions, and lastly secretory elements, the cellular membranes are fragile and vulnerable. The first ionic and metabolic disturbances of cerebral ischemia, as well as the hypoxia and edema which are its corollaries, are located there. Any damage to cerebral circulatory integrity inevitably is reflected through changes in the cellular membranes: vascular, platelet, and neuronal.(19)

Among the substances capable of injuring the membranal structures, oxygenated free radicals appear to be the most harmful.(16) Although these are formed in such quantities that they overwhelm the enzymatic defense systems (superoxide dismutase, catalase, and peroxidase), the result is spatial disorganization of the structures, and severe disturbances in enzymatic, ionic, and molecular functioning of the cellular membranes. The responsibility of the free radicals engendered during phases of metabolic distress, in particular in all ischemic situations, seems now to be well established.(10, 11, 16, 17, 30) *Figure 2* describes the sequence of the principal metabolic, cellular, and molecular events which lead to the production of oxygenated free radicals at the time of a tissular ischemic situation.

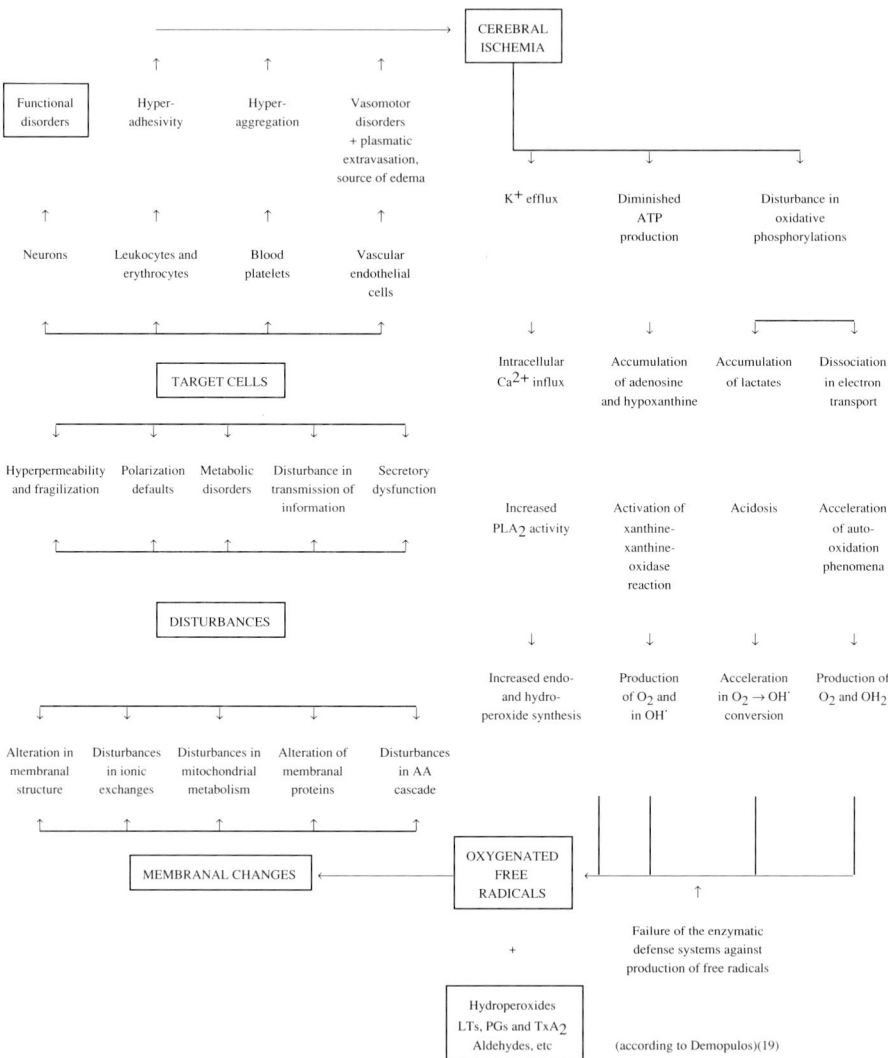

Figure 2: Sequence of the principal molecular events which link cerebral ischemia to the production of oxygenated free radicals and which explain the membranal and cellular effects thereof.

The effects of Ginkgo biloba extract on free radicals and on the membranal changes which they induce have been demonstrated at the molecular, membranal biochemical, cellular, tissular, and functional levels. At the molecular level, the formation of free radicals by the action of adriamycin(17) on the microsomes is combined with emission of a specific signal (sign of appearance of an oxygenated free radical) which can be revealed by electronic paramagnetic resonance. Ginkgo biloba extract suppresses the appearance of the signal, proof of elimination of the free radicals as soon as they are formed.(38) With respect to membranal biochemistry, the antiradical properties of Ginkgo biloba extract have been explored by measuring the electro-retinogram on a rat retina *in vitro*.(20) The retina, like all of the noble tissues, is particularly vulnerable to the deleterious effects of peroxidizing agents. Very rich in membranes, the retinal cells are the site of intense metabolic activity, from which come significant quantities of unsaturated fatty acids and a danger of biochemical imbalance causing hyperproduction of larger free radicals. At the time of a change in the retinal membranal structures through experimental peroxidation obtained *in situ* with a mixture of ferrous sulfate and sodium ascorbate, severe disturbances are found in the electroretinogram, revealed by flattening and even disappearance of the positive wave, and the survival time of the retina is greatly shortened. In this model, Ginkgo biloba extract is clearly opposed to the electroretinographic disturbances of the membranal peroxidation and significantly prolongs retinal functional capacities.

Ginkgo biloba extract protects the erythrocytes from loss of intracellular K^+ consecutive to membranal lipoperoxidation linked to production of superoxide ion by phenazine methosulfate.(36)

The effects of Ginkgo biloba extract on the tissue impacts of free radicals have been explored *in vitro* on the metabolism of soluble collagen microfibrills from calf skin(6) and *in vivo* with respect to rat paw tissue edema induced by adriamycin.(25)

The oxygenated free radicals produced by the xanthine-xanthine-oxidase reaction disturb anabolism and catabolism of the collagen microfibrils by causing cleavage of their helicoidal structure. Ginkgo biloba extract, even at low concentration (80 µg/mL) opposes this phenomenon.(6) This effect is directly linked to scavenging of free radicals.

Adriamycin, in subplantar injection into the rat paw, causes the appearance of biphasic inflammatory tissue edema: the first phase is early and corresponds to the release of mediators specific for inflammation; the second, later (lag time of five days) corresponds to peroxidation of membranal lipids. In fact, adriamycin possesses a quinonic cycle capable of accepting an electron which it will transmit to the molecular O_2 in order to produce superoxide ions, initiators of lipoperoxidation. Ginkgo biloba extract, administered orally, protects the rats against the appearance of the second phase of subplantar edema induced by adriamycin, which corresponds to the tissue effects of free radicals.(25) No antiinflammatory component is involved, since Ginkgo biloba extract has no effects on the first phase of edema.

Finally, the injection of sodium arachidonate in rats induces the appearance of a cerebral infarction with retention of water and Na^+, loss of K^+, and development of edema in the cerebral tissue, the results of production of free radicals via the cascade of arachidonic acid. Ginkgo biloba extract prevents the appearance of these ionic and tissue disturbances, its effects being related to a distinct diminution in the peroxidation index.(10)

Ginkgo biloba extract and cerebral aging

The phenomena accompanying or characterizing cerebral aging are not manifested equally in all species or in all individuals in the same species. In this field, it seems that the rat is a model whose cerebral hemodynamic, metabolic, and biochemical disturbances related to aging are relatively similar to those found in man.

Thus, three types of essential disorders in the course of aging have been demonstrated in elderly rats at the cerebral level: diminution in the circulatory flows, mainly in the hippocampus, the caudate nucleus, and the thalamus,(42) a diminution in the potential for uptake of glucose by the cerebral cells,(42) a deficit in activity of certain neurotransmitters, in particular dopamine, acetylcholine, and noradrenalin.(41)

Continella and Drago(15) showed that Ginkgo biloba extract, in oral treatment for one week, would improve the mnesic potentials of elderly rats subjected to the passive avoidance reaction test, without modifying the performances of young rats, thus excluding a psychotropic component. These results confirm that Ginkgo biloba extract assures normal function restoration for rats whose behavioral performances have been diminished by age.

They may be explained, at the tissular, cellular, and molecular levels, by the fact that Ginkgo biloba extract preferentially increases the flows in some cerebral areas, such as the hippocampus and the thalamus, which are most affected by cerebral aging.(39) Ginkgo biloba extract also improves dopamine turnover(39) and increases the density of the muscarinic acetylcholine receptors(45) in the hippocampus of elderly rats. These mechanisms probably contribute to the therapeutic effects of Ginkgo biloba extract in mnesic deficits and behavioral disorders of senescence.

Conclusions

Treatment for any ischemia, whether it is cerebral or peripheral, acute or chronic, is based in terms of functional recovery. The restoration of neuronal function, in the case of cerebral ischemia, will be more rapid and more significant with a multiple-impact drug. In fact, the processes of installation of cerebral insufficiency are numerous. They are of vascular, metabolic, and rheological origin, and today it appears clear that the physiopathological denominators common to all of these parameters are located in the membranes of the involved target cells.

Ginkgo biloba extract presents a very broad spectrum of pharmacological actions: its impacts are vascular, hemorheological, and metabolic all at the same time. In the classification of cerebrovascular drugs by Spagnoli(43) (*Table 2*), it alone, with co-dergocrine, possesses these characteristics. Ginkgo biloba extract thus exerts tissue-irrigating effects which it focuses preferentially in the ischemic areas by means of a direct vascular impact which is arterial and venous, as well as capillary. At the arterial level, this impact involves the endothelium, the smooth muscle layer, and the adventitia. It relieves the spasm but also combats postischemic vasoparalysis which is reflected by maintenance of effective tissue perfusion pressure. For the capillaries, it increases resistance and diminishes hyperpermeability, the source of the plasmatic extravasation which generates tissue edema, and limits anastomosic hemodiversion. In the veins, it reinforces vascular tonus and restores to the return circulation its efficacy in cleansing the metabolic waste products from hypoxia and acidosis.

Table 2

Tissular, cellular, and molecular impacts of several drugs with vascular, cerebral and peripheral orientations

Drug	Vascular impact	Metabolic activation	Hemorheological effects	Interactions with neurotransmitters
Almitrine		•		
Buflomedil	•			
Cetiedil	•			
Cinnarizine	•			
Cyclandelate	•	•		
Dihydroergocristine	•	•	•	•
Eburnamonine		•		
Flunarizine	•			
Ginkgo biloba	•	•	•	•
Ifenprodil	•	•		
Isoxuprine	•			
Naftidrofuryl	•	•	•	
Nicergoline	•	•	•	
Papaverine	•			
Pentoxyfilline	•		•	
Piribedil		•		•
Raubasine	•			
Vincamine		•		

Ginkgo biloba extract also exerts cellular metabolic effects, in addition to those which are the result of a better energy supply and better cleansing of metabolic wastes from tissular hypoxia. They are shown concretely through an increase in glucose uptake, maintenance of mitochondrial metabolic efficacy, and production of ATP by improvement in Na⁺K⁺ATP-asic yield, and by inhibition of uncoupling of oxidative phosphorylations. As to the hemorheological effects, we found a decrease in platelet hyperaggregability, antagonism toward experimental thrombo-embolisms of the arteries and cortical veins, diminution of aggregability of the erythrocytes, and protection against erythrocytic osmotic lysis.

The functional consequences are illustrated by the restoration of a normal neurological index both in models of experimental ischemia induced by ligation in gerbils and by embolization in rats, and in triethyletain-induced cytotoxic edema in rats.

The basic mechanisms are located, for the most part, at the membranal level. There is involved essentially the maintenance of the ultrastructural integrity of the membranes faced with the assault of oxygenated free radicals produced in the course of tissular ischemia, of interaction with the membranal ionic pumps, in particular Na⁺K⁺ATP-ase, often disturbed at the time of a deficiency in metabolic supply, of modulation in the activity of certain membranal or intracellular enzymes, in particular COMT, PDE, and lysosomial proteases.

There is also direct or indirect activity on the adrenergic system, physiological vasoregulator of the cerebral circulation and protector of the integrity of the blood-brain barrier, and stimulation of release in the vascular endothelium of vasorelaxant endogenous substances such as EDRF and prostacyclin.

Although we have pinpointed the principal cellular and membranal targets of substances which Ginkgo biloba extract contains, others still remain to be discovered. Thus, the discovery by P. Braquet et al.(12) of the specific antagonism manifested by certain ginkgolides toward the PAF-acether opens new pathways for research in the field of allergy and of respiratory or cardiovascular anaphylactic shocks.

The future of therapeutic research is found today more than ever in animal and vegetable nature. The use of natural sources thus makes possible the discovery of new structures which inspire chemists to new syntheses, an eminently fertile source for therapeutic research.

References

1. Allard M.: Traitement des troubles du vieillissement par extrait de Ginkgo biloba. De la pharmacologie à la clinique. *Presse Méd.*, 1985, *15*, 1540-1545.

2. Auguet M., Clostre F.: Effects of an extract of Ginkgo biloba and diverse substances on the phasic and tonic components of the contraction of an isolated aorta. *Gen. Pharmac.*, 1983, *14*, 277-280.

3. Auguet M., Hellegouarch A., Delaflotte S., Baranes J., DeFeudis F.V., Clostre F., Braquet P., Drieu K.: Effects of Ginkgo biloba extract on rabbit blood vessels. *In: Cerebral ischemia*. Bes A., Braquet P., Paoletti R., Siesjö B.K., Eds., *Excerpta Medica*, Amsterdam, 1984, 347-354.

4. Auguet M., Delaflotte S., Hellegouarch A, Clostre F.: Bases pharmacologiques de l'impact vasculaire de l'extrait de Ginkgo biloba. *Presse Méd.*, 1986, *15*.

5. Borchardt R.T., Huber J.A.: Catechol O-Methyltransferase-5 structure activity relationships for inhibition by flavonoids. *J. Med. Chem.*, 1975, *18*, 120-122.

6. Borel J.P., Braquet P., Monboisse J.C., Maquart F.X., Randoux A.: Effects of oxygen radicals, PAF-acether and leukotrienes on collagen metabolism. *In:* Oxy Radicals and their scavenger systems, R.A. Greenwald, G. Cohen, Eds., vol. II., *Excerpta Medica*, Amsterdam 1983, 334-338.

7. Borzeix M.G., Weber S., Akimjak J.P.: Cerebral edema induced by triethyltin (TET) in the rabbit and in the rat. *In:* Proc. of the 7th international Congress of Pharmacology, Satellite Symposium of Reims 1978.

8. Borzeix M.G., Labos M., Hartl C.: Recherches sur l'action anti-agrégante de l'extrait de Ginkgo biloba. Activité au niveau des artères et des veines de la pie-mère chez le lapin. *Sem. Hôpitaux*, 1980, *56*, 393-398.

9. Borzeix M.G.: Effect of Ginkgo biloba extract on 2 types of cerebral edema. *In:* Effects of Ginkgo biloba extract on Organic Cerebral Impairement, Agnoli A., Rapin J.R., Scapagnini V., Weitbrecht W.V., Eds., *John Libbey*, London, 1985.

10. Braquet P., Braquet M., Deby C.: Oxidative damages induced by cerebral ischemia: protective role of some radical scavenger and related drugs. *J. Cerebral Blood Flow Metabolism*, 1983, *3*, suppl. 1, 564-565.

11. Braquet P., DeFeudis F.V., Deby C., Braquet M.: Involvement of oxygen free radicals in biologic and pathologic processes. *In:* Cerebral Ischaemia, Eds. A. Bes, P. Braquet, R. Paoletti, B.K. Siesjö, *Excerpta Medica*, Amsterdam, 1984, 265-283.

12. Braquet P., Spinnewyn B., Braquet M., Bourgain R.H., Taylor J.E., Etienne A.,

Drieu K.: BN 52021 and related compounds: a new series of highly specific PAF-acether receptor antagonists isolated from Ginkgo biloba. *Blood and Vessels*, 1985, *16*, 558-572.

13. Chatterjee S.S.: Effects of Ginkgo biloba extract on cerebral metabolic processes. *In:* Effects of Ginkgo biloba extract on organic cerebral impairment. Agnoli A., Rapin J.R., Scapagnini V., Weitbrecht W.V., Eds., *John Libbey*, London 1985, 5-15.

14. Cohadon F.: Physiopathologie de l'œdème cérébral ischémique. *Circulation et Métabolisme du Cerveau.* 1983, *1*, 45-54.

15. Continella G., Drago F.: Behavioral effects of Ginkgo biloba extract. *In:* Effects of Ginkgo biloba on organic cerebral impairment, Agnoli A., Rapin J.R., Scapagnini V., Weitbrecht W.V., Eds., *John Libbey*, London 1985.

16. Deby C., Pincemail J., Hans P., Braquet P., Lion Y., Deby-Dupont G., Goutier R.: Mechanism of free radicals production in the arachidonic cascade and role of antilipoperoxydants and free radical scavengers. *In:* Cerebral ischemia, Bes A., Braquet P., Paoletti R., Siesjö B.K., Eds., *Excerpta Medica*, Amsterdam, 1984, 249-258.

17. DeFeudis F.V., Auguet M., Delaflotte S., Hellegouarch A., Baranes J., Chapelat M., Braquet M., Etienne A., Drieu K., Clostre F., Braquet P.: Some *in vitro* and *in vivo* actions of an extract of Ginkgo biloba (GBE 761). *In:* Effects of Ginkgo biloba extract on organic cerebral impairment. Paris, Londres, *John Libbey*, 1985, pp. 17-29.

18. Delaflotte S., Auguet M., DeFeudis F.V., Baranes J., Clostre F., Drieu K., Braquet P.: Endothelium – dependant relaxations of rabbit isolated aorta produced by carbachol and by Ginkgo biloba extract. *Biomed Biochim. Acta,* 1984, *43,* 5212-5216.

19. Demopoulos H., Seligman M., Schwartz M., Tomasula J., Flamm E.: Molecular pathology of regional cerebral ischemia. *In:* Cerebral ischemia, Bes A., Braquet P., Paoletti R., Siesjö B.K., Eds., *Excerpta Medica*, Amsterdam, 1984, 259-264.

20. Doly M., Bonhomme B., Braquet P., Meyniel G.; Electro-physiological study of lipid peroxydation on isolated rat retain. *In:* Oxy Radicals and their scavenger systems, Greenwald R.A., Cohen G., Eds., vol II, *Elsevier*, Amsterdam, 1983, 330-333.

21. Edvisson L.: Vascular autonomic nerves and corresponding receptor in brain vessels. *Path. Biol.*, 1982, *30,* 261-268.

22. Ernst E.: Hemorheological effects of standardized Ginkgo extract *in vitro. In:*

Effects of Ginkgo biloba extract on organic cerebral impairment, Agnoli A., Rapin J.R., Scapagnini V., Weitbrecht W.V., Eds., *John Libbey*, London, 1985.

23. Etienne A., Baranes J., Hecquet F., Hellegouarch A., Clostre F.: Effet stabilisateur de membrane d'un extrait de Ginkgo biloba. *Planta Medica*, 1980, *39*, 237.

24. Etienne A., Hecquet F., Clostre F., DeFeudis F.V.: Comparaison des effets d'un extrait de Ginkgo biloba et de la chlorpromazine sur la fragilité osmotique, *in vitro*, d'érythrocytes de rat. *J. Pharmacol.* (Paris), 1982, *13*, 291-298.

25. Etienne A., Chapelat M., Braquet M., Clostre F., Drieu K., DeFeudis F.V., Braquet P.: In vivo studies of free radical scavenging activity; relation to cerebral ischaemia. *In:* Cerebral ischaemia, Bes. A., Braquet P., Paoletti R., Siesjö B.K., Eds., *Excerpta Medica*, Amsterdam, 1984, 379-384.

26. Fieschi C., Lenzi G.L.: Experimental models of focal cerebral ischemia. *In:* Cerebral ischemia, Bes A., Braquet P., Paoletti R., Siesjö B.K., Eds., *Excerpta Medica, Amsterdam,* 1984, 56-62.

27. Furchgott R.F.: The role of endothelium in the responses of vascular smooth muscle to drugs. *Ann. Rev. Pharmacol. Toxicol.*, 1984, *24*, 175-197.

28. Gabard B., Chatterjee S.S.: Cerebral edema induced by briethyltin in the rat: effects of an extract of Ginkgo biloba. *Naunym Schmiedeberg's Arch. Pharmacol.*, 1980, 311 (suppl.) R 68.

29. Garay R.P., Meyer P.: A new test showing abnormal net Na^+ and K^+ fluxes in erythrocytes of essential hypertensive patients. *Lancet,* 1979, 349-353.

30. Hillered L., Ernster L., Arfors K.E.: Brain Ischemia and oxygen radicals. *In*: Cerebral Ischemia, Bes A., Braquet P., Paoletti R., Siesjö B.K., Eds., *Excerpta Medica*, Amsterdam, 1984, 293-300.

31. Karcher L., Zagermann P., Krieglstein J.: Effect of an extract of Ginkgo biloba on rat brain energy metabolism in hypoxia. *Naunym-Schmiedeberg's Arch. Pharmacol.*, 1984, *327*, 31-35.

32. Lagrue G., Baillet J., Behar A.: Activité d'un extrait végétal complexe dans les œdèmes idiopathiques orthostatiques. *Sem. Hôpitaux,* Paris, 1978, *54*, 214-217.

33. Larssen R.G., Dupeyron J.P., Boulu R.G.: Modèle d'ischémie cérébrale expérimentale par microphère chez le rat. Etude de l'effet de deux extraits de Ginkgo biloba et du naftidrofuryl. *Thérapie*, 1978, *33*, 651-660.

34. Le Poncin Lafitte M., Rapin J.-R.: Effect of Ginkgo biloba on changes induced by quantitative cerebral micro-embolization in rats. *Arch. Int. Pharmacodyn.*, 1980, *243*, 236-244.

35. Le Poncin Lafitte M., Martin P., Lespinasse P., Rapin J.-R.: Ischémie cérébrale

après ligature non simultanée des artères carotides chez le rat: effet de l'extrait de Ginkgo biloba. *Sem. Hôp., Paris*, 1982, *58*, 403-406.

36. Maridonneau I., Braquet P., Garay R.P.: Na⁺ and K⁺ transport damage induced by oxygen free radicals in human red cell membranes. *J. Biol. Chem. Chem.*, 1983, *256*, 3107-3113.

37. Mueller S.M., Ertel P.J., Felten D.L., Overhage J.M.: Sympathetic nerves protect against blood-brain barrier disruption in the spontaneously hypertensive rat. *Stroke*, 1979, *13*, 83-88.

38. Pincemail J., Deby C.: Propriétés antiradicalaires de l'extrait de Ginkgo biloba. *Presse Méd.*, 1986, *15*, 1475-1479.

39. Rapin J.R., Le Poncin-Lafitte M.: Modèle expérimental d'ischémie cérébrale. Action préventive de l'extrait de Ginkgo biloba. *Sem. Hôp.*, Paris, 1979, *55*, 42-43.

40. Rapin J.R., Duterte D., Le Poncin-Lafitte M.: Hypoxie normobare et activité cérébrovasculaire chez la souris. *J. Pharmacol*, 1980, *11*, 101.

41. Samorajski T.: Normal and pathologic aging of the brain in brain neurotransmitters and receptors in aging and age-related disorders. *In: Aging, vol. 17*. Enna S.J. et coll Eds., *Raven Press*, New York, 1981, 1-12.

42. Sokoloff L.: Effects of normal aging on cerebral circulation and energy metabolism. *In:* Brain function in old age. Evaluation of changes and disorders, Hoffmeister F., Müller C. Eds., *Springer-Verlag*, Berlin-Heidelberg-New York, 1979, 367.

43. Spagnoli A., Tognoni G.: Cerebroactive drugs. Clinical pharmacology and therapeutic role. *In: Cerebrovascular disorders drugs*, 1983, *26*, 44-69.

44. Spinnewyn B., Blavet N., Clostre F.: Effets du Ginkgo biloba sur l'ischémie cérébrale expérimentale chez la gerbille. *Presse Méd.*, 1965, *15*, 1511-1515.

45. Taylor J.E.: The effects of chronic, oral Ginkgo biloba extract administration on neurotransmitter receptor binding in young and aged «Fischer 344» rats. *In:* Effects of Ginkgo biloba extract on organic cerebral impairment. Agnoli A., Rapin J.R., Scapagnini V., Weitbrecht W.V., Eds., *John Libbey*, London, 1985.

CLINIC

Treatment of Old Age Disorders with Ginkgo Biloba Extract
From Pharmacology to Clinic

M. Allard

IPSEN, 30, rue Cambronne. F 75015 Paris

Summary

Ginkgo biloba extract is prescribed in psychic and behavioural disorders of the elderly, in peripheral vascular deficiency and in functional disorders of ischaemic origin in the E.N.T. and eye areas.

Numerous controlled clinical trials justify these prescriptions and are in agreement with the pharmacological data currently available. Experimentally, Ginkgo biloba extract has proved active on the circulatory and rheological functions, on neuronal metabolism threatened by ischaemia or hypoxia, on neurotransmission and on membrane lesions caused by free oxygenated radicals.

Concerning Alzheimer's disease and dementia, no firm conclusion can be drawn for the time being due to the lack of animal model. However, experimental data suggest that the product may act on a number of major elements of these diseases.

From what is already known about Ginkgo biloba extract, it appears that it fulfills the conditions laid down by the W.H.O. concerning the development of drugs effective against cerebral ageing.

The principal indication for Ginkgo biloba extract (EGb 761, Rökan®, Intersan) deserves throughtful consideration. The rather vague expression "psycho-behavioral disorders of senescence" should disappear; it should be replaced by another, but any rate, the patients and their complaints will always be there. In 1979 it replaced other labels, in particular "cerebral vascular insufficiency" or "cerebral circulatory insufficiency", since it was rather general, in order to correspond to the state of knowledge of that time.

The clinical entity which this term covers is still poorly defined and not well known. However, it is a preoccupation of our contemporaries, both physicians and patients, which is increasing. It is currently one of the most frequent reasons for consulting a physician. That is why the group of products including Ginkgo biloba extract is one

Rökan (Ginkgo Biloba). Recent Results in Pharmacology and Clinic
Edited by E.W. Fünfgeld
© Springer-Verlag Berlin Heidelberg New York 1988, pp. 201-211

of the most widely used in the entire therapeutic armamentarium to which the presciber has access: approximately 4% of prescriptions(13).

Also, a dual change in thinking is taking place and is forcing us to interest ourselves more in intellectual decline. First, senile dementia – a disease in the course of which the symptomatic description outlined above is particularly marked – is now experienced less as a natural event, in the normal order of things, a distressing way to end one's life, but more as a "disease". On the other hand, the health requirements of each person, both for himself and for those close to him, have increased, whereas the acceptance (or tolerance) by the entourage and its availability are decreasing, even when the disturbances are mild; this phenomenon is related at least partially to increasing urbanization.

From cerebral circulatory insufficiency to Alzheimer's disease

The entire symptomatology could correspond to several different clinical entities, and there is a great variety in more or less similar synonyms, some more specific than others, the sometimes guarded usage of which to define either identical diseases, or related or more advanced disorders. Several terms can thus be applied to the same illness: chronic cerebral insufficiency, cerebral circulatory insufficiency, cerebrovascular deficit, cerebrovascular diseases, chronic cerebral ischemia, "functional" disorders of (old) age, chronic mental deficit condition, intellectual weakening or deterioration, mental impairment, intellectual decline (or deficit), cerebral involution, cerebral aging or senescence, idiopathic cerebral degeneration of elderly persons, benign amnesiac deficit associated with senescence, changes in the cognitive and emotional functions, mental disorders related to age, senile dementia, mild, moderate, or severe demential syndrome, Alzheimer's disease, dotage, senility, and so forth.

These names are often accompanied by symptomatological details: disorders of memory, mood, concentration, or even headaches, tinnitus, vertigo, instability or drunken sensations, etc. Numerous authors recognize the entity "benign forgetfulness of age" or "benign mnesic weakening of aging" . The World Health Organization (WHO) sometimes prefers the obviously outdated expression "other and poorly defined cerebrovascular diseases" with chronic cerebral ischemia (code 437 and 437.1 of the CIM), but also the term "neuronal aging" or "intellectual deterioration" (30, 31).

It is found that these definitions are articulated because of extremely variable taxinomic or terminological principles based on symptoms or on various etiopathogenic hypotheses (in particular, ischemic vascular deficit and aging), or on the deficit of an organ, a system, a function, or even when we speak of cardiac or renal insufficiency.

Although the condition or conditions treated with Ginkgo biloba extract are difficult to outline, the deficiency in the matter pertains as much to knowledge of the disease (or of aging) as to knowledge of the drug. Although the mode of action of the latter is only partially known, this comes first, since the etiopathogenesis of the conditions to which it is addressed is still a mystery for the most part. It has always been thus, for most drugs.

It is actually very difficult to define aging precisely in comparison with dementia (or with Alzheimer's disease). "Does Alzheimer's disease represent an exaggeration of normal aging?" L. Berg(4) believes that it is impossible to answer this question.

Furthermore, even if it were possible (or when it becomes possible) to establish this distinction from a fundamental standpoint, how do we make the differential diagnosis between the two conditions when faced with the clinical picture presented by a patient? Or again, if the hypothesis of a continuum or of varied clinical forms of the same disease is selected, for lack of known predictive criteria, how do we give a prognosis in practice?

Without approaching the preventive aspect of the therapy, what is the degree of disorders which justifies treatment (or a therapeutic trial) or, inversely, at what stage does recourse to treatment become illusory?

This comment takes on particular acuity if we consider the possibility of a "threshold" effect, beyond which a demential syndrome would become irreversible or a benign deterioration would become malignant. Alzheimer's disease is mentioned when we are faced with a patient presenting with primary dementia, after having eliminated the more specific causes such as the often curable depressive syndromes and secondary dementias. Two principal forms must be considered, either separately or together: a vascular form and a degenerative form. The first represents approximately 20% of the cases, the other 50%, and mixed forms, ten to 20%(23).

It has long been considered that the degenerative form had a presenile predilection (called Alzheimer's disease), and the vascular form was globally defined as senile dementia. It was considered that signs of dementia after 65 years of age were directly due to vascular disturbances in particular, "arteriosclerosis", hence the terms "cerebral ischemia", or "circulatory insufficiency", which have long prevailed.

The histopathological changes observed in the course of senile dementia are usually the same as those described by Alois Alzheimer in presenile dementia(38): overall atrophy of the cortex with deepening of the grooves and increase in size (or dilatation) of the cerebral cavities, diminution in the number of neurons, neurofibrillar conglomerates, granulo-vacuolar degeneration, and senile plaques made up of amyloid protein substance. Also, significant changes are frequently observed in the vascular walls.

All of these histopathological signs are not specific for severe forms of dementia, since they are encountered, to a lesser degree it is true, in elderly persons without demonstrable cognitive changes or "with mild psychocognitive disorders". This could be an argument in favor of a continuum ranging from the unaffected person to the person with severe senile dementia.

The distinction is made on the basis of the severity of these lesions, their density, and their distribution.

Therefore a similarity is observed in the ensemble of the phenomena of aging, particularly neuronal, with Alzheimer's dementia, from both the clinical and physiopathological standpoints.

Possible mechanisms of effect of Ginkgo biloba extract

From the etiopathogenic standpoint, as to the origin of dysfunction or neuronal disappearance, several explanations have been suggested to explain cerebral aging and Alzheimer's disease. Thus, genetic, toxic, circulatory, metabolic, membranal, infectious, immune, or cholinergic causes have been evoked one by one.

In the current state of our knowledge, it appears unlikely that Ginkgo biloba extract acts on genetic or toxic (aluminum) factors of the disease. Antiviral activity is improbable, although it has been shown that Ginkgo biloba contains antiviral substances(3). Activity on the immune system cannot be completely excluded, since recently one of the novel specific substances in Ginkgo has been shown to be, in both oral and injectable administration, one of the most potent inhibitors of the "platelet-activating factor" (PAF), a substance which appears to be increasingly important in the mechanisms of platelet aggregation, inflammation, allergy, and shock, as well as in the rejection of grafts(7).

We shall retain essentially the physiopathological standards in which pharmacological intervention is plausible or reasonably envisageable in the current state of our knowledge.

Cerebral blood circulation

Numerous case histories using very advanced methods of investigations have shown that in patients suffering with Alzheimer's disease there is a significant reduction in cerebral blood flow. Similar diminutions seem to exist in elderly persons apparently suffering with demential syndrome, but they are definitely more marked in Alzheimer's disease (and in senile dementia). These disturbances are perhaps only the reflection or the result of other disorders: simple general disappearance of neurons with diminution in requirements, or of the specialized nerve structures responsible for regulation of flow, or even disorders of the vasoactive neuromediators, for example(20).

As there are no satisfactory animal models for Alzheimer's disease, studies have been made particularly of models that simulate human aging, which is accompanied by vascular disorders and a decrease in flow comparable to that observed in man.

This approach involves either isolated vessels and the microcirculation, or intact organisms in which ischemia is induced by suppression or reduction of the blood supply. Since this disturbance causes symptoms reminiscent of those of aging and since a decrease in flow is observed in man, the effects of the therapy on these parameters have been particularly studied.

EGb exerts a *vasoregulating activity on the entire vascular tree:* arteries, capillaries, veins. This activity is dose-dependent and can vary considerably depending upon the nature, the size, and the tissue origin of the vessel, but also its basic tonus and its physiological or pathological condition(1).

EGb opposes arterial spasm and exerts a vasodilatating action on the veins; it regulates venous capacity, combats capillary hyperpermeability, and reinforces capillary resistance(22, 25).

The result of this ensemble of activities is an overall increase in blood flow, which is also due to a rheological change which can be definitely individualized.

The *rheological effects* of EGb have been studied *in vitro* and *in vivo*(5, 7, 14) in platelet and erythrocytic hyperaggregation and the thrombotic processes of the microcirculation. Although this increase in flows is easier to demonstrate in acute or exaggerated conditions, it has been verified both in man and in animals at different levels.

From the hemodynamic standpoint, the effects of EGb have been evaluated by cerebral circulation time(18, 37) xenon 133 clearance(21), plethysmography, thermometry(10), reactive hyperemia, measurement of distal perfusion pressures, and measurement of arterial compliance(27).

Another histological change encountered in Alzheimer's disease involves the vascular wall more directly. This is cerebral vascular amyloidosis, indicated by congophilic angiopathy and dyshoric angiopathy. It is also observed to a lesser degree in elderly persons who are not manifesting clinical signs of intellectual deterioration, but it is much more frequently encountered in the course of Alzheimer's type dementias, as well as in trisomia(21). It is possible that this protein accumulation in the vessel walls is related to abnormal passage of substances from the vessel toward the nerve tissue, an indicator of a breakdown of the blood-brain barrier. On this subject, let us note that, in an experimental model, Ginkgo biloba extract exerts protective effects against precocious rupture of the blood-brain barrier in the rat(19).

Metabolic changes

Changes in the neuron metabolism are partially correlated with changes in cerebral blood flow. Decreased glucose uptake and oxygen usage, with the fall in energy which arises therefrom, are consistent in patients presenting with Alzheimer's disease.

The protective effect of EGb versus these phenomena is shown objectively by the survival rate of animals subjected to experimental ischemia or hypoxia(24), through improvement in the cortical area in levels of ATP and lactates, and by better glucose and oxygen uptake(28).

Several studies have demonstrated the protective effects of EGb toward cellular metabolism and more particularly toward the cerebral cells. These effects have been verified in various severe experimental models involving ischemia or cerebral anoxia: cerebral embolization by microspheres or by ligation of the carotids(28), normobaric and hypobaric hypoxia(24), traumatic triethyletain-induced edema(17).

Also in man, cerebral metabolism has been very particularly explored in the course of a study in patients having had a cerebral vascular accident and retaining a moderate neuropsychic deficit(21, 37). The clinical improvement was correlated with better use of O_2 and glucose. This model is far removed from degenerative dementias, but it is given as a pharmacological demonstration with reservations as to its perfect extrapolation.

Neurotransmission disturbances

Numerous biochemical disturbances have been described in the brains of patients presenting with Alzheimer's disease, in particular with respect to the neurotransmittors. The best studied is the significant decrease in cortical cholineacetyltransferase (CAT) activity, more distinct in the hippocampus. These modifications can be correlated either with the severity of the clinical disturbances or with the degree of histological damage and are partially found in elderly persons(26).

Recently, a significant decrease has been found in the number of cerebral acetylcholine receptors (muscarinic receptors), which control the release of neuromediators from the cholinergic nerve endings. This decrease or even disappearance of receptors may explain the decrease in CAT. In long-term treatment in rats, it was possible to show that EGb induces a distinct increase in the number of muscarinic acetylcholine receptors in the hippocampus in elderly animals in comparison with control animals in which a decrease on the order of 20% was found in bonding capacity(36).

Furthermore, changes in other neurotransmittors have just been demonstrated. Studies conducted with Ginkgo biloba extract have shown (under notably different physiopathological conditions) an improvement in the rate of synthesis of cerebral catecholamines. The administration of EGb and of a dopamine precursor tagged with C^{14} brings about an increase in the index of dopamine and noradrenalin formation, provided that these animals have undergone ischemia.

Membranal damage and intervention of free radicals

This involves an etiopathogenic hypothesis common to aging and to senile dementia of Alzheimer type. The radical theory of aging incriminates the deleterious effects of free radicals, which would be responsible for the processes of cytological degradation which in their turn would bring about functional disorders. The cellular membranes, but also nucleic acids and cytoplasmic proteins, are particularly sensitive to these substances(6, 8, 12, 15, 35).

It has been shown that EGb would exert a marked antiradical activity both *in vitro* in purely chemical reactions, and in experimental cellular models, even on entire organisms(15).

Clinical applications

This ensemble of pharmacological properties could explain why EGb exerts a considerable antiedematous activity and a beneficial effect in all other cases in which an ischemic process is implicated:
- in the treatment of certain peripheral vascular disorders, clinical manifestations of arteriopathy of the lower extremities (intermittent claudication syndrome);
- in ORL, in the treatment of certain vertiginous syndromes, tinnitus, certain losses of auditory acuity;
- in ophthalmology, in retinal deficits, probably of ischemic mechanism.

While restricting ourselves to therapeutic trials conducted in double-blind and comparatively, both in France and abroad, we found that there is statistically significant activity in *arteriopathies*(11, 16, 32). The latest study(2) was conducted according to a strict methodology corresponding to the most recent European recommendations as to selection of patients and criteria for evaluation of efficacy.

Although pharmacological experimentations in animals are also rare in this field, the clinical and paraclinical parameters are precise and recognized, and the process of evaluation well controlled. The principal criterion of efficacy is still walking distance on the treadmill under standardized conditions until the appearance of pain, then of functional impotence with plethysmographic control of the perfusion pressures.

Various studies all conclude there is a statistically significant improvement in patients under the influence of Ginkgo biloba extract in comparison with placebo or with a comparison product.

As to neurosensorial disorders, these include functional deficits in sight, equilibrium, and hearing, which are not obviously linked to objective major lesions of the eye or ear.

The various embryological, histological, and neurobiochemical relationships of the eye and inner ear with the brain permit us to understand that the pharmacological results obtained in these organs could often be similar.

Experiments relative to retinal changes in the rat rendered diabetic by alloxane(12) or to edema after laser photocoagulation in the rabbit show the activity of Ginkgo biloba extract. The same is true with respect to the study of isolated organs or tissues, such as the retina submitted to various aggressions, by free radicals, for example.

In ophthalmology, the first clinical studies were conducted in the open(33); they involve degenerative maculopathies, retinal disorders related to glaucoma, diabetic retinopathy, or various phenomena of vascular occlusion.

The same approach resulted in proposing and using Ginkgo biloba extract in ORL disorders which appear to be correlated with degenerative conditions or with ischemic disturbances of the sensory organs of the ear, the frequency of which is strongly related to increasing age. Although the definition of these disturbances and their etiopathogenic relationship also seems difficult to pinpoint, the essential element of the pathology is represented by vertiginous syndromes and secondly by tinnitus and hypoacousia (often of presbyacousic type).

Various clinical studies have been conducted with Ginkgo biloba extract in these conditions, versus either placebo or comparison products(21, 29); the results have always been good. Electronystagmography(34) and craniocorpography(9) have permitted a more objective evaluation of the therapeutic benefit in a field in which the clinical manifestations appear to be mainly subjective.

Discussion and Conclusion

Although we might wish to become involved in the four directions indicated by WHO for the purpose of controlling neuronal aging by pharmacological means and of elaborating a rational policy for prevention and treatment, it would be necessary, "in order to act on the intrinsic cause of aging, to act on the extrinsic, circulatory and metabolic, causes of neuronal aging, to facilitate and reinforce the functioning of the altered neurotransmitter systems, to improve the symptoms caused by neuronal aging" (31).

For Ginkgo biloba extract, there is good coherence between the pharmacological and clinical data. The mechanisms of effect are exerted at different levels, and EGb supplies at least a partial response to the afore-cited points and to several practical problems in geriatric pathology (perhaps because of the multiplicity of its components and of their different impacts). Of course, the heterogeneity of all of these disturbances, the intrication of the factors, the multiplicity of causes, the nosological haziness, the difficulties in establishing a consensus on evaluation criteria and tools for unquestionable clinical evaluation, make evaluation of a product such as Ginkgo biloba extract difficult.

It is certain that the statistically significant difference demonstrated in various clinical studies on disorders of senescence, whether cerebral, neurosensorial, or distal, is in many cases inadequate to return a patient to normal. It can nevertheless have basic value for him, as for an amblyopia patient changing from 2/10 to 4/10 is much more important than changing from 8/10 to 10/10. This gain can transform the life of a patient and is sufficient to put him over a critical threshold, to allow him to recover a portion of his autonomy or to delay institutionalization.

References

1. Auguet M., Clostre F.: Effects of an extract of Ginkgo biloba and diverse substances on the phasic and tonic components of the contraction of an isolated rabbit aorta. *Gen. Pharmacol.*, 1983, *14*, 277-280.

2. Bauer U.: L'extrait de Ginkgo biloba dans le traitement de l'artériopathie des membres inférieurs. *Presse Méd.*, 1986, *15*, 1546-1549.

3. Beladi I., Pusztai R., Mucsi I., Bakay M., Cabor M.: Activity of some flavonoïds against viruses. *Ann. N. Y. Acad. Sci.*, 1977, *284*, 358-364.

4. Berg L.: Does Alzheimer's Disease represent an exageration of normal aging? *Arch. Neurol.*, 1985, *42*, 737-739.

5. Borzeix M.G., Labos M., Hartl C.: Recherches sur l'action antiagrégante de l'extrait de Ginkgo biloba. Activité au niveau des artères et des veines de la pie-mère chez le lapin. *Sem. Hôp. Paris.*, 1980, *56*, 393-398.

6. Braquet P., Braquet M., Deby C.: Oxidative damages induced by cerebral ischemia: protective role of some radical scavengers and related drugs. *J. Cereb. Blood Flow Metab.*, 1983, *3*, Suppl. 1, 564-565.

7. Braquet P., Etienne A., Touvay C., Bourgain R.H., Lefort J., Vargaftig B.B.: Involvement of platelet activating factor in respiratory anaphylaxis, demonstrated by PAF-acether inhibitor BN 52021. *Lancet*, 1985, *1*, 1501.

8. Clairambault P., Magnier B., Droy-Lefaix M.T., Manier M., Pairault C.: Effet de l'extrait de Ginkgo biloba sur les lésions induites par une photocoagulation au laser à l'argon sur la rétine de lapin. *Sem. Hôp. Paris.*, 1986, *62*, 57-59.

9. Claussen C.F.: Etude randomisée, conduite en double insu, des effets de l'extrait de Ginkgo biloba et du placebo. La craniocorpographie montre une réduction statistiquement significative de la symptomatologie vertigineuse et ataxique. *Arztl. Praxis*, 1984, *36*, 1.

10. Clement J.L., Livecchi G., Jimenez C., Morino S., Drevard R., Eclache J.: Modifications à des conditions thermiques défavorables: méthodologie et résultat de l'étude de l'extrait de Ginkgo biloba. *Actua. Angéiol.*, 1982, *7*, 3-8.

11. Courbier R., Jausseran J.M., Reggi M.: Etude en double insu croisée du Tanakan dans les artériopathies des membres inférieurs. *Méd.*, 1977, *126*, 61-64.

12. Doly M., Droy-Lefaix M.T., Bonhomme B., Braquet P.: Effets de l'extrait de Ginkgo biloba sur l'activité électrophysiologique de la rétine isolée de rat diabétique. *Presse Méd.*, 1986, *15*, 1480-1483.

13. *Dorema*: Etude permanente de la prescription. Classes thérapeutiques, Automne 85, T1.

14. Ernst E.: Hemorheological effects of standardized Ginkgo extract in vitro. *In:* Effects of Ginkgo biloba extract on organic cerebral impairment, Agnoli A., Rapin J.R., Scapagnini V., Weitbrecht W.V., Eds., *John Lbbey*, London, 1985, 57-62.

15. Etienne A., Chapelat M., Braquet M., Clostre F., Drieu K., De Feudis F.V., Braquet P.: *In vivo* studies of free radical scavenging activity: relation to cerebral ischemia. *In:* Cerebral Ischemia., A. Bes., P. Baquet, R. Paoletti, Bo. K. Siesjö, Eds., *Excerpta Medica.*, Amsterdam, 1984, 379-384.

16. Frileux Cl., Copé R.: L'extrait concentré de Ginkgo biloba dans les troubles vasculaires périphériques. *Cah. Artériol. Royat.*, 1975, *3*, 117-122.

17. Gabard B., Chatterjee S.S.: Cerebral edema induced by triethyltin in the rat: Effect of an extract of Ginkgo biloba. *Naugn Schmiedebers Arch. Pharmacol.*, 1980, *311*, (suppl.), R68.

18. Galley P., Safi N.: Tanakan et cerveau sénile. Etude radiocirculographique. *Bordeaux Médical.*, 1977, *10*, 171-176.

19. Grosdemouge C., Le Poncin Laffitte M., Rapin J.R.: Effets protecteurs de l'extrait de Ginkgo biloba sur la rupture précoce de la barrière hémoencéphalique chez le rat. *Presse Méd.*, 1986, *15*, 1502-1505.

20. Gustafson L., Risberg J.: Regional cerebral blood flow measurements by the ^{133}Xe inhalation technique in differential diagnosis of dementia. *Acta. Neurol. Scand. Suppl.*, 1979, *60* (suppl. 72), 546-547.

21. Heiss W.D., Zeiler K.: Medikamentöse Beeinflussung der Hirndurchblutung. *Pharmacotherapie*, 1978, *1*, 137-144.

22. Hellegouarch A., Baranes J., Clostre F., Drieu K., Braquet P., De Feudis F.V.: Comparison of the contractile effects on an extract of Ginkgo biloba and some neurotransmitters on rabbit isolated vena cava. *Gen. Pharmacol.*, 1985, *16*, 129-132.

23. Jellinger K.: Neuropathological aspects of dementia resulting from abnormal blood and cerebrospinal fluid dynamics. *Acta. Neurol. Belg.*, *76*, 83-102.

24. Karcher L., Zagerman P., Krieglstein J.: Effect of an extract of Ginkgo biloba on rat brain energy metabolism in hypoxia. *Naunyn-Schmiedeberg's Arch. Pharmacol.*, 1984, *327*, 31-35.

25. Lagrue G., Baillet J., Behar A.: Activité d'un extrait végétal complexe dans les oedèmes idiopathiques orthostatiques. *Sem. Hôp. Paris.*, 1978, *54*, 214-217.

26. Lamour Y.: Systèmes cholinergiques centraux et démences de type Alzheimer. *In:* Maladie d'Alzheimer et autres démences séniles. Fondation nationale de Gérontologie, 1985, 18-29.

27. Le Devehat C., Lemoine A., Zoubenko C., Cirette B.: Mode d'action des médicaments vasoactifs dans les artériopathies diabétiques. Etude critique des explorations fonctionnelles vasculaires. *Mises à Jours Cardiologiques,* 1980, *9,* 1-8.

28. Le Poncin-Laffitte M., Martin M., Lespinasse P., Rapin. J.R.: Ischémie cérébrale après ligature non simultanée des artères carotides chez le rat: effet de l'extrait de Ginkgo biloba. *Sem. Hôp. Paris.,* 1982, *58,* 403-406.

29. Natali R., Rachinel J., Pouyat P.M.: Essai comparatif croisé en O.R.L. de deux médications vaso-actives. *Cah. d'ORL,* 1979, *14,* 185-190.

30. OMS - CIM: Manuel de la classification statistique internationale des maladies, traumatismes et causes de décès. O.M.S., Vol. 1, Genève, 1977, 271.

31. OMS: Le vieillissement des neurones et ses implications en neuropathologie humaine. Série des rapports techniques., n° 665-881.

32. Salz H.: Zur Wirksamkeit eines Ginkgo biloba Präparats bei arteriellen Durch-blutungsstörungen der unteren Extremitäten. Kontrollierte Doppelblind-Cross-Over-Studie. *Therapie der Gegenwart,* 1980, *II,* 1345-1356.

33. Saracco J.B., Estachy G.: Etude du Tanakan sur la microcirculation oculaire. *Med. Prat.,* 1980, n° 4, 67-72.

34. Schwerdtfeger F.: Traitement des vertiges par l'extrait de Ginkgo biloba, contrôles électronystagmographiques. *Therapiewoche,* 1981, *31,* 8658-8667.

35. Sinex F.M., Merril C.R.: Alzheimer disease, Down's syndrome and aging. *Ann. N. Y. Acad. Sci.,* 1982, *396,* 1-190.

36. Taylor J.E.: The effects of chronic, oral Ginkgo biloba extract administration on neurotransmitter receptor binding in young and aged "Fisher 344" rats. *In:* Effects of Ginkgo biloba extract on organic cerebral impairment, Agnoli A., Rapin J.R., Scapagnini V., Weitbrecht W.V., Eds., *John Libbey,* London, 1985, 31-34.

37. Tea S., Celsis P., Clanet M., Marc-Vergnes J.P.: Effets cliniques hémodynamiques et métaboliques de l'extrait de Ginkgo biloba en pathologie vasculaire cérébrale. *Gaz. Méd. France,* 1979, *86,* 4149-4152.

38. Tomlinson B.F., Blessed G., Roth M.: Observation on the brains of demented old people. *J. Neurol. Sci.,* 1970, *11,* 205-242.

Ginkgo Biloba Extract in the Treatment of Arteriopathy of the Lower Limbs
Sixty-Five Week Study

U. Bauer

Département de Chirurgie, Service des maladies vasculaires. Maria Hilf-Krankenhaus Dahlienweg 3. D-5483 Bad Neuenahr-Ahrweiler 1. Federal Republic of Germany

Summary

Thirty-six patients with arteritis were treated with Ginkgo biloba extract for sixty-five weeks. For the first six months of the treatment period, these patients participated in a double-blind randomised comparison with 35 well-matched patients taking placebo. Subsequently, those patients taking Ginkgo biloba extract were given the option to continue treatment on an open basis with follow-up at regular three-monthly intervals. Ginkgo biloba extract therapy gave significantly greater pain relief and walking tolerance than the placebo after six months of treatment, and this improvement continued throughout the whole duration of the study. This symptomatic and measurable improvement was combined with excellent tolerance of the drug.

The evaluation of a drug in the treatment of arteriopathy of the lower limbs is delicate. The great variability in symptomatology, the spontaneous temporary remissions related to a strictly controlled dietary regimen are well known. This trial was conceived and conducted according to the current methodological rules recommended for clinical research in this field(9, 10) in such a way as to carry out a high-quality study. The Ginkgo biloba extract (EGb 761, Rökan®, Intersan) is a standardized and titrated extract of Ginkgo biloba leaves. The beneficial effects of this medication have been demonstrated pharmacologically(1, 2, 3, 14) and clinically(4, 8, 11, 13).

Patients and Methods

The patients had had dominant unilateral pain for more than 12 months, with arteriographic proof of a unilateral occlusion of the superficial femoral artery and symptoms corresponding to Stage IIb of Fontaine's classification(6). The impact on

Rökan (Ginkgo Biloba). Recent Results in Pharmacology and Clinic
Edited by E.W. Fünfgeld
© Springer-Verlag Berlin Heidelberg New York 1988, pp. 212-220

the other arteries (deep femoral, iliac) was not considered as a criterion for exclusion from the study, insofar as these lesions did not aggravate the hemodynamic parameters. Patients with other disorders capable of interfering with walking perimeter (effort angina, respiratory insufficiency, arthritis) were excluded. The selection of patients was rigorous, for the purpose of obtaining a homogeneous group with respect to the location and severity of the lesions. Any associated treatments were evaluated carefully in order to eliminate any vasoactive, psychotropic, antihistaminic, beta-blocking, calcium antagonist, platelet antiaggregant, and anticoagulant drugs.

Before final admission to the study, the patients underwent therapeutic weaning for six weeks, during which they received placebo. Their dietary regimen was adjusted and tobacco use reduced to a maximum of five cigarettes per day. Those who had been unable to conform to this restriction by the end of this period were excluded. The same was true for patients with an increase in their walking perimeter of more than 30%, or those capable of walking a distance of more than 300 meters at the end of this placebo period.

After six weeks of weaning on placebo, the patients were divided at random into two therapeutic groups. One group received 40 mg EGb three times a day (that is, a daily dose of 120 mg), and the others, the corresponding placebo. Throughout the duration of the trial, no walking training program was implemented.

At the end of this 24-week double-blind treatment period, the randomization code was disclosed and a preliminary statistical analysis was performed(5). It was then decided to continue treating the EGb group for a longer period, but in an open study. Data were collected first at the time of selection (week -6), at the end of the drug-weaning period (week 0), then in the 6th, 12th, 24th, 52nd, and 65th weeks of treatment. Each evaluation comprised a subjective estimate of the pain by means of a 10-cm visual vertical analog scale, and an objective measurement of walking tolerance (treadmill, standard conditions of 3 km/hr), maximal distance of 600 meters, 10% inclination, temperature 20°C, in the afternoon. The distance covered before the appearance of pain was noted, as was the total distance covered. All of these data were correlated with the blood pressure at the ankle after effort. Furthermore, a plethys-mograph was taken with venous occlusion by a pneuomatic cuff inflated for three minutes, as well as a Doppler test at rest and immediately after effort.

Heart rate, blood pressure, weight, and side effects were regularly noted. The hematological and biochemical parameters were evaluated at weeks 0, 24, and 52. Both the patient and the investigator were asked to give their overall evaluation of the treatment, using the terms "very good", "good", "moderate", or "poor". Because of the length of the study, adherence was attentively monitored by verifying the content of the bottles. Any patient having forgotten or refused to take 10% or more of the prescribed treatment throughout the duration of the test was eliminated. In conformity with the Helsinki agreement, an informal verbal consent to the therapeutic trial was obtained from each patient.

Statistical analysis

A preliminary analysis was made at the end of the 24th week of the double-blind trial(15). An additional analysis was done after 35 weeks, then a third at the end of the total 65-week period. Furthermore, a two-factor analysis of variance (ANOVA) was performed, taking the drug treatment as probability for one factor and the successive test periods as the probability for the other factor. The method adopted was that of the least squares, and the Newman-Keuls model was selected for the test *a posteriori,* by considering a probability of less than 0.01 as being the level of significance, these two techniques being recommended by Kirk(12). In the final analysis, the orthogonal polynomial coefficients were used to test the linearity of all tendencies apparent over time, while following the methods recommended by Kirk(12). The Student t-test was used to analyze the results recorded in the course of the paramedical investigations.

Results

From the 80 patients recruited at the time of the dual initial phase of this study, one was excluded for nonconformity to the criteria for inclusion, 44 were treated with EGb, and 35 with placebo. The variables (sex, age, weight, height, diabetic or not, location of the lesions and pain) did not show significant differences between the two groups. However, despite the randomization, the group treated with EGb seemed to present a more severe symptomatology. Forty-one of the 44 patients treated with EGb choose to continue taking the drug during a long-term open study, and 36 patients (average age 60.7-1.3 years) were followed for 65 weeks. Five of the 41 patients were eliminated from the study for medical reasons which were not related to the drug treatment: one accidental wound, one cerebral vascular accident, one pulmonary carcinoma, one myocardial infarction, one congestive cardiac insufficiency. The mean body weight remained unchanged for the patients treated regularly with EGb (72.7 kg ± 1.8 kg).

Visual analog scale

The pain, as it was subjectively experienced and reported on this 10-cm scale, diminished in both groups throughout each study period, as shown in *Table 1*. The preliminary statistical analysis made at 24 weeks showed a highly significant reduction (P < 0.01) in pain over the course of time in the group treated with EGb. The improvement was almost four times that obtained with placebo. This improvement was confirmed in the 39 patients who continued the therapy for 54 weeks, and the 36 who continued for 65 weeks.

Walking perimeter

The results on walking perimeter before the appearance of pain and on the maximal distance covered, is reported in *Figure 1*.

In the EGb group, at the 24th, 52nd, and 65th weeks, a statistically significant gradual improvement was found ($P < 0.01$) with respect to the distance covered before the appearance of pain and in that for the total distance covered. The placebo group also showed a significant improvement ($P < 0.05$) in distance covered before the painful sensation, but the increase in total distance covered was not significant. In the placebo group, one patient had to undergo an operation in week 12, and there were therefore not enough data available at week 24. In another patient the total distance covered could not be measured in week 24 because of an angina pectoris.

In the group treated with EGb, as time passed it was found that an increasing number of patients were capable of covering the total distance of 600 meters: seven patients (15.9%) at week 24, seven (17.9%) at week 52, and nine (25%) at week 65. In the placebo group, only two patients (5.7%) were able to cover the distance of 600 meters at week 24. In fact, as early as the 24th week, the improvement in the EGb group, calculated in percentage, was spectacular, and this continued until the 65th week.

Plethysmography

The plethysomograph gives a significant advantage ($P < 0.01$) to the EGb group over the placebo group at week 24, if we consider both mean blood circulation and maximal circulation in the more severely affected member. However, the time required in order to reach maximal circulation did not vary notably.

Table 1

Results from subjective evaluation of pain according to the Visual Analog Scale.

Average distance measured	Weeks of Treatment			
in mm from 0 cm (represent-ing absence of pain)	0	24	52 (n=39)	65 (n=36)
Placebo s.e. (n=35)	59.6 2.0	57.7 2.1 n.s.	–	–
EGb s.e.	64.8 1.9	43.3 2.7 $P < 0.01$	37.9 2.3 $P < 0.01$	28.6 3.44 $P < 0.01$

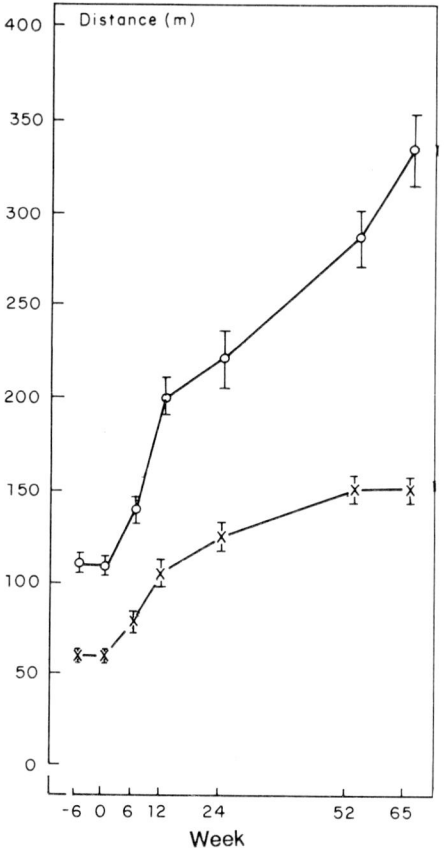

Figure 1: Results of exercise on the treadmill. Walking perimeter as a function of distance covered before the appearance of pain (x–x) and average total distance covered (o–o). (The bars represent the standard error.)

Doppler test

The Doppler resting test was not improved in either of the two groups. After effort, in the EGb group only, a slow improvement was noted, which became significant in the 52nd week (P < 0.05) and in the 65th week (P < 0.01).

In a majority of the patients the pressure at the ankle immediately after effort was below 60 mmHg, which confirms the ischemic origin of the pain.

Clinical and biological parameters

No special effects on blood pressure or heart rate were recorded, and the results from the hematological and biochemical examinations showed no adverse effects on renal and hepatic functions. The increase in cholesterol level, observed in both groups at week 24, was not maintained in Group EGb, the levels having returned to the initial values at week 52.

Tolerance, observance, and overall evaluation

EGb was well tolerated throughout the treatment period, which is indicated by the excellent observance on the part of the patients. No patient was eliminated from the study because of refusing or forgetting the treatment. At the end of the treatment period, an overall evaluation of "good" or "very good" was given by the investigator and by 31 patients.

Statistical analysis

The numerical irregularity of each treatment group in the first part of the study arose from human error made by the person responsible for distributing the treatments. Because of this unfortunate error, and in order to avoid poor interpretation of the results, a separate but identical statistical analysis was made on the first 47 patients (23 placebo and 24 EGb) who were admitted to the study before the error in randomization had been made. This analysis confirms the overall results on all points, with the same profile of improvement, in particular with respect to tolerance to walking.

Discussion

It has long been known how difficult it is to conduct a controlled clinical trial in intermittent claudication. A certain number of possible explanations may be advanced to explain either subjective or objective clinical improvement. Among these is found variability in the history and potential for spontaneous improvement or even improvement resulting from regular exercise or from stopping smoking. The greatest care has been applied to the methodology of this study, and everything has been done in order to comply as completely as possible with the recently published recommendations on this subject(9,10).

Ginkgo biloba extract has already been tested in arteriopathies of the lower extremities(4, 8, 11, 13, 15) and the results have confirmed the efficacy of this drug in various forms of distal circulatory insufficiency.

The clinical improvement recorded, both from the standpoint of improvement in pain and from that of increased walking perimeter, is in perfect agreement with the overall evaluation as expressed by both the patients and the investigator. Most of the patients admitted to this study were smokers, but all of these who were incapable of limiting their consumption to fewer than five cigarettes per day were dropped at the end of the six-week pre-inclusion period (therapeutic weaning and observation). The good observance of this prescription was verified at each consultation. This reduction in tobacco, and perhaps a consecutive increase in dietary intake, might explain the increase in blood cholesterol recorded in both therapeutic groups in the course of the first part of the trial. A significant decrease in triglycerides ($P < 0.05$ at the 65th week), as well as a return of the HDLs to normal was obtained in patients treated long-term, and perhaps resulted from the restriction of tobacco and alcohol during the trial. Furthermore, no prescription was given for walking practice.

These findings are in agreement with those of Widmer et al(16), who concluded that the major risk factors in peripheral arteriopathies are tobacco, hypertension, and an elevation of beta-lipoproteins. All of our patients benefited from treatment with Ginkgo biloba extract, regardless of their type of arteriopathy, diabetics included, and regardless of the severity of their condition.

The suggested mechanism of action for EGb is an improvement in cellular metabolism, particularly in the hypoxic and ischemic areas. This could be demonstrated by measuring oxygen and glucose consumptions(14); but it was also necessary to take into consideration a capacity for "scavenging" free radicals(7). Quite as important is the action of the drug at the vascular level, which is reflected by an increase in blood flow(1, 2, 3). The mechanisms brought into play are in agreement with the results of this study; they confirm that in this type of disease, Ginkgo biloba extract is an important and effective therapy.

Conclusion

The elimination of risk factors is a therapeutic solution that is rarely adequate in arteriopathies of the lower extremities. An additional therapy – in the form of a drug which is active orally – is necessary in the face of reparative surgery. In this long-term trial comprising an initial phase conducted in double-blind, EGb made it possible to obtain both subjective and objective improvements from the standpoint of the painful sensations and from that of improvement in walking perimeter. These beneficial effects, which were shown to be stable over time, as well as the absence of significant side effects, in our opinion make Ginkgo biloba extract a drug of choice among agents administered orally in the treatment of arteriopathies of the lower limbs.

References

1. Auguet M., DeFeudis F.V., Clostre F., Deghenghi R.: Effects of an extract of Ginkgo biloba on rabbit isolated aorta. *Gen. Pharmacol.*, 1982, *13*, 225-230.

2. Auguet M., DeFeudis F.V., Clostre F.: Effects of Ginkgo biloba on arterial smooth muscle responses to vasoactive stimuli. *Gen. Pharmacol.*, 1982, *13*, 169-171.

3. Auguet M., Clostre F.: Effects of an extract of Ginkgo biloba and diverse substances on the phasic and tonic components of the contraction of an isolated rabbit aorta. *Gen. Pharmacol.*, 1983, *14*, 277-280.

4. Bastide G., Montsarrat M.: Artérite des membranes inférieurs. Intérêt du traitement médical après intervention chirurgicale. Analyse factorielle, *Gazette Médicale de France*, 1978, *15*, 4523-4526.

5. Bauer U., Six months double-blind randomised clinical trial of Ginkgo biloba extract versus placebo in two parallel groups in patients suffering from peripheral arterial insufficiency. *Arzneimittel - Forsch/Drug Res*, 1984, *34*, 716-720.

6. Becker F.: Exploration de la fonction artérielle dans l'artériopathie chronique oblitérante des membres inférieurs par les méthodes non invasives d'exploration fonctionnelle vasculaire. Corrélation avec la classification de Leriche et Fontaine. *Lyon Médical*, 1983, *250*, 87-94.

7. Braquet P., Braquet M., Deby C.: Oxidative damage induced by cerebral ischaemia: protective role of some radical scavengers and related drugs. *J. Cereb. Blood Flow Metab.*, 1983, *3* (Suppl. 1) 564-565.

8. Courbier R., Jausseran J.M., Reggi M.: Etude à double insu croisée du Tanakan dans les artériopathies des membres inférieurs. *Méditerranée Médicale*, 1977, *126*, 61-64.

9. Cristol R., Serradimingi A.: Evaluation de l'efficacité des traitements médicaux de la claudication intermittente. 18e Congrès français de pathologie vasculaire, Paris, 14-16 mars 1984, pp., 12-18.

10. EG-Richtlinien: Vorschlag für eine Empfehlung des Rates zu den Versuchen mit Arzneispezialitäten im Hinblick auf deren Inverkehr bringen. *Pharm. Ind.*, 1984, *46*, 1123-1141.

11. Frileux C., Cope R.: L'extrait concentré de Ginkgo biloba dans les troubles vasculaires périphériques. *Cahiers d'Artériologie de Royat*, 1975, *3*, 117-122.

12. Kirk R.E.: Experimental design: procedures for the behavioural sciences. *Brooks-Cole Publishing Co.*, Belmont, California, 1968.

13. Le Devehat C., Lemoine A., Zoubenco C., Cirette B.: Etude du Tanakan dans les artériopathies diabétiques distales. Etude critique des explorations fonctionnelles vasculaires. *Mise à jour Cardiologiques,* 1980, *IX,* 1-8.

14. Le Poncin-Lafitte M., Martin P., Lespinasse P., Rapin J.R.: Ischémie cérébrale après ligature non simultanée des artères carotides chez le rat: Effet de l'extrait de Ginkgo biloba. *Semaine des Hôpitaux de Paris,* 1982, *58,* 403-406.

15. Salz H.: Zur Wirksamkeit eines Ginkgo biloba-Präparats bei arteriellen Durchblutungsstörungen der unteren Extremitäten. Kontrollierte Doppelblind-Cross-over-Studie. *Therapie de Gegenwart,* 1980, *119,* 1345-1356.

Idiopathic Cyclic Edema
Role of Capillary Hyperpermeability and its Correction by Ginkgo Biloba Extract

G. Lagrue, A. Behar, M. Kazandjian, K. Rahbar

Service de Néphrologie, Hôpital Henri Mondor, F 94010 Créteil

Summary

Idiopathic cyclic oedema is a frequent and often unrecognized condition in young women. It is characterized by water and sodium retention with secondary hyperaldosteronism due to capillary hyperpermeability.

Treatment is not easy. It includes spironolactone, sometimes sympathomimetics and hygienic-dietetic measures. Thiazide diuretics and laxatives must be avoided. Correcting the capillary defect is of paramount importance. This defect is detected and measured by Landis' labelled albumin test.

The authors have tried Ginkgo biloba extract administered orally or by intravenous infusion. Full correction of the biological anomaly was obtained in 10 cases in which Landis' test was performed before and after oral treatment, and in the 5 cases treated by intravenous infusion.

The syndrome of orthostatic idiopathic edema described by Mach in 1955(6) is a frequent condition which has long been unrecognized. It occurs in women of childbearing age; it is frequently combined with endocrine-gynecological disorders(1, 2).

Physiopathological review

Clinically, the idiopathic edema syndrome is characterized by diurnal weight gain, rapid and labile, with swelling of the legs and ankles. This weight gain, which causes weight variations of more than 1.5 kg in a day's time, is related to diffuse swelling involving the skin and the hypodermis as well as the muscles. All of these disorders are maximal in prolonged standing position, and they are consistently aggravated by heat and improved by decubitus and simple rest at night(3, 4, 6). The condition evolves by recrudescence, with the edema regressing only incompletely as it becomes permanent. The edematous flare-ups are often accompanied by polydipsia, oliguria, asthenia, effort dyspnea, constipation, and headaches.

Rökan® (Ginkgo Biloba). Recent Results in Pharmacology and Clinic
Edited by E.W. Fünfgeld
© Springer-Verlag Berlin Heidelberg New York 1988, pp. 221-227

After several years, a chronic edematous condition has become installed, punctuated by more acute outbursts.

From the biological standpoint, the orthostatic idiopathic edema syndrome is characterized by water-sodium retention in orthostatism with secondary hyperaldosteronism related to exaggeration of capillary permeability(4). This hyperpermeability, which extends to the lymphatic vessels, constitutes the essential physiopathological element and explains the loss of water and proteins from the vascular sector and the diminution in volemia. Luteal insufficiency is very often present and intervenes at least partially in the genesis of the capillary permeability disorder(5).

Treatment is difficult. Maintenance psychotherapy is indispensable, but it should be covertly performed, without ever letting it be known that the disturbances experienced are excessive. First of all iatrogenic complications must be avoided, such as the abuse of laxatives and/or saluretics. In order to limit secondary hyperaldosteronism, diets too low in sodium must be avoided, and moderate doses of spironolactone (100 to 300 mg/day) should be added in order to prevent the patients, yearning for the spectacular effects of diuretics on the edema and of laxatives on their constipation, from becoming addicted again to these medications.

This treatment is effective, but is still purely symptomatic; the disturbances reappear little by little after suspension of the treatment.

Some, on the basis of the hypothesis of a lack of venous vasoconstriction, suggest the use of sympathomimetics. The administration of dihydroergotamine also seems to reduce the effects of orthostatism. The use of an elastic restraint bandage on the lower limbs is useful, since it partially reduces the effects of orthostatism(3). Physical measures are also recommended which, when practiced regularly, contribute to improvement in the swelling syndrome: elevating the foot of the bed; performing gymnastics while lying down (mainly pedaling movements); avoiding prolonged standing, and, if possible, the harmful effects of heat; among sports, swimming is certainly one of the most beneficial.

Administration of progestationals in the second part of the cycle is an indispensable element in all cases where luteal insufficiency exists(5).

Finally, an attempt must be made to correct the disturbed capillary permeability, the essential physiopathological element in this syndrome.

Patients and methods

The capillary permeability disorder can be evaluated by the following methods:

After the injection of radio-iodinated albumin, the radioactivity curve shows the loss of albumin from the vascular sector, mainly in orthostatism. Serial measurements are taken, by successive blood samples, of the radioactivity in the circulating blood during the first two hours.

The Landis isotopic test is both simpler and more accurate. After i.v. injection of albumin tagged with technetium (99 mTc), the radioactivity of the circulating blood is measured on the forearms externally by use of a gamma camera. A cuff is placed on one of the arms, exerting pressure of 80 mmHg for ten to 12 minutes; the cuff is then removed and the measurement is continued for approximately ten minutes. Under normal conditions, the elevation in venous pressure in the forearms has the result of blood stasis with increased radioactivity. If capillary permeability is normal, there is little diffusion of albumin outside of the vessels, and, after removal of the cuff, radioactivity falls rapidly, returning to its previous level within several minutes (*Figure 1*).

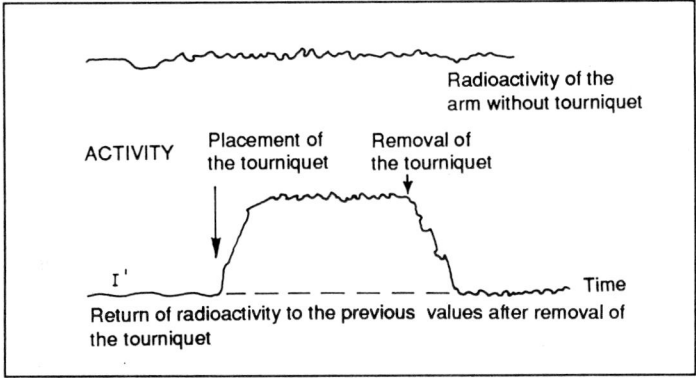

Figure 1. Normal subject. No retention of tagged albumin.

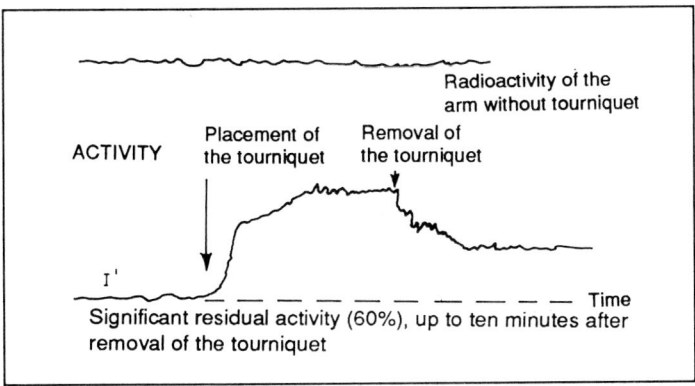

Figure 2. Pathological subject. Retention of tagged albumin.

In the case of abnormal capillary permeability, the increase in venous pressure is accompanied by diffusion of the tagged albumin into the interstitial spaces. When the cuff is removed, radioactivity falls more slowly than in the normal subject and stabilizes at a level higher than the initial level. There is retention of the tagged albumin (*Figure 2*). The percentage of albumin thus retained is a function of the intensity of the capillary permeability disorder. It is calculated as a function of the number of impulses (IPM).

$$\frac{C - A}{B - A} \times 100 = \text{percent retention.}$$

A being baseline radioactivity, B being radioactivity attained at balance under the cuff, C being radioactivity measured six minutes after removal of the cuff (*Figures 2 and 3*).

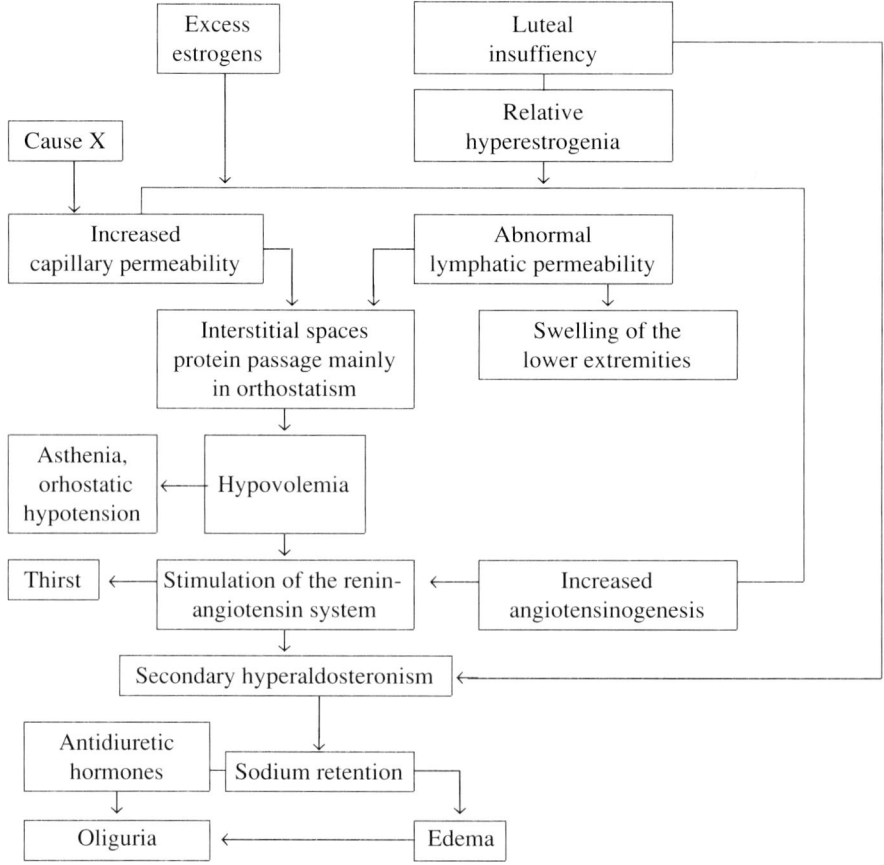

Figure 3: Diagram of the physiopathology of idiopathic cyclic edema syndrome.

In 30 cases of clinically definite orthostatic idiopathic edema, a disturbance in capillary permeability was present in all cases with retention ranging from 10% to 40% (N <8%). The magnitude of the retention figure obtained by isotopic counting reflects the intensity of the edematous syndrome. On the contrary, in edema secondary to the abuse of diuretics and laxatives, the capillary permeability test was always normal, even in the presence of edema.

The properties of Ginkgo biloba extract led us to use it in order to attempt to correct the disturbance in capillary permeability and to study its effect on the chronic symptoms of the syndrome. Ginkgo biloba extract was used:

- either as an oral solution administered for durations of one to six months at the dose of 4 to 6 mL/day (or 160 to 240 mg of dry extract);

- or as the injectable preparation, lyophilized extract (IPS 200, Rökan®, Intersan, not marketed) administered every day at the dose of four to six bottles, that is, 200 to 300 mg lyophilized extract in slow infusion for one hour in 250 mL isotonic glucose solution, four to five days in succession.

The treated patients were all suffering with a clinically proven orthostatic idiopathic edema syndrome, confirmed by a positive Landis isotopic test, a index of 10 to 30%.

Group I: 11 women were treated orally and the Landis test was given before and after four to eight weeks of treatment. At the same time studies were made of capillary resistance (in five cases), blood pressure, weight and magnitude of the edema, and tolerance.

Group II: five patients received the treatment by infusion in the course of hospitalization required by a particularly intense edematous flareup. The Landis isotopic test was performed before and after five days of infusion.

Results

Group I

Complete correction of the physical abnormality was obtained: the tests which were all initially disturbed became normal after one to two months of treatment in the ten cases in which the test could be given before and after treatment.

Parallel with the changes in capillary permeability, capillary resistance was distinctly improved in the cases in which the study could be made before and after treatment.

One of the 11 women treated interrupted the treatment on the tenth day because of unconvincing symptoms which she attributed to the test product.

In the other ten patients we obtained the following modifications in the so-called cyclic edema syndrome (weight, diuresis) in comparison with the treatment which had been followed (antialdosterone):

– three very good results (disappearance of the edema),
– six good results (improvement in the edema),
– one fairly good result.

Blood pressure, initially low in most cases, was moderately increased, which is a logical result of reduction in capillary permeability, and therefore of correction of the hypovolemia.

Let us note also in one case the disappearance of constipation.

Overall tolerance was good. In only two cases out of 11, some disorders were attributed to Ginkgo biloba extract but without the responsibility of the product having been proved. For one of these, muscular cramps were involved, not requiring suspension of treatment, and for the other patient palpitation and insomnia which resulted in interrupting the treatment on the tenth day.

Group II

In the five patients treated with IPS 200 infusion, the capillary permeability test repeated at the end of treatment was normal; at the same time an increase was noted in water-sodium diuresis, with a weight loss of 2 to 5 kg. Local and systemic tolerance were generally excellent. The treatment was then continued orally.

Discussion

Disturbance in capillary permeability has as a consequence stereotyped clinical symptoms, particularly exacerbation of orthostatism disorders and orthostatic hypotension. The causes and mechanisms of capillary hyperpermeability are certainly multiple and within the framework of this syndrome several entities probably exist, some of which have recently been identified, such as Gleich's syndrome (cyclic edema with hypereosinophilia, concerning which we recently reported a case history), and cyclic shock syndrome with monoclonal gammapathy, one case of which is reported in this same issue.

When the cause or mechanism of the capillary permeability disorder is unknown, the syndrome is called idiopathic; its occurrence exclusively in women suggests the role of hormonal factors and, in particular, of luteal insufficiency, since the correction of the latter by progesterone improves the capillary permeability disturbance. But other factors probably play a part, as indicated by the action of substances with Vitamin P activity (flavonoids, diosmine, anthocyanosides, rutin, etc.), and in particular that of Ginkgo extract.

In summary, in women suffering with orthostatic idiopathic edema, it is necessary first of all to avoid therapeutic errors, the sources of iatrogenic complications (use of thiazide diuretics, abuse of laxatives). The results obtained by the various methods which we have reviewed are encouraging: some unquestionable improvements have been observed, but at the cost of very long-term treatment, the multiplicity and magnitude of the subjective disorders often making evaluation of the clinical results difficult.

References

1. Behar A., Baillet J., Lagrue G.: Une nouvelle méthode de mesure de la per-méabilité capillaire par méthode isotopique. *J. Mal. Vasc.*, 1977, *2*, 101-104.

2. Gleich G., Schroeter A., Marcoux J.P. et coll.: Episodic angioedema associated with eosinophilia. *N. Engl. J. Med.*, 1984, *310*, 1621-1626.

3. Kuchel O., Horry K., Gregorova I., Marek J., Kopecka J., Kobilkova J.: Inap-propriate response to upright posture: a precipitating factor in the pathogenesis of idiopathic edema. *Ann. Intern. Med.*, 1970, *73*, 245-251.

4. Lagrue G., Weil B., Behar A.: Le syndrome d'œdèmes idiopathiques orthosta-tiques. *J. Mal. Vas.*, 1977, *2*, 93-100.

5. Lagrue G., Behar A., Morville R.: Etude de la fonction ovarienne au cours des œdèmes idiopathiques orthostatiques. *Presse Méd.*, 1983, *12*, 2859-2862.

6. Mach R., Fabre J., Mullera J., Neher R., Borth R.: Œdème idiopathique par rétention sodique avec hyperaldostéronurie. *Bull. Soc. Med. Hop.*, Paris, 1955, *106*, 726-736

Recurrent Shock Associated with Monoclonal Gammopathy
Acute and Chronic Treatment with Oral and Parenteral Ginkgo Biloba Extract

G. Lagrue, K. Rahbar, A. Behar, A. Sobel, J. Laurent

Service de Néphrologie, Hôpital Henri Mondor, F 94010 Créteil

Summary

In a rare but severe case of hypovolaemic shock related to monoclonal gammopathy, intravenous infusion of Ginkgo biloba extract resulted in dramatic recovery. Treatment was pursued with the oral form.

In the group of capillary hyperpermeability syndromes, cyclic shock syndrome with monoclonal gammopathy stands out. Since the first observation by Clarkson in 1960 and the first French case history by Larcan in 1969, 15 case histories have been published; the relationship between monoclonal gammopathy and capillary permeability disturbance is still a mystery, and no therapy has yet proved effective(1, 2, 3, 4).

This syndrome comprises recurrent shock conditions, very severe, very difficult to treat, related to increased capillary permeability and characterized by an increase in hematocrit and a decrease in albuminemia, a dissociation which signals vascular hyperpermeability with vascular extravasation of proteins.

Case history

This involves a woman born in 1938; the condition started suddenly in November 1975 with a major state of shock, with hypovolemia and hemoconcentration (hematocrit 67%), very difficult to control and lasting more than 30 hours. In the course of ten years of later evolution, the following observations were made:

– Existence of monoclonal gammopathy of benign type with a kappa IgG peak between 5 and 10 g/L, combined with a moderate decrease in C3 (63 to 80 mg/L) and in C4 (10 to 16 mg/100 mL).

Rökan (Ginkgo Biloba). Recent Results in Pharmacology and Clinic
Edited by E.W. Fünfgeld
© Springer-Verlag Berlin Heidelberg New York 1988, pp. 228-230

– Demonstration of a disturbance in capillary permeability by the Landis isotopic test. This abnormality exists permanently to various degrees; in the course of primary shock, the retention index is 55%, a very high level (N < 7%). In the absence of treatment, the index varies between 25 and 40%. This capillary permeability disorder is accompanied by chronic clinical signs, comparable to those of idiopathic edema: diffuse edema and swelling, predominant in the lower extremities, aggravated by standing, with chronic asthenia, rapid weight variations, orthostatic hypotension. These manifestations had been in existence for several years when the first shock occurred. The capillary permeability disorder was corrected more or less completely, with the indices returning to less than 20% with the administration of IPS 200 (Rökan®, Intersan, not marketed): either by infusion (six 50-mg bottles every day for five days) resulting in transitory normalization of the Landis test; or orally, at high dosage (400 mg of pure extract per day). This treatment, given continuously, was shown to be the only one to produce a definite clinical (sic).

In the course of the evolution, two new episodes of cyclic shock occurred: one took place in August 1978, several days after several plasma exchange sessions which had brought about transitory normalization of capillary permeability, with the same difficulties in resuscitation; the other occurred in June 1985, with the same prodromic signs as the first two times: sudden exacerbation of the edema with diarrhea and hypotension. Treatment by infusions of Ginkgo biloba extract (400 mg of extract in two hours) was followed by a spectacular improvement in all of the signs.

Comments

Capillary permeability disorder is easily demonstrated and measured by the Landis isotopic test. By means of this test it is possible to evaluate the magnitude of the disorder, to follow its variations, and to study the influence of various therapies.

The edematous syndrome with disturbed capillary permeability is present outside of crises, with a symptomatology that is entirely comparable to that of idiopathic cyclic edema.

The link between monoclonal gammopathy and disturbed capillary permeability was confirmed by the evolution after plasmapheresis: we observed transitory disappearance of the capillary permeability disorder parallel to the decrease in the monoclonal peak (from 8 to 4 g/L) with secondarily a rebound and occurrence of severe shock. But the mechanism leading to increased capillary permeability is still under debate.

The permanent presence of a decrease in C3 and C4, found in our patient, has been reported in other observations(1); the mechanism of this abnormality and its role in the capillary permeability disorder are unknown.

Lastly, this observation allows us to emphasize the favorable effects of Ginkgo biloba extract in this condition for which no treatment was known until now: rapid regression of a state of shock, and thanks to prolonged treatment, improvement in the capillary permeability disorder with parallel diminution of the various associated clinical signs. Whereas the spontaneous prognosis is usually very gloomy (four deaths among ten cases in less than three years), the current survival time of our patient is more than ten years.

References

1. Atkinson J.P., Waldmann T.A., Stein S.F., Gelfand J.A., Mc Donal W.J., Heck L.W., Cohen E.L., Kaplan A.P., Franck M.M.: Systemic capillary leak syndrom and monoclonal IgG gammopathy. *Medicine*, 1977, *56*, 225-239.

2. Clarkson B., Thompson D.K., Horwirth M., Luckey E.H.: Cyclical edema and shock due to increased capillary permeability. *Am. J. Med.*, 1960, *29*, 193-216.

3. George C., Regnier B., Le Gall J.R., Gastine H., Carlet J., Rapin M.: Hypovolemic shock with oedema due to increased capillary permeability. *Intensive Care Med.*, 1978, *4*, 159-163.

4. Larcan A., Calamai M., Heully M.C., Helmer J.: Choc cyclique par exagération de la perméabilité vasculaire. *Presse Méd.*, 1969, *77*, 1931-1934.

Treatment of Senile Macular Degeneration with Ginkgo Biloba Extract
A Preliminary Double-Blind Study Versus Placebo

D. A. Lebuisson, L. Leroy, G. Rigal

Centre Médico-Chirurgical Foch. F 92151 Suresnes Cedex

Summary

Senile macular degeneration is a frequent cause of blindness for which there is no satisfactory medical treatment. A double-blind trial comparing Ginkgo biloba extract with a placebo was conducted in 10 out-patients at the Hôtel Foch. Drug effectiveness was assessed on the results of fundoscopy and of measurements of visual acuity and visual field.

In spite of the small population sample, a statistically significant improvement in long distance visual acuity was observed after treatment with Ginkgo biloba extract. The assumed pathogenesis of senile macular degeneration is discussed with emphasis on free oxygenated radicals.

Senile macular degeneration is a frequent clinical entity. Unfortunately, to give such a diagnosis often amounts to a finding of failure resulting in a gradual and irreversible loss of central visual acuity.

Its pathogenesis is still poorly defined: there has been agreement for several years in acknowledging its multifactorial origin. An attempt has been made to individualize the various factors implicated in order to suggest appropriate therapeutic approaches, but at the present time no medical treatment has proved to be clinically effective.

Ginkgo biloba extract (EGb 761, Rökan®, Intersan) having shown in numerous pharmacological studies some protective properties toward the membranes and cellular metabolism, it seemed legitimate to test it in human pharmacology in this indication, while conforming to a currently well-structured methodology: a randomized double-blind study in comparison with placebo.

Rökan (Ginkgo Biloba). Recent Results in Pharmacology and Clinic
Edited by E.W. Fünfgeld
© Springer-Verlag Berlin Heidelberg New York 1988, pp. 231-236

Methods

This clinical trial combines 20 case histories of senile maculopathy followed in consultation at the Foch Medico-Surgical Center.

Criteria for selection

The patients, more than 55 years of age, had recent senile maculopathy (diagnosed for less than one year), confirmed by angiography, without any detectable abnormality other than arteriosclerosis related to age, and distant visual acuity of more than one-tenth.

Excluded were patients not meeting these criteria for inclusion because of another ophthalmological impairment such as diabetic or hypertensive retinopathy, chorioretinitis, chronic glaucoma, maculopathy of other origin (congenital, infectious, inflammatory, or myopic). The same was true for patients having opacification of the transparent media of the eye, making angiographic exploration impossible, as well as those suitable for ophthalmological surgery or laser photocoagulation in the course of the trial, or who could not interrupt a treatment which might skew analysis of the results, in particular drugs of the same therapeutic class as Ginkgo biloba extract, anticoagulants, and platelet antiaggregants.

Establishing the diagnosis

The diagnosis was performed by the ophthalmologist as a function of examination of the fundus of the eye with the three-glass test which evaluated particularly the magnitude of the areas of ischemia, edema, and hemorrhages; fluoresceine angiography, which made it possible to confirm the diagnosis and to the analyze the lesions; measurement of distant and near visual acuity for each eye with correction; analysis of the visual field according to the technique of Friedmann.

Monitoring of the evolution was based upon examination of the fundus of the eye, measurement of distant and near visual acuity, and analysis of the visual field.

Conduct of the test

After verification of the selection criteria, the patients received a case history number which governed the treatment group to which they were assigned. A balanced distribution of the patients between the two groups was carried out before the beginning of the study by means of a permutation table. The consent of each patient had been obtained before inclusion in the trial, after which the purpose and method were explained to them.

Drug treatments in progress were continued only insofar as they were absolutely necessary and had been prescribed for more than three months.

For the therapeutic study, the patients received either Ginkgo biloba extract or placebo of the same appearance, same odor, and same taste at the dosage of 2 mL twice a day, that is, for Ginkgo biloba extract, 80 mg morning and evening.

The therapeutic study lasted for six months, and the same parameters were measured in the same paraclinical tests performed at the end of treatment.

For the statistical analysis, the Student t-test was used for the quantitative variables, and the χ^2 test for the qualitative variables.

Results

Before treatment, the two groups presented no significant difference; average age EGb 64.7 ± 9.5 years; placebo 67.5 ± 8 years.

On distance visual acuity (Table 1)

Under the influence of the treatment, the two study groups evolved in significantly different manners. Visual acuity in the most affected eye gained 2.3/10 in the group of patients treated with Ginkgo biloba extract. The evolution of the control group was not significant. It was noted that at the time of inclusion in the study, the patients on EGb had less visual acuity than those in the placebo group (difference not statistically significant).

Table 1

Acuity of distant vision: evolution at the end of six months of treatment

Treatment	EGb	Placebo
Number of patients	10	10
Most affected eye at time of inclusion (1/10)	3.8 ± 0.6	4.8 ± 0.9
Six months later (1/10)	6.1 ± 0.8	5.4 ± 1.06
Gain	2.3 ± 0.7	0.6 ± 0.37
Significance	Student t-test: $P < 0.05$	NS
	intergroup analysis, Student t-test: $P < 0.09$	

On near visual acuity

Near visual acuity, measured with the Parinaud scale, improved, but in a non-statistically significant manner. the same was true for analysis of the visual field according to the technique of Friedmann.

The overall evaluation by the physician, based on all of the clinical data, is shown in *Table 2*. It was found that there is a difference between the two groups ($\chi^2 = 12.05$; 2 degrees of freedom $P < 0.01$); it is definitely in favor of EGb (nine out of ten patients were improved or very improved).

Table 2

Clinical opinion of the practitioner. Code: 1 = definite exacerbation; 2 = slight exacerbation; 3 = stabilization; 4 = slight improvement; 5 = distinct improvement.

Scoring (from 1 to 5)	1	2	3	4	5
Placebo (No. of patients)	3	1	4	2	0
EGb (No. of patients)	0	0	1	6	3

Discussion

These results, although limited, should be analyzed in the light of what is known about the pathogenesis of senile macular degeneration in order to be better understood. Different authors have attempted to outline the various pathogenic factors.

They have been able to emphasize the role of primary subretinal hemorrhages(3), damage to the vessels, to the choriocapillary, and the retina(4, 7), an inflammatory reaction in the choroid(6), appearance of a vaso-proliferative factor following localized destruction of the choriocapillary(5), the existence of histological precursors(1) (accumulation of hyalin material between the basal of the pigmental epithelium and Brüch's membrane, the appearance of drüsen, disorganization of Brüch's membrane, and a functional alteration in the pigmented epithelium).

In this pathogenic chain, everything happens as if these successive changes accumulate in order to promote the appearance of subretinal neovessels at a later stage.

Some exogenous factors have also been reported(8). In particular, excessive exposure to light could play a role in senile macular degeneration: heating of the retina would play a part, but cooling at the time of irrigation (normally very important) becomes deficient and the action directs light rays onto the photoreceptors. In subjects of the White race, the paucity of retinal pigmentation has been mentioned as a promoting factor. In fact, the pigmental epithelium and the photoreceptors of the macular area would be more exposed by the reflection of photons on the sclera, with this bombardment by photons bringing about in the saccules of the photoreceptors in the retina, a very oxygenated tissue, the production of free radicals with a change in the biological membranes.

Physiologically, the pigmented epithelium phagocytes the waste material from the photoreceptors. The photochemical aggression contributes to the accumulation of lipofuchsines in the pigmented epithelium. In senile macular degeneration, cellular debris would no longer be digested by the epithelial cells, causing the appearance of histological stigmata.

Recent pharmacological studies(8) showed that the acquisition of a free radical scavenger protects the neurosensorial retina at the time of continuous luminous trauma. The oxygenated free radicals are not only a subproduct of the action of light on the retina. Their role in situations of tissue ischemia has been shown. The variability of tissue oxygen concentrations in the course of these situations promotes the genesis of toxic forms of oxygen, dangerous for the cellular membranes, which promote the formation of retinal edema. Ginkgo biloba extract, which has proved its capacity for scavenging free radicals(2) and its good retinal concentration, merits use in human pharmacology.

Conclusion

This therapeutic trial, although including a limited number of case histories, seems to us to furnish proof of the value of Ginkgo biloba extract in the treatment of recent senile macular degenerations. In fact, after six months of treatment, a significant improvement was found in acuity of distance vision, which for the patient is obviously an essential criterion in his life relationships.

Such a result in these degenerative diseases is encouraging, even though the ophthalmoscopic signs did not show a significant evolution; the therapeutic objective in these maculopathies most often being to obtain stabilization of the lesions and improvement of the visual deficit.

References

1. Coscas G.: Pathogénie de la dégénérescence maculaire sénile. *Bull. Soc. Belge Ophtal.*, 1984, *209,* 117-127.

2. Doly M., Braquet P.: Effet des radicaux libres oxygénés sur l'activité électro-physiologique de la rétine isolée de rat. *J. Fr. Ophtalmol.*, 1985, *8,* 273-277.

3. Gass J.D.M.: Pathogenesis of disciform detachment of the neuro-epithelium. *Am. J. Ophtalmol.*, 1967, *63,* 573.

4. Kornzweig A.L.: Changes in the choriocapillaris associated with senile macular degeneration. *Annal. Ophtalmol.*, 1977, *9*, 753-764.

5. Ryan S.J.: Subretinal neo-vascularization after argon laser photocoagulation. *Arch. Klin Ophtalmol.*, 1980, *215*, 29-42.

6. Sarks S.H.: Drusen and their relationship to senile macular degeneration. *Austral. J. Ophtalmol.*, 1980, *8*, 117-130.

7. Toczynski E., Tso M.O.M.: The architecture of the choriocapillaris at the posterior pole. *Am. J. Ophtalmol.*, 1976, *81*, 428-440.

8. Tso M.: Pathogenic factors of aging macular degeneration. *Ophtalmology.*, 1985, *92*, 628-635,

Therapeutic Trial in Acute Cochlear Deafness
Comparative Study with Ginkgo Biloba Extract and Nicergoline

C. Dubreuil

Service du Pr A. Morgon, Hôpital Edouard Herriot, F 69000 Lyon

Summary

Ischemia and the metabolic disorder it entails would seem to be the pathogenic mechanism behind acute cochlear deafness, irrespective of the triggering process.

The prognosis is entirely dependent on the rapid initiation of an effective treatment. At the end of a double-blind therapeutic trial comparing Ginkgo biloba extract and a standard alpha blocker (nicergoline), a significant recovery was observed in both therapeutic groups, but improvement was distinctly better in the Ginkgo biloba group.

Ischemia of the cochlea is the histopathogenic hypothesis most frequently evoked to explain the sudden onset of perception deafness which usually appears without an obvious precipitating cause. The rapidity of institution of treatment governs the quality of recovery and seems to be an essential factor in the chronicity or non-chronicity of an auditory deficit.

This study had the purpose of comparing treatment with Ginkgo biloba extract (EGb 761, Rökan®, Intersan) to treatment with an α-blocker (nicergoline) commonly prescribed in the same indication.

Methodology

Criteria for selection

In order to be admitted to the study, the patients had to present acute cochlear deafness, partial or complete, appearing less than one week earlier. This could be idiopathic sudden deafness, or deafness due to sound trauma or to barotrauma.

Excluded were deafness of gradual onset, deafness of bacterial, toxic, neoplasic, or iatrogenic origin, or deafness related to a central neurological disease, as well as traumatic deafness due to a direct lesion (fracture of the petrous portion of the temporal

Rökan (Ginkgo Biloba). Recent Results in Pharmacology and Clinic
Edited by E.W. Fünfgeld
© Springer-Verlag Berlin Heidelberg New York 1988, pp. 237-244

bone, foreign body, rupture of the eardrum). Also, all patients who were receiving treatment impossible to interrupt and capable of interfering with evaluation of efficacy were not admitted to the study.

Criteria for judgment

Upon admission to the study, all patients were given an initial complete ORL examination including clinical and otoneurological examination, impedancemetry, electronystagmography with a caloric test and auditory evoked potentials, all tests necessary in order to verify the conditions for admission and to confirm the diagnosis.

Monitoring of the progress of the patients, as well as evaluation of therapeutic efficacy, was based on tonal audiometry, supplemented by vocal audiometry. During the hospitalization phase, that is to say until the tenth day, the audiograms were taken every two days. A final control evaluation after 30 days of treatment verified the stability of the results obtained.

In case of associated vertigo or of labyrinthic damage, the caloric tests were repeated at the end of treatment.

Conduct of the trial

After verification of the criteria for admission, the patient received a case history number which determined the treatment which he received. Treatments were distributed before the initiation of the study by balanced randomization with the assistance of random numbers.

The consent of each patient was requested before admission to the study, which was explained to him along its major outlines.

The treatments were either Ginkgo biloba extract (EGb) at the dosage of 4 mL b.i.d., or nicergoline (NCG), two tablets t.i.d., which corresponds for both products to a dosage double that ordinarily prescribed. The duration of treatment was 30 days. No other therapy was prescribed: steroid, anticoagulant, hyperbaric chamber, vasoactive treatment, etc.

Twenty patients were admitted to the study and divided into two equal groups. Two cases (one in each group) were excluded for nonobservance of the protocol (time before starting the treatment exceeded in one case, prohibited drug combination in the other).

Comparability of the groups

Both groups were strictly comparable in the beginning, with respect to the clinical data and the audiometric data.

At the time of admission, the overall average tonal audiometry deficit was:

EGb, 385.5 ± 38.9 decibels per patient, or an average loss of 64.25 decibels in the six frequencies tested.

NCG, 369.9 ± 22.9 decibels per patient, or an average loss of 61.65 decibels in the six frequencies tested.

The average age of the patients was 48 years for EGb and 51.1 years for NCG.

The average time before starting treatment was the same in both groups, 4.4 days.

Results

Tonal audiometry

This was the principal test for monitoring the evolution of the patients having acute cochlear deafness. *Table 1* presents the results for the frequencies tested at the time of the evaluations made on the tenth and 30th days. Examination of this Table will show that all of the patients at the time of their admission to the study had "severe" deafness corresponding to a mean deficit of 60 dB per frequency.

On the tenth day, a significant difference was found between the two treatment groups (*Figure 1*). In fact, from this date onward, the group treated with EGb recovered a good auditory capacity corresponding to an average gain of 30 decibels per frequency, whereas the group treated with NCG gained 21 decibels. In the EGb group this improvement continued, and at the time of the evaluation made on Day 30, the patients had gained 34 decibels per frequency on the average (NCG group 23 dB).

The relative improvement, which takes into consideration the auditory deficit measured at the time of admission before treatment was started, confirms the crude data (*Table 2, Figure 2*). The results for the EGb group are distinctly better than those for the other group. Also, between the two audition evaluations (Day 10 and Day 30), the improvement on EGb treatment continued, unlike that which was obtained with the α-blocker.

Thus, after one month of treatment, the patients in the EGb group registered a total gain which exceeded that of the NCG group by 67 dB: the difference amounted to 6 to 15 decibels, depending upon the frequencies (*Table 3*).

Table 1

Evolution of tonal audiometry as a function of frequency and treatment (nine patients per group), at the time of the various evaluations: gains on Day 10 and Day 30, frequency by frequency. Total deficit in all frequencies. Average loss per frequency.

Treatment	Frequency	Audiogram			Gain on D10	Gain on D30
		D0 decibels	D10	D30		
Ginkgo biloba extract	250 Hz	− 53.3	− 30.0	− 28.3	+ 23.3 db	+ 25 db
	500 Hz	− 57.8	− 27.2	− 25.5	+ 30.6 db	+ 32.3 db
	1000 Hz	− 62.2	− 33.9	− 30.5	+ 28.3 db	+ 31.7 db
	2000 Hz	− 64.4	− 33.9	− 31.1	+ 30.5 db	+ 33.3 db
	4000 Hz	− 66.7	− 33.9	− 30.5	+ 32.8 db	+ 36.2 db
	8000 Hz	− 81.1	− 48.9	− 35	+ 32.2 db	+ 46.1 db
	Total deficit	− 385.5	− 207.8	− 180.9	+ 177.7 db	+ 204.6 db
	Average deficit by frequency	− 64.2 (per freq.)	− 34.6 (per freq.)	− 30.1 (per freq.)	+ 30 db (per freq.)	+ 34.1 db (per freq.)
Nicergoline	250 Hz	− 40.5	− 27.2	− 28.3	+ 13.3 db	+ 12.2 db
	500 Hz	− 48.3	− 32.8	− 30.5	+ 15.5 db	+ 17.8 db
	1000 Hz	− 55.5	− 32.8	− 32.8	+ 22.7 db	+ 22.7 db
	2000 Hz	− 61.1	− 35.6	− 36.7	+ 25.5 db	+ 24.4 db
	4000 Hz	− 76.7	− 50.5	− 46.7	+ 26.2 db	+ 30 db
	8000 Hz	− 87.8	− 63.9	− 56.7	+ 23.9 db	+ 31.1 db
	Total deficit	− 369.9	− 242.8	− 231.7	+ 127.1 db	+ 138.2 db
	Average deficit by frequency	− 61.6 (per freq.)	− 40.4 (per freq.)	− 38.6 (per freq.)	+ 21.2 db (per freq.)	+ 23 db (per freq.)

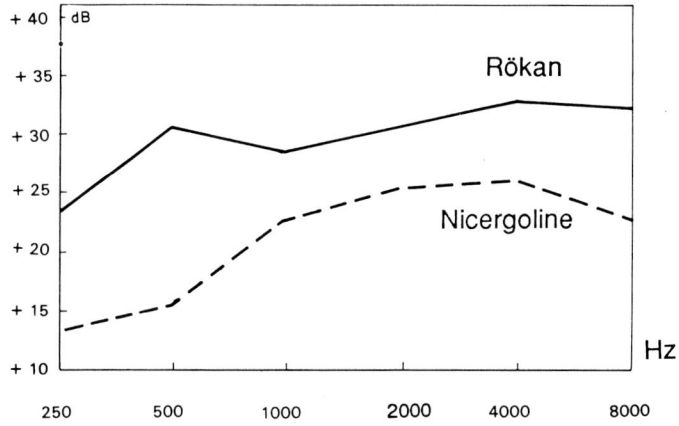

Figure 1: Average gain on Day 10

Table 2

Relative improvement, frequency by frequency, on Day 30, and relative average improvement on Day 10 and Day 30, calculated from the deficit found at the time of admission for the two treatments studied.

Frequency	Relative improvement on Day 30	
	EGb	NCG
250 Hz	38.9%	22.6%
500 Hz	52.3%	34.4%
1000 Hz	49.4%	39.1%
2000 Hz	49.7%	39.4%
4000 Hz	53.6%	41.0%
8000 Hz	58.6%	39.1%
Overall relative improvement		
Average on D10	47.5%	35.5%
Average on D30	52.3%	37.8%

Vocal audiometry

Analysis of vocal audiometry involved three parameters:
– the threshold of 50% intelligibility,
– the appearance of the curve,
– the distortion phenomena.

At the time of admission, the amplitude of the perception deafness was confirmed, and investigation of the existence of distortion. At the end of the study it was found that distortion had almost totally disappeared in both groups. Analysis of the 50% threshold of intelligibility gave the following results (on the average): EGb, 33.7 dB; NCG, 42 dB.

This corroborates the results from the tonal audiometry, since the auditory threshold was 30.1 dB in the EGb group and 38.6 dB in the NCG group.

Thus, comparison of both groups of patients by means of objective and reliable criteria demonstrated the much greater efficacy of the Ginkgo biloba extract treatment. It appears important to continue the treatment for several weeks, since it was found that audition continued to improve between the tenth and 30th days, which was not the case with the comparison treatment.

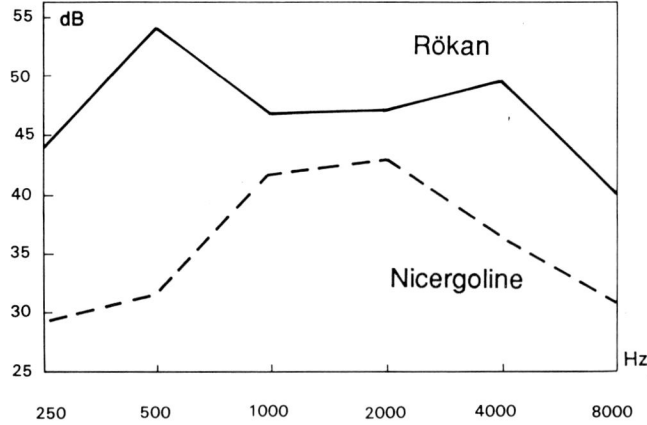

Figure 2: Relative improvement on Day 10

Associated ORL symptomatology

Labyrinth tests: the vestibular test and the caloric tests showed that all patients in the group treated with EGb (9/9) had normal tests at the end of the trial, whereas in the group treated with nicergoline, the tests remained disturbed in one-third of the patients (3/9).

As for the tinnitus, in the EGb group it was noted that all patients had recovered with the exception of two patients (one partially improved and one failure). In the NCG group, two patients recovered, and three were not improved, and two patients had only partially improved.

Overall evaluation of the ORL expert investigator

After 30 days of treatment, the ensemble of the clinical and paraclinical results as well as the complaints of the patients showed a much larger number of very good results, one moderate, one failure), than in the control group (three very good, two average, and four failures).

Tolerance

Clinical and laboratory tolerance (complete blood count, ionogram, creatinine, transaminases, platelet aggregability) were excellent in both therapeutic groups. Platelet aggregability was the subject of careful monitoring (PRP aggregometry); in the initial evaluation performed on the day of hospitalization, no platelet hyperaggregability was noted, unlike what has sometimes been described.

Table 3

Therapeutic efficacy. Audiometric gain, frequency by frequency, for both treatments studied, and difference in gain by frequency between these two groups (EGb – NCG).

Frequency	Gain on D30 EGb group	Gain on D30 NCG group	Difference between the two groups EGb – NCG
250 Hz	+25 db	+12.2 db	+12.8 db
500 Hz	+32.3 db	+17.8 db	+14.5 db
1000 Hz	+31.7 db	+22.8 db	+ 8.9 db
2000 Hz	+33.3 db	+24.4 db	+ 8.9 db
4000 Hz	+36.2 db	+30 db	+ 6.2 db
8000 Hz	+46.1 db	+31.1 db	+15 db
Total	+204.6 db	+138.3 db	+66.3 db

Discussion and Conclusion

The results obtained in the course of this therapeutic trial are in favor of the etiopathogenic hypothesis of ischemic distress of the sensorial cells in the cochlea. This hypothesis was postulated for any acute cochlear deafness, whether sudden idiopathic deafness or deafness due to sound trauma or barotrauma was involved. The better results observed in the group treated with Ginkgo biloba extract are proportional to its complex mechanism of effect. In fact, in addition to hemodynamic properties, particularly on the microcirculation of ischemic tissues, it has metabolic properties which protect the anoxic cells from the deleterious consequences of anoxia, particularly lipid peroxidation. The small number of patients included in this study makes it possible to draw only a cautious conclusion. The comparative study which we conducted in a homogenous group of recent acute cochlear deafness cases, however, does allow us to demonstrate a much greater efficacy of Ginkgo biloba extract in comparison with the comparable α-blocker. Usually the therapeutic result was obtained as early as the tenth day; in order to consolidate the result obtained, it seems that it would be necessary to continue the treatment for several weeks.

A Multicenter Randomized Double-Blind Study of Ginkgo Biloba Extract Versus Placebo in the Treatment of Tinnitus

B. Meyer

Service d'Oto-Rhino-Laryngologie, Hôpital Saint-Antoine, F 75012 Paris

Summary

This important multicenter study of 103 tinnitus out-patients during a 13-month treatment period was carried out by ten E.N.T. specialists, using the double blind, drug versus placebo method. The results were conclusive as regards the effectiveness of Ginkgo biloba extract and made it possible to determine the prognostic value of different parameters. Of special importance among these parameters were site and periodicity of the disease. However, the Ginkgo biloba extract treatment improved the condition of all the tinntius patients, irrespective of the prognostic factor.

Tinnitus, a very frequent symptom, troublesome both for the patient and for the physician who has difficulty – when he is able to do so – in being explicit about the physiopathological mechanism and lacks certainty as to what therapeutic posture to adopt.

The fact that tinnitus is relatively benign when present alone explains why it is encountered most frequently in everyday practice. In order to study tinnitus cases of recent onset, that is, less than a year old, it was necessary to carry out a private study, despite the complexity of organization.

This study had the purpose of quantifying the efficacy of treatment of recent tinnitus with Ginkgo biloba extract (EGb 761, Rökan®, Intersan), a product widely prescribed in this indication because of the etiopathogenic hypotheses considered. Ginkgo biloba extract (EGb) has been found active in ischemic processes, in membranal exchanges, and on certain neurotransmitters. This study also sought to demonstrate prognostic factors making it possible to determine profiles for patients responding to the treatment.

Rökan (Ginkgo Biloba). Recent Results in Pharmacology and Clinic
Edited by E.W. Fünfgeld
© Springer-Verlag Berlin Heidelberg New York 1988, pp. 245-250

Methodology

Ten otorhinolaryngology specialists in private practice participtated in the study and contributed 103 case histories in 12 months. After randomization, the patients were treated in double-blind for three months either with EGb or with a placebo strictly identical in appearance. The dosage was 4 mL/day in two doses. The duration of treatment could not be less than one month in order to draw conclusions as to a possible therapeutic failure.

The patients included had recent tinnitus, that is, appearing less than a year earlier.

Excluded from the study were patients suitable for surgical or anti-infectious treament, those suffering with acute inner or middle ear infections (otitis, eustachian salpingitis), or associated pathological disorders capable of skewing analysis of the results.

Also excluded were patients already under treatment and for whom the evolution was favorable, as well as those who required medical treatment which might interfere with evaluation of the results.

The criteria for establishment of the diagnosis and for monitoring were esentially clinical and comprised the definition of the patients and description of the tinnitus: timbre, schedule, rhythm, impairment, intensity, overall evolution, and time before disapearance; other associated ORL symptoms such as vertigo and hypoacousis were routinely investigated.

The paraclinical examinations comprised essentially tonal audiometry performed at the time the diagnosis was given and possibly repeated on the basis of the clinical condition. The performance of other tests (impedancemetry, electronystagmography) were left to the discretion of the physician.

Statistical analysis was by means of the χ^2 test for the qualitative variables and the Student t-test for the quantitative variables. In order to evaluate the influence of the various parameters on the evolution, a step-by-step decreasing logistic regression was done.(2)

Results

Comparability of the groups at the time of admission

After breaking of the double-blind, both treatment groups were analyzed in order to verify comparability at the time of admission to the study; 161 variables were analyzed.

The mean value of severity, graded from 1 to 4, was identical in both groups, but distribution by class presented a slight difference. This corresponds to a broader distribution within the placebo group, and more centered around the values of 2 and 3 in the EGb group. Therefore one group was not more severely affected than the other.

The intensity of the tinnitus, graded from 0 to 3, was comparable in the two groups. Impairment, coded from 0 to 3, was also comparable in both groups (*Table 1*).

Table 1
Comparison of the groups at the time of admission

Criteria	Grade	Placebo	Ginkgo biloba extract	Statistical calculation
Severity	1 (Mild)	8	3	$\chi^2 = 8.956$ $P < 0.03$ 3 degrees of freedom
	2 (Moderate)	11	25	
	3 (Troublesome)	21	27	
	4 (Severe)	4	1	
	Average =	2.47	2.46	
Intensity	0	0	0	$\chi^2 = 0.708$ 3 degrees of freedom – not significant
	1	9	9	
	2	30	37	
	3	4	9	
Impairment	0	2	1	$\chi^2 = 0.578$ 2 degrees of freedom – not significant
	1	16	18	
	2	20	29	
	3	7	10	

Both groups were also comparable for length of time the syndrome had been present, age, and sex:
- time syndrome had been present: EGb, 127 days; placebo, 143 days; t = 0.67;
- age: EGb, 50.97 years; placebo, 49.76 years; t = 0.39;
- sex: EGb, 29 men, 29 women; placebo, 25 men, 20 women ($\chi^2 = 0.31 - 1$ degree of freedom).

Table 2
Overall evolution

Patient condition	Ginkgo biloba extract	Placebo
1-2	0	0
3	16	14
4	6	12
5	9	7
6	22	11
7	2	1

1-2 = exacerbation; 3 = no change; 4 = slightly improved;
5 = improved; 6 = much improved; 7 = suspension because of intolerance.

Table 3
Percent of good evolution

Prognostic classification	Placebo	Ginkgo biloba extract
Class 1, old, bilateral, intermittent	50%	75%
Class 2, recent, unilateral, permanent	66%	75%
Class 3, recent, bilateral, permanent	33%	80%
Class 4, old, unilateral, permanent	29%	46%
Class 5, old, bilateral, permanent	11%	20%

There was also no difference with respect to the consumption of tobacco or alcohol, the ORL history (effect on the middle ear, barotrauma, phonotrauma, ototoxic involvement), and the associated syndromes (vertigo, hypoacousis).

Analysis of the tonal audiometry performed at the time of admission to the study also showed no difference between the two groups.

Analysis of therapeutic efficacy

Overall evolution: comparison of the two groups showed a significant difference in favor of the EGb group ($\chi^2 = 4.44 - 2$ degrees of freedom, P = 0.05) (*Table 2*).

Time before disappearance, or distinct improvement: there is a statistically significant difference in favor of the group treated with EGb, the evolution of which was much faster ($\chi^2 = 3.90 - 1$ degree of freedom, unilateral test P = 0.03).

Thus, the median, that is to say the time before the disappearance or distinct improvement in 50% of the tinnitus cases, was 70 days in EGb group and 119 days in the placebo group.

Evolution of intensity of the tinnitus between the first and last consultations: this appeared to be statistically better in the EGb group. Difference in intensity: EGb = 1.00; placebo = 0.67; Student t-test = 1.79; unilateral P test = 0.03.

Decrease in impairment between the first and the last consultations: this was greater for the treated group (0.84) than for the control group (0.59); this difference is at the limit of significance (Student t-test = 1.38; unilateral P test = 0.08).

Study of the prognostic variables

Statistical analysis showed that three variables have prognostic value: the history of the disease (more than 30 days, less than 30 days), the site (unilateral, bilateral), and periodicity (permanent, intermitent).

Study of the links among these three variables made it possible to demonstrate five different prognostic classes (*Table 3*).

Conclusion

This multicenter study, performed by ORL specialists in private practice, with a rigorous methodology, despite the difficulties which this includes in a field in which the subjective component is significant, as it confirms the results of treatment with placebo, brought together 103 case histories of recent tinnitus. It was thus possible to meet the two objectives established:

– to verify the efficacy of treatment with EGb;(1)
– to analyze the prognostic value of the various parameters by demonstrating those whose influence was determinant (history, site, and periodicity), as well as to specify the modalities of their interaction.

Tinnitus characterized as recent, unilateral, and intermittent, has a good prognosis. Treatment with EGb improves the evolution of the tinnitus regardless of its prognostic factors.

References

1. Meyer B: Etude multicentrique des acouphènes, épidémiologie et thérapeutique. *Annal. ORL* 1986, *103*, 185-188.

2. Nakache J.P., Gueguen A., Pierart H.: Utilisation du modèle logistique dans l'étude de l'influence des variables initiales et du traitement sur l'évolution de l'acouphène. *Revue de Statistique Appliquée* (sous presse).

Diagnostic and Practical Value of Craniocorpography in Vertiginous Syndromes

C.F. Claussen

Institut de Recherche Neuro-otologique, D-8730 Bad Kissingen
Federal Republic of Germany

Summary

Sensations of rotation or dizziness and nausea are the subjective symptoms characteristic of vertiginous syndromes; nystagmus and oscillations of the head and body are the objective signs. Craniocorpography is a method for recording and measuring these oscillations. Rapidly and inexpensively it provides easier diagnosis, follow-up, and measurement of therapeutic effectiveness. In this double-blind trial, the author has demonstrated the beneficial effects of Ginkgo biloba extract in vertiginous syndromes without obvious anatomical localisation.

Equilibrium disorders present four major categories of elements having diagnostic value. Vertigo and nausea constitute the significant subjective symptoms; nystagmus and oscillations of the head and body reflect objective sensorimotor disturbances. There is a simple relationship between nystagmus and vertigo, while the relationships between nausea and oscillations can be represented only by means of complicated models. In order to develop an optimal appropriate therapy, it is important to exploit quantitatively and in a standardized manner the paraclinical tests which make it possible to refine the study of these symptoms.

Equilibrometry has the purpose of studying the mechanisms involved in balance. The essential components of equilibrometry are analysis of the head and body movements by craniocorpography (CCG) and study of the nystagmic movements of the eyes by the electronystagmogram (ENG). In conformity with the neurosensorial diagram shown in *Figure 1* (diagram of entry and exit) for the sensorimotor correspondences, a vestibular stimulus is conveyed from the vestibule to the median longitudinal bundle. This corresponds to the sensorial component of the measuring system. The measurable response which follows is either a motor reaction in the eye such as nystagmus, called oculovestibular, or reactions of positioning of the head and body. The latter correspond to the vestibulomedullary component of the system.

Rökan (Ginkgo Biloba). Recent Results in Pharmacology and Clinic
Edited by E.W. Fünfgeld

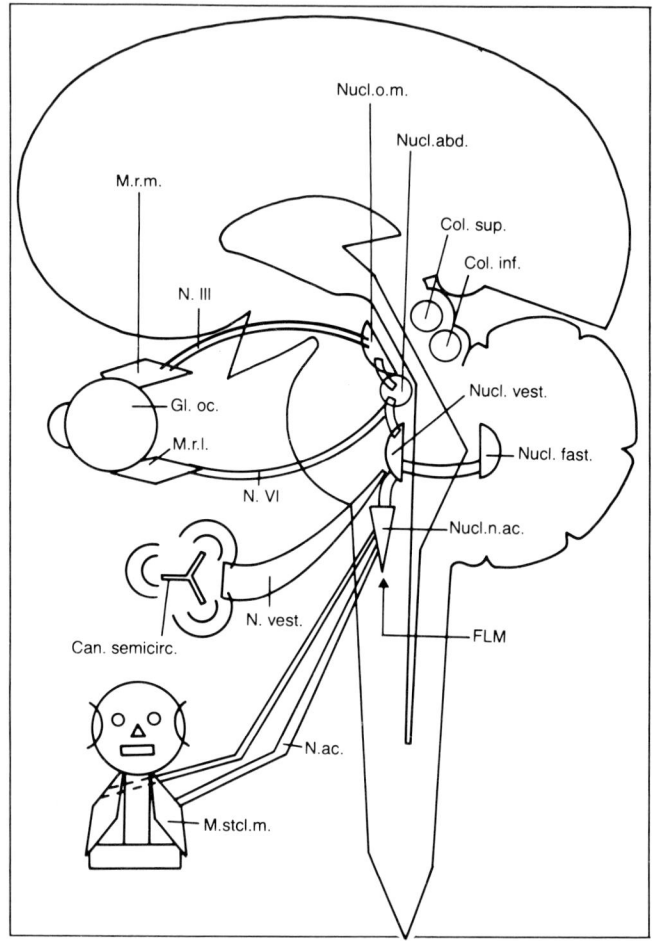

Figure 1: Neurosensorial diagram of balance. RSM = right superior muscle. O.M. nucl. = oculomotor nucleus. Abd. nucl. = abductor nucleus. Sup. col. = anterior quadrigeminal tubercle. Inf. col. = posterior quadrigeminal tubercle. Oc. gl. = eyeball. REM = right external muscle. Vest. nucl. = vestibular nucleus. Fast. nucl. = fastigien nucleus. Semicir. can. = semicircular canal. Vest. nucl. = vestibular nucleus. MLB = median longitudinal bundle. Ac. n. = accessory nerve. Stclm. m. = sternocleidomastoid muscle.

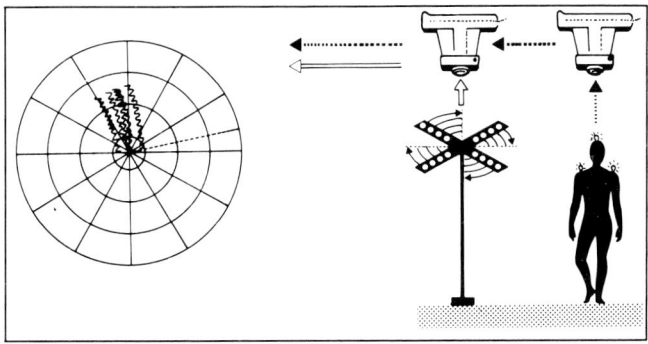

Figure 2: Craniocorpography technique.

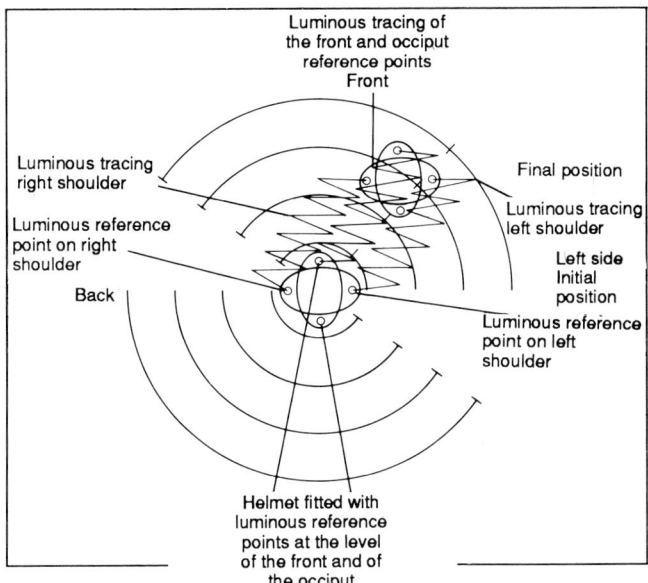

Figure 3: Diagramatic representation of the results obtained by craniocorpography in Unterberger's walking-in-place test.

By comparing the contents of the vestibulo-ocular, vestibulomedullary, and retino-ocular regulation circuits, and the reactions of the auditory pathways, an ensemble of topofunctional and neuro-otological analyses is obtained which makes it possible to locate and to treat specifically the disturbances localized in the receptors or in the central nervous system, or in both.

Electronystagmography is a refined test, irreplaceable, but it requires impeccable instrumentation and technique. It also requires an adequate lapse of time.

Craniocorpography

Craniocorpography (CCG) is a procedure for photographic registration of body and head movements.(1),(5) It serves for the objective recording of vestibulome-dullary tests of the balance function. By analogy with mass audiometric recording, in Germany, craniocorpography is now considered in industrial medicine as an exploratory test prior to hiring persons who will perform duties which could engender vertigo, or even could simply compromise their safety when they are already presenting with a deficiency in balance.

Bases

Craniocorpography is a photo-optical method to record movements of the head and shoulders as seen from above. In order to do this, the head and shoulders are equipped with luminous reference points (*Figure 2*). The light tracings are recorded by means of an instantaneous device (Kodak or Polaroid type) which allows several exposures on the same sensitive surface. In order to be able to use quantitatively the tracings of movments of the head and shoulders, a rotating screen placed just above the head of the patient turns; the patient is also fitted with luminous reference points; at the time of a second flash, this permits projecting a system of polar coordinates. The cra-niocorpogram thus obtained corresponds to a radar image of the movements of the head and body in space.

The most sensitive vestibulomedullary test is walking in place (Unterberger and Fukuda). The patient must take 80 to 100 steps, with the arms extended. During the test his eyes are covered with a band in order to suppress visual stimulations which would permit him to correct his orientation. This examination reflects the vestibular disturbances with the greatest sensitivity and makes it possible to record them (*Figure 3*).

The parameters analyzed in the walking-in-place test are the following:
– the magnitude of shift between the initial position and the final position;
– the angle of deviation between the departure direction and the final direction, that is, the angular deviation;
– rotation of the body around its own axis;

– the magnitude of oscillation of the head at each step, in other words, the lateral amplitude of the oscillations.

In combination with this test, the Romberg test is used, which is, however, much less sensitive to disturbances of vestibular origin. The patient is asked to remain standing in an absolutely upright position, for three minutes if possible, with the eyes bandaged.

Analysis of the Romberg test uses the following parameters:

– the magnitude of the oscillations in the antero-posterior direction;
– the amplitude of the lateral oscillations;
– the rotation of the axis of the head in relation to the axis of the shoulders, sometimes improperly called "torticollis angle";
– typical configuration of the luminous tracings of the head and shoulders.

It should be reported that, for this last parameter, there is a diagram typical of Parkinson's disease, in which the oscillations of the head in the antero-posterior direction are accentuated and exaggerate the shaking of the head. The antero-posterior oscillations of the luminous tracings coresponding to the shoulder movements are much weaker.

Topodiagnostic analysis

The clinical studies as well as analysis of the histological sections and the neuroradiological, neurosurgical, and otosurgical examinations show that the typical craniocorpogram diagrams (walking-in-place or Romberg) can be defined in peripheral and central vestibular pathology.

The vestibular pathological symptoms are diagrammed (*Figure 4*) beside a neuroanatomical representation of the structures involved in balance. In the anatomical sketch, the fourth ventricle with its four vestibular nuclei (on the edges, at right and left) will be recognized in the middle of the diamond; above, in the median longitudinal bundle, the oculomotor nuclei; below, also in the median longitudinal bundle, the accessory nuclei.

Laterally, beside the diamond are found the archeocerebellar nuclei, essentially the fastigien nuclei. Collaterally, in the pontocerebellar angle, the vestibular nerves range from the vestibular organs of the cup to the vestibular nuclei. The vestibular peripheral zone is demarcated from the center to the vestibular nuclei by the passage from the first to the second vestibular motoneuron.

A disturbance affecting for example the cupulovestibular complex is reflected in the craniocorpographic image (*Figure 4D*) by a deviation of the luminous tracing toward the right, corresponding to the movements of the head and body. The lateral deviation is again within the norms; in this case, the oscillation is slighter than the normal interval included between the different standard circles on the craniocorpogram.

In cases in which the archeocerebellum or the median or inferior cerebellar peduncles are affected unilaterally, in addition to an increase in lateral oscillation, an increase is found in lateral deviation which exceeds the accepted norms. This almost "reversed" lateral deviation historically described as Barré's disharmony, unlike peripheral vestibular disturbances, is directed not to the side of the lesions, but in the reverse direction (*Figure 4E*).

Barré's disharmony is demonstrated by comparing the craniocorpogram with the walking-in-place and the caloric "butterfly" diagram.

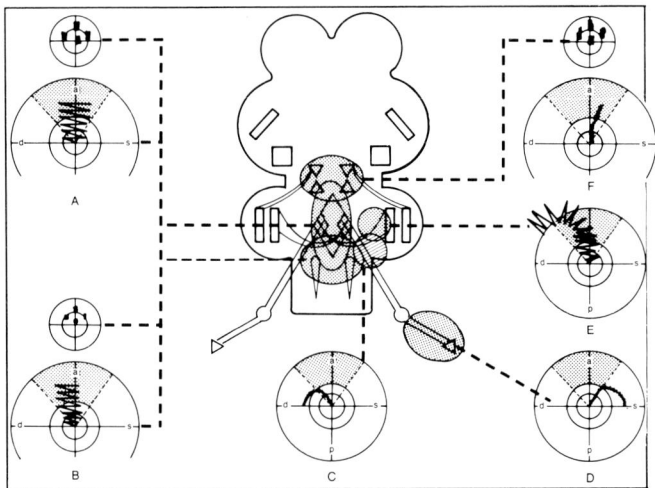

Figure 4: Topodiagnostic diagrams of craniocorpography outside of the walking-in-place test or in upright posture.
A: extensive diffuse lesions of the brain stem;
B: vestibulobulbar disturbances;
C: Barré's disharmony due to peripheral and central lesion; difference in comparison with the healthy side with normal lateral deviation;
D: peripheral disturbances;
E: Barré's cerebellar-type disharmony; difference in comparison with the healthy side with considerable lateral deviation;
F: central disturbances with participation of the anterior cerebellar peduncles or of the red nuclei or of the locus niger.

In rare cases of neurinoma, the CPG is modified during evolution, the deviation changes in direction and is then oriented toward the side opposite the lesion, which signals the onset of compression of the justarestiform tract (*Figure 4C*).

If the vestibulomedullary disturbances orginate in the lower portion of the fourth ventricle, more precisely in the medulla oblongata, a normal craniocorpogram is usually obtained in the Romberg test. The craniocorpogram corresponding to walking-in-place reveals a central disturbance and shows a striking accentuation in lateral oscillations (*Figure 4B*).

Cerebellar or peripheral lesions, in which the floor of the fourth ventricle is untouched, give isolated disturbances in the Romberg-method craniocorpogram, while the CCP by walking-in-place remains normal (*Figure 4F*).

In central disturbances of the posterior cranial fossa with vertigo and dizziness, extensive lesions are often involved, related to a cerebral vascular accident, to a disturbance in tissue exchanges, or to cranial injury. It is in these cases that the combination of the two pathological craniocorpographic diagrams is observed. Whether walking-in-place or Romberg, the craniocorpogram is disturbed (*Figure 4A*).

This combination is statistically more frequent than isolated abnormalities in the Romberg-method craniocorpogram, but less frequent than isolated abnormalites in the craniocorpogram (walking-in-place).

Practical value in therapy: trial with Ginkgo biloba extract

Pharmacotherapy given sytemically for neurotological disturbances is sure to develop rapidly. As the differential diagnosis is constantly refined, therapy can only improve and become differentiated in its turn.

A simple and practical test, easy to use, craniocorpography lends itself wondrously well to investigative tests of the "mass examination" type; but it can also be used as a statistical and discriminating test making it possible, to a certain degree, to evaluate the short-term efficacy of drugs prescribed for patients presenting with a vertiginous or ebrious syndrome. We verified it in a therapeutic study conducted in double-blind in 33 elderly patients presenting with vertigo and ataxia and treated with Ginkgo biloba extract (EGb 761, Rökan®, Intersan) in comparison with placebo.

The craniocorpographic examination was made before the initiation of treatment with 120 mg EGb per day or the corresponding placebo. The same test was repeated after six and 12 weeks of treatment. All of the patients underwent a thorough ORL examination which as a whole showed nothing in particular. In adddition to collection of objective data, the patients were questioned concerning the subjective evolution of their vertiginous syndrome.

Subjectively, according to the interrogation, the vertigo regressed at the end of 12 weeks in 20% of the patients having received placebo and in 50% of the patients treated with EGb. No side effects were reported throughout the treatment with either of the therapies (*Figure 5*).

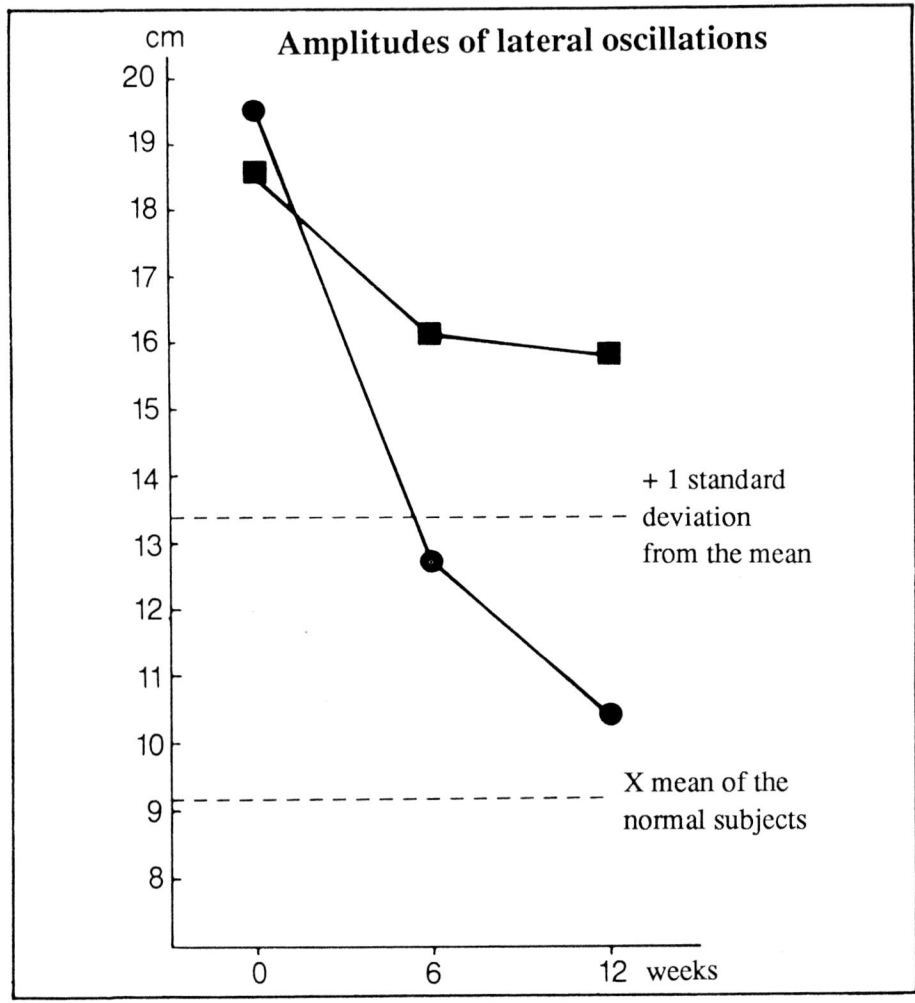

Figure 5: Amplitude of the lateral oscillations. Significant diference in favor of Ginkgo biloba extract: P < 0.02 at the end of six weeks of treatment and P < 0.005 at the end of 12 weeks.

Conclusion

This therapeutic trial showed us that craniocorpography is an easy and inexpensive test often making it possible to outline the lesional topography, to follow the evolution of a vertiginous syndrome, or to verify the effects of a therapy.

Applied to the study of Ginkgo biloba extract, this test has made it possible to demonstrate a very significant improvement in comparison with placebo.

References

1. Claussen C.F., Aust G., Hortmann G., Müller-Kortkamp M: Praktikum der Elektronystagmographie. Bd. 2 der Verhlg. der GNA, *Edition medicin et pharmacie*, Frankfurt, 1975.

2. Claussen C.F., Lühmann M.V.: Das Elektronystagmogramm und die neurootologische Kennliniendiagnostik. *Edition medicin et pharmacie*, Hamburg und Neu-Isenburg, 1976.

3. Claussen C.F.: Schwindel – Ein Leitfaden für Klinik und Praxis. *Edition medicin et pharmacie*, Dr. Werner Rudat and Co., Hamburg, 1981.

4. Claussen C.F.: Schwindel im Alter – Neue Möglichkeiten einer neurootologischen Differentialdiagnose und Differentialtherapie. *In*: Therapie im Alter, Bergener M., Kark B., *Steinkopf-Verlag*, Darmstadt, 1984.

5. Claussen C.F.: Presbyvertigo, Presbytaxie, Presbytinnitus. *Springer-Verlag*, Berlin, Heidelberg, New York, Tokyo, 1985.

Treatment of Disturbed Equilibrium with Ginkgo Biloba Extract
Multicenter Double-Blind Study Versus Placebo

J.P. Haguenauer[1], F. Cantenot[2], H. Koskas[3], H. Pierart[4]

(1) Service Pr. Gaillard, Hôpital de la Croix Rousse. F 69000 Lyon
(2) Service du Pr. Lafon, CHU de Besançon. F 25000 Besançon
(3) Service du Pr. Garcin, Hôpital Ste Marguerite. F 13000 Marseille
(4) Institut I.P.S.E.N., 30, rue Cambronne, F 75737 Paris Cedex 15

Summary

This study, conducted in three centers, included 70 patients with vertiginous syndrome of recent onset and undetermined origin treated in a double-blind trial for three months with Ginkgo biloba extract versus placebo.

The results show that the effectiveness of Ginkgo biloba extract on the intensity, frequency, and duration of the vertigo was statistically significant. At the end of the trial, 47% of the treated patients were free of their symptoms, as against 18% of those who received placebo.

Regardless of location – vestibular system or central nervous system – ischemia is the most frequently invoked hypothesis in disturbances of equilibrium without obvious medical or surgical etiology. Clinical and pharmacological studies have demonstrated the hemodynamic and metabolic properties of Ginkgo biloba extract (EGb 761, Rökan®, Intersan) in ischemic tissues. Its efficacy on the functional pathology of the auditory system has already been demonstrated in the course of prior clinical studies. However, we can contrast with these the very subjective character of equilibrium disturbances.

This is why we decided to implement a multicenter study according to a strict methodology, double-blind versus placebo.

Methodology

General conditions

This study combined 70 case histories of patients suffering with equilibrium disturbances of recent onset. Three centers participated:

Rökan (Ginkgo Biloba). Recent Results in Pharmacology and Clinic
Edited by E.W. Fünfgeld
© Springer-Verlag Berlin Heidelberg New York 1988, pp. 260-268

– the Service of Pr. Gaillard, Hôpital de la Croix-Rousse, Lyon, who gathered 40 case histories;

– the Service of Pr. Garcin, Hôpital Sainte Marguerite, Marseille, who contributed 12 case histories;

– the Service of Pr. Lafon, CHU de Besançon, who contributed 18 case histories.

Inclusion began in the spring of 1984 and lasted for one year.

Criteria for selection

In order to be admitted to the study, the patients had to have a vertiginous syndrome confirmed by clinical examination, persistent and recent, that is, active for less than two years.

Excluded were patients suffering with paroxysmal vertigo falling into the classification of Ménière's disease; "false vertigo" reflecting another disease: orthostatic hypotension; height vertigo; hematological, metabolic, or neurological disorders. Also excluded were patients with vertigo of tumoral, inflammatory, infectious, or toxic etiology, or vertigo due to direct trauma or vertigo related to disturbed vision or disturbed deep sensitivity.

The same was true for patients having a disease which could interfere with interpretation of the results, and those who could not interrupt a treatment which might skew the evaluation of therapeutic efficacy, in particular drugs of the same therapeutic class as Ginkgo biloba extract and histamine analogs.

The diagnosis, essentially clinical, was given by the ORL investigator as a function of the interrogation which specified the type of vertigo, circumstances of onset, and possibly the associated symptomatology: tinnitus, hypoacousis, nausea, headaches, etc. It was also based on a complete otoneurological examination and an electronystagmogram, with caloric tests. This evaluation was supplemented by a tonal audiometry.

Criteria of efficacy

Monitoring of the evolution and evaluation of drug efficacy were based on the following criteria:

– the data from the interrogation: intensity, frequency, and duration of the vertiginous attacks and the associated signs.

– an analog visual scale allowing the patient to quantify the overall severity of the disorder at each consultation. The scale ranged from 0 (absent) to 100 (extreme).

– an otoneurological examination including investigation of deviation of the indices, a Romberg sign, blind compass gait (Babinski-Weill test), pathological nystagmus.

– overall evalution by the clinician who evaluated the improvement in the patient as a function of the initial condition according to the following code: disappearance of the vertigo (0), good improvement (1), slight improvement (2), stabilization (3), exacerbation (4).

Conduct of the trial

After verification of the criteria for admission and exclusion, the patients received a case history number which governed the treatment batch which was assigned to them. The groups were divided before the beginning of the test by means of a table of random numbers so that the groups were balanced.

Each patient's consent was sought before his admission into the study, which was explained to him along its major outlines.

Treatments in progress were continued only to the extent that they were necessary and had been prescribed for more than three months. Their nature and their dosage was transcribed into the case history file.

The treatments were either EGb or placebo strictly identical in appearance. The dosage was 2 mL b.i.d., which corresponds in the EGb group to 160 mg per day Ginkgo biloba extract.

After admission, the patients were reviewed after 30 days, 60 days, then 90 days of treatment. At each consultation, adherence to the treatment was detailed, and omissions were noted in the case history notebook.

Biological tolerance was verified at the time of admission and at the end of the study; it comprised a complete blood count, uricemia, transaminases, cholesterolemia, triglyceridemia, creatininemia.

Population studied

Among the 70 patients admitted to the study, three were not seen again after the first consultation. Two belonged to the placebo group and one to the EGb group. The analysis therefore involved 67 case histories, 34 EGb and 33 placebo.

The principal data describing the study population appear in *Table 1*. It was found that more than 70% of the patients (48/67) had no ORL history.

Table 2 summarizes the essential characteristics of the disturbances in equilibrium compiled from the interrogation; the vertigos were, on the average, recent (four months), almost all precipitated by movement of the body or the head (59/67 cases). In more than two-thirds of the cases, the vertigo was rotary, intermittent, accompanied by hypoacousis, tinnitus, and/or neuroautonomic signs (nausea, vomiting, headaches).

In half of the cases the vertigo was becoming worse during the period preceding admission, in the other half it was stable (*Table 3*).

On the analog visual scale which quantifies the overall severity of the disorders experienced by the patient, the figures on Day 0 are practically identical for EGb (= 53.1 ± 3.4) and for *placebo (= 52 ± 4.2)*.

At the clinical examination, the signs did not orient the etiology of the e*quilibrium disorder*s (*Table 4*) toward a precise topographical diagnosis. The criteria for exclusion having eliminated the patients for whom the cause could be specified, the study included patients suffering with an equilibrium disorder without a defined etiopathogenesis.

Statistically, analysis of all of these data showed no significant difference between the two groups.

Table 1

Description of the population

Characteristics	EGb	Placebo
Number of patients	34	33
Age	52 ± 2.5	46.4 ± 2.4
Sex	16 M/18 F	18 M/15 F
ORL history		
• acoustic trauma	6	5
• barotrauma	0	1
• infectious pathology	3	0
• tympanic rupture	1	1
• ototoxic lesion	1	1
Non-ORL history		
• cervical trauma	7	6

Table 2

Description of the disturbance in equilibrium upon admission
(characteristics, circumstances of onset, and accompanying signs)

Elements of comparison	EGb	Placebo
Mean chronicity (in weeks)	19 ± 6.2w	22.7 ± 6.4w
Number of patients	34	33
Circumstances of onset • mobilization • rotation of the head • position of the head	13 14 5	16 10 1
Vertigo • rotary • oscillating • permanent/intermittent	20 14 3/27	29 6 5/27
Accompanying signs • hypoacousis • tinnitus • headaches • nausea/vomiting	20 20 4 20	15 17 6 17
Overall mean impairment upon admission Analog visual scale coded from 0 to 100 mm	62 ± 3.7 mm	67 ± 4.4 mm

Table 3

Evolutive tendency of the vertigo in the course of the period preceding admission

Parameters	EGb group	Placebo group
Number of patients	34	33
Exacerbation	15	16
Stable	18	15
Improvement	1	1
Unknown	–	1

Table 4
Otoneurological examination before and after treatment

Examination signs	EGb		Placebo	
	D0	D90	D0	D90
Deviation of the indices				
• harmonious deviation	4	0	9	2
• nonharmonious deviation	2	0	1	0
Blind Babinski gait				
• generalized deviation	2	0	4	0
• titubatory deviation	6	3	5	2
Romberg test				
• inclination	9	2	13	3
Horizontal nystagmus	8	1	9	1

Results

On the vertigo

Each of the parameters (intensity, frequency, and duration of the vertigo) was scored as a function of the preceding consultation in the following manner:

disappeared 0, diminished 1, stable 2, exacerbated 3. Thus an improvement is reflected by decrease in this score. The means of the results appear in *Table 5*. These show that the vertiginous symptomatology decreased more in the Egb group than in the control group.

At the end of the trial, the overall score, varying from 0 (disappeared) to 9 (exacerbated) totals the results obtained in the three consultations. It demonstrates a significantly greater mean improvement in the Egb group with respect to intensity, frequency, and duration of the vertigo (Student t-test: $P < 0.05$) (*Table 5*).

On the analog visual scale

This scale, filled in by the patient at each consultation, allowed him to quantify the impact of the vertigo on his daily life.

The relative improvement was expressed as percentage. It is equal to the difference between the values at time t (Day 30, Day 60, Day 90) less that on Day 0, divided by the measurements on Day 0 (*Table 6*).

The improvement experienced by the subjects in the group treated with EGb was significant as early as the first month of treatment and increased in the course of successive evaluations, to reach 75% at the end of the study. The difference from the placebo group is very significant (comparison of percentage, Student t-test).

Table 5

Mean total score obtained from the sum of the sources on Day 30, Day 60, and Day 90, scored at each consultation from 0 (disappeared) to 3 (exacerbated). The mean total score could then vary from 0 to 9.

Mean total score	EGb	Placebo	Significance
Intensity	3.37	4.46	P = 0.02
Frequency	3.24	4.20	P = 0.02
Duration	3.33	4.50	P = 0.03

Table 6

Visual analog scale filled out by the patient. It expresses the impairment due to the disorders in balance. The reults correspond to the relative improvement as a function of the initial values.

Time	EGb	Placebo	Significance (Student t-test)
D30	43.4%	−5.7%	0.02
D60	60.1%	15.7%	0.01
D90	74.7%	18.3%	0.01

Associated symptomatology

In both groups, the clinical signs and the symptoms accompanying the vertigo (hypoacousis, tinnitus, headaches, nausea) scarcely changed during the follow-up period.

Supplemental tests

Upon electronystagmography, the caloric tests measured at the time of admission were disturbed in 50% of the patients (EGb 16/34, placebo 19/33), a comparable manner in both groups (χ^2 = 1.33, 1 degree of freedom).

At the end of treatment it was found that the two groups had developed differently. In the EGb group the tests were normal in 80% of the cases (27/33), whereas in the placebo group this rate was only 57% (19/33). This difference in evolution is significant (χ^2 = 3.33, 1 degree of freedom: P = 0.06).

As to the tonal audiometry, it did not vary notably in the two groups during the study.

Overall evaluation

The number of patients recovered (*Figure 1*) was significantly greater in the EGb group at each consultation.

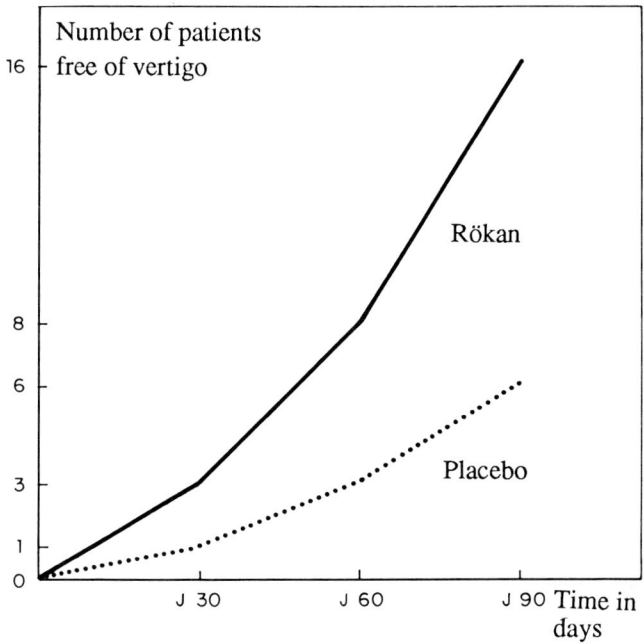

Figure 1: Evolution of the number of recovered patients; at the end of the trial, 47% of the subjects treated with Ginkgo biloba extract had recovered, as opposed to 18% in the placebo group.

Table 7
Overall evaluation of the efficacy of the treatment by the physician at the end of the study

Evaluation	EGb	Placebo
Exacerbation	0	1
Stabilization	0	14
Slight improvement	5	4
Good improvement	13	8
Disappearance	16	6
Number of patients	34	33

It was 47% against 18% at the end of the study.

On the other hand, the overall evaluation made by the ORL investigator demonstrated the difference in improvement between the two groups (*Table 7*). In the group treated with Ginkgo biloba extract, the number of patients recovered or much improved is twice as great as in the placebo group and reached 85% at the end of treatment ($\chi^2 = 17.5$, 3 degrees of freedom: $P < 0.001$).

As to clinical and biological tolerance, these were excellent in both groups.

Conclusion

Disturbances in equilibrium are frequently encountered in ORL or general daily practice and often it is not possible to specify the etiology. Functional tests make it possible to evaluate the severity with difficulty, and the sole element in monitoring the evolution is the complaints expressed by the patient.

The lack of objectivity of this criterion requires recourse to a strict methodology in order to evaluate the genuine efficacy of a treatment: double-blind, versus placebo, in groups very comparable at the start.

Under these conditions, after three months of treatment, Ginkgo biloba extract proved its efficacy; both from the standpoint of the patient and from that of the investigator, a distinct improvement was found in 85% of the patients.

Effect of Ginkgo Biloba Extract on the Endocrine Parameters

J.P. Felber

Laboratoire d'Endocrinologie et de Biochimie Clinique, Département Médecine Interne C.H.U.V., 1011 Lausanne, Switzerland

Summary

In order to find out whether Ginkgo biloba extract has an influence on endocrine balance, seven male volunteers (mean age: 26.1 years) received twice the usual dose of the drug for eight weeks.

Various hormonal assays and stimulation tests with LHRH and TRH were performed before treatment and after four and eight weeks of treatment.

No significant change or tendency to change was observed. The other, usual blood tests also were unmodified.

In the course of the last 15 years, much interest has been taken in the problem of possible relationships between neuroendocrine symptoms and psychiatric disorders. Not only are neuroendocrine disturbances found in various mental diseases,(2) but it has been shown that certain treatments can appreciably modify endocrine balance. In senile dementia, it is necessary to differentiate pseudodementia of organic origin (for example, hypothyroidism) from "idiopathic organic cerebral impairment."(1) This is why we decided to investigate whether or not Ginkgo biloba extract (Rökan®, Intersan), a product widely used in this indication, could act directly on endocrine function. The study was conducted in healthy volunteers.

Methodology

Subjects

The subjects selected were seven healthy male volunteers from 20 to 35 years of age (average age 26.1 years); the purpose and the methodology of the trial were explained to them and their consent was obtained.

Rökan (Ginkgo Biloba). Recent Results in Pharmacology and Clinic
Edited by E.W. Fünfgeld
© Springer-Verlag Berlin Heidelberg New York 1988, pp. 269-273

Conduct of the study

This was an open study, lasting for two months, on the effects of a moderately high dose (twice the usual dose) of Ginkgo biloba extract. The various tests were given before the trial began and at the end of the first and second months of treatment. The product was administered in three daily doses (3x 80 mg), and good observance was verified at each control (Week 0, Week 4, Week 8). The tests made and the methods used are summarized in *Table 1*.

Table 1
Laboratory tests performed for the seven volunteers

Parameters	Method of assay	Normal values
Blood glucose (fasting)	Glucose oxidase, Beckman	3.9-5.6 mM/l
White cells	standard	4-10 10 (12)/l
Red cells	standard	4.4-5.8 10 (9)/l
Hemoglobin	standard	133-177 g/l
Hematocrit	standard	0.40-0.52
Proteins	standard	63-78 g/l
Sedimentation rate	standard	–
Uric acid	standard	140-460 µM/l
Immunoreactive insulin	RIA-Herbert	5-20 µU/ml
STH	RIA	0.5-4 µU/ml
T3	RIA	1.5-3.3 nmol/l
T4	RIA	60-150 nmol/l
TBG	RIA	15-20 µg/ml
ACTH	Berson-Yellow 1968	8-85 pg/ml
Cortisol	standard	0.1-0.7 µM/l
Calcium	standard	2.15-2.55 mM/l
Cholesterol	standard	3.1-6.5 mM/l
HDL Cholesterol	standard	0.78-1.81 mM/l
Triglycerides	standard	0.84-1.94 mM/l

LHRH TRH stimulation was also done, as well as the corresponding assays of FSH, LH, PRL, TSH.

Statistical analysis

Statistical analysis was done on the IBM PC XT using Statpro software (Wadsworth Factory Inc.). A two-way analysis of variance was made for the equal and unequal samples according to the results using a multiple regression program.

Results

All of the volunteers finished the study. One of them did not undergo the second control: in the analysis of variance, his values for this control were established on the basis of the mean of the first and third controls, except for the stimulation tests. In one of the subjects, the STH level is missing for the first control; it was therefore deleted from the final analysis with respect to this factor. The various results are summarized in *Tables 2 and 3*.

Table 2

Mean results (MSI) for the laboratory parameters

Parameters	Week 0		Week 4		Week 8		P
Red cells	5.1	(0.3)	5.3	(0.4)	5.2	(0.5)	n.s.
White cells	6.3	(2.4)	7.1	(3.0)	6.7	(2.5)	n.s.
Hemoglobin	149.9	(7.7)	159.3	(8.0)	151.7	(13.7)	n.s.
Hematocrit	0.4	(0.02)	0.5	(0.02)	0.4	(0.04)	n.s.
Proteins	66.1	(3.6)	66.8	(3.9)	66.0	(6.0)	n.s.
Sedimentation rate	2.7	(1.7)	2.5	(1.5)	2.7	(1.8)	n.s.
Uric acid	338.4	(48.9)	306.5	(72.8)	314.0	(100.8)	n.s.
Glucose	97.7	(7.7)	101.4	(20.3)	85.0	(7.4)	n.s.
IR insulin	18.2	(17.9)	26.4	(18.0)	9.1	(5.8)	n.s.
STH	0.7	(0.7)	0.5	(0.5)	0.7	(0.8)	n.s.
T3	2.8	(0.3)	2.8	(0.2)	2.7	(0.5)	n.s.
T4	91.1	(19.7)	93.3	(14.3)	86.6	(17.0)	n.s.
T3/T4	0.031	(0.003)	0.032	(0.004)	0.031	(0.006)	n.s.
TBG	14.8	(2.2)	17.3	(3.1)	15.0	(2.0)	p=0.048
ACTH	18.6	(12.2)	25.3	(13.7)	20.9	(7.0)	n.s.
Cortisol	0.38	(0.11)	0.46	(0.08)	0.44	(0.08)	n.s.
Calcium	2.3	(0.1)	2.4	(0.1)	2.3	(0.1)	n.s.
Cholesterol	5.1	(1.1)	4.9	(0.8)	4.7	(0.9)	n.s.
HDL Cholesterol	0.9	(0.2)	0.9	(0.1)	0.9	(0.1)	n.s.
Triglycerides	0.9	(0.5)	1.2	(0.4)	1.3	(0.6)	n.s.

Table 3
Mean results from the stimulation tests

Parameters	Week 0	Week 4	Week 8	P
FSH – 15'	2.2 (1.0)	2.5 (1.1)	2.2 (1.2)	
0	2.1 (0.9)	2.4 (1.0)	2.1 (1.1)	
15'	4.1 (2.6)	4.8 (2.4)	4.0 (2.1)	
30'	4.7 (3.2)	5.8 (3.2)	4.8 (2.7)	n.s.(0.65)
60'	4.8 (2.8)	5.6 (2.4)	4.9 (2.6)	
120'	4.2 (2.7)	4.9 (2.3)	4.1 (1.9)	
LH – 15'	5.0 (1.5)	5.4 (1.9)	5.5 (2.0)	
0	4.8 (1.5)	5.4 (1.9)	4.9 (1.9)	
15'	25.1 (16.0)	30.3 (20.4)	19.6 (6.4)	
30'	28.3 (15.8)	36.0 (24.6)	21.9 (6.4)	n.s.(0.61)
60'	22.6 (11.9)	29.4 (19.8)	22.1 (9.1)	
120'	15.2 (8.0)	18.7 (10.4)	12.2 (1.2)	
PRL – 15'	6.0 (1.4)	7.5 (2.3)	6.2 (1.3)	
0	5.4 (1.5)	6.6 (1.8)	5.3 (1.1)	
15'	25.3 (4.7)	24.9 (5.8)	24.5 (4.7)	
30'	22.7 (3.7)	19.6 (3.0)	21.3 (2.8)	n.s.(0.12)
60'	14.9 (1.4)	12.1 (1.6)	14.0 (1.5)	
120'	7.7 (0.9)	6.3 (1.5)	7.7 (1.3)	
TSH 0	1.7 (1.1)	1.7 (0.7)	1.4 (0.5)	
30'	9.6 (3.5)	9.5 (3.6)	10.0 (5.9)	n.s.(0.55)

Discussion and Conclusion

These results show that no characteristic tendency stands out for any of the parameters examined. No statistically significant difference was found for TGB, but here also no significant tendency appeared. All of the parameters tested remained within the range of normal values, except for several variations in glucose and insulin level, which are due to nonobservance of the conditions of strict fasting by two of the subjects. At any rate, long-term clinical studies have already established that Ginkgo biloba extract has no effect on fasting glucose blood level.

No side effects were reported, aside from a subjective effect of "improved memory", reported spontaneously by one of the subjects at the end of four weeks of treatment.

Despite the small number of subjects studied, we could conclude that Ginkgo biloba extract, administered at moderately high doses for two months, in no way modified endocrine balance and that from this standpoint the product may be considered as entirely safe. It can also be concluded that the mechanism of effect does not occur directly through a hormonal mechanism. The only remaining possibility is "restoration" of disturbed hormonal activity in dementia, but this requires detailed investigations in patients.

References

1. American Psychiatric Association: Diagnostic and statistical manual of mental disorders. 3rd Edition, Washington D.C.: APA, 1980.

2. Carroll B.J.: Neuroendocrine Function in Psychiatric Disorders. *In*: Psychopharmacology: A generation of progress, Lipton, Di Mascio, Killiam (Eds.), *Raven Press*, New York,1978, 487-497.

Development of a Model for Study of the Antiedematous Properties of Ginkgo Biloba Extract

D. Hannequin[1], A. Thibert[2], Y. Vaschalde[1]

(1) Clinique Neurologique (Pr Samson), Hôpital Charles Nicolle. 1, rue de Germont
  F 76000 Rouen
(2) IPSEN. 30, rue Cambronne, F 75737 Paris Cedex 15

Summary

The vasogenic edema observed after irridation of the brain represents a new and interesting model for studying the antiedematous properties of a drug. We have just completed a first clinical study of injectable Ginkgo biloba extract, with the dual purpose of establishing criteria for simple and nontraumatic quantification of edema.

The results from this pilot study led us to continue this evaluation under strict methodological conditions, in view of their therapeutic and epidemiological value.

Two types of postradiotherapy edema(1),(3),(4),(6) may be distinguished. "Delayed" edema occurs more than a month after radiotherapy; its pathogenesis is complex and can involve cellular necrosis and inflammatory cellular infiltration. "Early" edema occurs less than a week after radiotherapy; this is vasogenic edema. The primary lesion consists of a functional change in the capillary endothelium, which is particularly sensitive to radiation. Electron microscope studies(1) have shown increased pinocytosis activity of the endothelial cells, their distortion, an enlargement in the perivascular spaces. Changes in permeability of the blood-brain barrier are indicated, as early as six hours after exposure, by intercellular edema of the white substance; the edema is maximum around 48 hours and regresses before the sixth day.

Early postradiotherapy edema can be a model for study of the antiedematous properties of a drug in human clinical practice.

The purpose of this study was to contribute to the development of this model and to confirm the value in this indication of Ginkgo biloba extract (EGb, Rökan®, Intersan), the antiedematous properties of which have been well established in animal pharmacology:(2)

– protection versus lipid peroxidation through an antiradical effect;

Rökan (Ginkgo Biloba). Recent Results in Pharmacology and Clinic
Edited by E.W. Fünfgeld
© Springer-Verlag Berlin Heidelberg New York 1988, pp. 274-277

– prevention of vasogenic edema by embolization with microspheres or arterial clamping;
– protection of the blood-brain barrier.

Patients and Method

Methodological problems

The clinical expression of early edema has not been studied adequately enough to disclose an accurate frequency rate, since there are numerous interacting variables. Two factors seem to promote it: chemotherapy, through the capillary fragility which it induces, and prior intracranial hypertension, which is difficult to quantify clinically.

The other essential elements are the nature of the tumor (glioblastoma/metasteses), its volume, the peritumoral edema, whether or not there has been prior surgery, the site of the tumor (a clinically "silent" area or not), its impact on the drainage pathways, the type of radiotherapy used, the associated treatment (steroids, barbiturates).

The "ideal" methodological conditions for quantifying early edema and its effects may be summarized as follows:

– clinical criteria for monitoring for 48 hours, making it possible to describe a symptomatology that is variable in intensity, ranging from nausea and non-incapacitating headaches to the extreme situations of encephalopathy or acute intracranial hypertension;
– homogenous groups acording to the criteria mentioned above (multicenter study);
– nontraumatic paraclinical methods to evaluate the precocious edema objectively (nuclear magnetic resonance);
– methods for evaluating the functional sequelae (electroencephalography/evoked potentials).(5)

Preliminary study

The "pilot" study in progress is for the purpose of testing the reliability of the medical protocol by using a simple clinical monitoring scale, before considering a study which would meet the other three conditions, much more difficult to fulfill.

This was therefore an open clinical study. The criteria for admission were absence of clinical intracranial hypertension, stability of the neurological semiology, stability of associated treatments for ten days, and patient consent.

The treatment consists of i.v. administration of 100 mg EGb (two bottles) diluted in 500 cc isotonic glucose serum infused in two hours. The infusion was given during the two hours preceding each of the first three radiotherapy sessions.

Clinical monitoring took place in several stages. The patient was examined by the neurologist immediately before the infusion in order to confirm his meeting the criteria for admission. The evaluation criteria were clinical: headaches, nausea, vomiting, drowsiness, exacerbation of the deficit, epilepsy attack. These were repeated in the course of the 24 hours following each radiotherapy session, by both the neurologist and the nursing personnel. The first four criteria were graded according to a four-point scale: absence, low intensity, moderate, severe.

Notes were made in the case history of the time the symptom occurred, its evolution, and the treatment prescribed. Blood pressure was taken before and after each infusion.

The patient was seen again at the end of the radiotherapy sessions given later without preventive treatment.

Results

Ten patients were included in the protocol at this date, six men and four women with an average age of 54 years. The diagnosis was glioblastoma for ten patients, and one out of two times in an initial picture of intracranial hypertension.

Surgery was performed for four of these tumors, and in two cases chemotherapy was added to the surgical exeresis. Radiotherapy had to be undertaken in all of these patients.

Five patients remained completely asymptomatic during radiotherapy, and four others presented with minor symptoms (headache or drowsiness, rapidly resolved without treatment). In the last patient (glioma of the corpus callosum with initial intracranial hypertension), headaches with drowsiness required the prescription of mannitol.

The method of intravenous administration caused no problems of intolerance, either venous or gastric.

Blood pressure was checked before and at the end of the infusions (37 EGb infusions for all ten patients). For each of the infusions, the "after treatment – before treatment" difference in systolic and diastolic pressures were established. Concerning systolic pressure, like diastolic pressure, the means of these differences, very slightly negative, were not significantly different from 0 (t-test for paired series). The case-by-case analysis showed no clinically significant pressure variation, with the exception of patient No. 4, whose systolic pressure, initially slightly elevated (150 to 170 mmHg), fell two to three points after each infusion, while the diastolic pressure remained stable.

Conclusion

At this stage of the study four points are obvious:

– the good tolerance of Ginkgo biloba extract;

– the simplicity of the clinical coding;

– the "drowsiness" criterion was found to be too inaccurate for reliably grading the "mild drowsiness" classification. It needs to be supplemented by a quantified and simple evaluation of the attention capacities of the patients;

– therapeutic efficacy could not, by definition, be tested at this phase of the study. The feasibility of such a protocol encourages proposing its extension in order to fulfill the methodological conditions (multicenter/doubl-blind/paraclinical, statics, and functional quantification methods). The therapeutic value is duplicated by an epidemiological value.

References

1. Csanda E.: Radiation brain edema. *Adv. Neurol.*, 1980, *28*, 125-146.

2. Etienne A., Hecquet F., Clostre F.: Mécanismes d'action de l'extrait de Ginkgo biloba sur l'œdème cérébral expérimental. *Presse Méd.*, 1986, *15*, 1506-1510.

3. Holdorff B.: Radiation damage to the brain. *In*: Handbook of Clinical Neurology, *North-Holland*, New York, 1975, *23*, 639-663.

4. Kingsley D.P., Kendall B.E.: CT of the adverse effects of therapeutic radiation of the central nervous system. *A.J.N.R.*, 1981, *2*, 453-460.

5. Maccolini E., Franzoni E., Vecchi V., Bravetti G.O., Guidelli Guidi S.: Visual evoked potentials in early and late CNS changes due to antileukemia treatment in children. Preliminary report. *Ital. J. Neurol. Sci.* 1982, *3*, 295-299.

6. Oliff A., Bleyer W.A., Poplack D.G.: Acute encephalopathy after initiation of cranial irradiation for meningeal leukaemia. *Lancet*, 1978, *ii*, 13-15.

Methodology of a Controlled Trial in Alzheimer's Disease

H. Dehen[1], G. Dordain[2], M. Allard[3]

(1) Clinique Neurologique, Hôpital Beaujon. 100, boulevard du Général Leclerc.
 F 92110 Clichy
(2) Service de Neurologie, Hôpital Nord. Route de Châteaugay, B.P. 145 Cebazat.
 F 63100 Clermont-Ferrand
(3) IPSEN. 30, rue Cambronne. F 75015 Paris

Summary

Various evaluation scales suggested for studying the clinical evolution of Alzheimer-type dementias are discussed, and the practical aspects of a controlled clinical trial are considered.

A tentative protocol has been designed, combining multiple independent evaluations with several validated scales and tests. This protocol is suitable for a multicenter study, since it includes only evaluation tools which are easy to handle and do not require too much time. It should permit the selection of a relatively homogenous group of patients and make it possible to quantify the course of Alzheimer's disease over a one-year period.

The discussion emphasizes the predictable difficulty of evaluating a therapeutic benefit based on our current incomplete knowledge about the natural evolution and prognostic factors of the disease.

Long considered as having an inexorable outcome, Alzheimer's disease has for several years been the subject of therapeutic investigation.(13),(16) Many clinical trials have been undertaken. A general review by Thomas Crook(7) gives a complete overview. It mentions controlled trials with various "vasoactive" drugs or with cholinergic substances. Currently, interest is directed toward neuropeptides, inhibitors of serotonin uptake, calcium inhibitors, aluminum chelators, etc. Therapeutic "cocktails" are in the process of development in accordance with multiple neurotransmitter deficits. The methodology is often different from one test to another. There is no single strategy.

Rökan (Ginkgo Biloba). Recent Results in Pharmacology and Clinic
Edited by E.W. Fünfgeld
© Springer-Verlag Berlin Heidelberg New York 1988, pp. 278-290

Evaluation scales

Among the numerous scales for evaluation of cognitive functions and behavioral modifications, none can be considered as the reference tool. The difficulties and criticisms derive partially from the fact that these scales were conceived and adapted by specialists belonging to such different disciplines as geriatrics, psychiatry, or neurology.(10),(15) In order to have a complete overview of the spectrum of possible choices, it is enough to consult the considerable studies made by Israel et al.(11) of most of the available tests and their suitability for a geriatric study.

It is scarcely possible to elaborate here on the relative advantages and drawbacks of these numerous evaluation instruments. We shall limit ourselves to a selection.

The Sandoz scale for clinical appreciation in geriatrics, the SCAG of Shader et al.,(19) does not seem to be suitable for studying the evolution of Alzheimer's disease. It includes only five items having the purpose of exploring cognitive functions, the others evaluating essentially depression and anxiety. This is a nonspecific scale conceived more for elderly subjects in general and the functional disorders of old age than for a precise and defined condition.

Some tests that are widely used because they are brief, the MSQ ten-point mental status questionnaire by Kahn et al.,(12) or the famous Mini-Mental Test by Folstein et al.,(8) often encounter the criticism that they are not sensitive enough instruments for the evaluation of moderate deficits.

The global deterioration scale (GDS) by Reisberg et al.,(17) also widely used, gives an excellent clinical description of the severity of the Alzheimer's disease, but essentially it evaluates cognitive decline by a code from one to seven (four being considered as the figure indicating the certainty of a demential state).

The scale proposed by Blessed et al.(4) has the advantage of measuring cognitive and noncognitive aspects and mainly of having been validated anatomically. Seventy-six neuropathological studies have established a relationship between the score on the evaluation scale and the number of senile plaques. Its limitation is perhaps the fact that it deals with very advanced Alzheimer's disease; we might ask whether or not its sensitivity and reliability are identical in early dementia.

We can also site the London Psychogeriatric Rating Scale (LPRS), the Extended Scale for Dementia (ESD), the Functional Dementia Scale (FDS), and Luria's battery of tests, etc.

The three evaluation scales which seem to us to be the most used are Folstein's Mini-Mental test,(8) the Reisberg global deterioration scale,(17) and the scale by Blessed et al.(4) In the recent study by Chui et al.,(5) studying the natural evolution of 146 cases of Alzheimer's disease, the three scales were used jointly, and a satisfactory correlation appeared among them. The recent scale of Rosen et al.,(18) specially designed to define initial severity and to quantify the evolution of Alzheimer's disease, seems to us to constitute an improvement in comparison with what has been proposed, but it has not been used enough for its exact value to be known.

Guiding principles

Although it seems difficult at present to select the ideal "measuring instrument" for Alzheimer's disease, it may be desirable to attempt to obtain a consensus on several basic points.

First, we believe that the scales specifically designed to judge a demential state should be differentiated from those used to evaluate functional disorders of old age (without any precise pathological state).

The tests proposed should be directed toward both the cognitive and non-cognitve (behavioral) aspects of the disease. It should be *realistic* by permitting demonstration of the subject's capacitites in coping with the activities of daily life: shopping, household tasks, keeping appointments, etc. It should avoid tests using senseless tasks, comprising, for example, forms selected at random.

These evaluation instruments should not require recourse to a psychologist or to very specialized personnel, but should be suitable for use by a clinician (neurologist, psychiatrist, geriatrician), and also by different medical teams, without special equipment, without any training other than their daily experience within the normal framework of the classical clinical examination. This condition is imposed by the necessity for resorting to multicenter studies, a requirement in order to assure an adequate recruitment, that is, several hundred patients having deterioration of equivalent severity and constituting a homogenous group.

Also, observation of this rule would make it possible to propose, generalize, extrapolate, or distribute the same protocol later on to other clinicians; it is then possible, within strict statistical and methodological limits, to establish comparisons with other studies performed in different countries or with different therapies.

It seems desirable to combine multiple independent evaluations from different compilations of data (combination of several scales).

To take into account the margin between the desirable and the feasible in a clinical trial, administration of the battery of proposed tests should require no more than a maximum of one hour. The patient with intellectual deterioration is a subject who tires easily, rapidly losing his motivation and becoming uncooperative. In addition, the examiner himself may also experience similar fatigue when faced with such an exhaustive battery of tests.

The duration of surveillance is often six months.(21) We may ask ourselves whether this period is long enough to demonstrate a difference in the evolution of a disease which lasts an average of eight years.(2)

Table 1
Dementia scale by Blessed et al.
First part: Scale A conerning interrogation of the entourage

Blessed's scale A (score from 0 to 28): Note: Circle the number corresponding to the answer obtained A. INTERROGATION OF THE ENTOURAGE I. *Changes in performance of daily activities*	YES- COMPLETE INCAPACITY	PERMANENT NONCAPACITY	±PARTIAL, VARIABLE, OR INTERMITTENT CAPACITY
1. Incapable of accomplishing daily tasks	1	0.5	0
2. Incapable of handling small sums of money	1	0.5	0
3. Incapable of remembering a short list of words, for example while doing errands	1	0.5	0
4. Incapable of finding his way around his apartment	1	0.5	0
5. Incapable of finding his way in familiar streets	1	0.5	0
6. Incapable of identifying the environment (as for example, knowing whether he is in a hospital or at home)	1	0.5	0
7. Incapable of remembering recent events (for example, recent trips, visits of parents or friends, the menu from the previous day)	1	0.5	0
8. Tendency to live in the past	1	0.5	0
TOTAL I			

II. *Changes in habits*	
9. Nutrition:	
Eats properly with appropriate cutlery	0
Eats sloppily, using only a spoon	1
Eats with hands	2
Must be fed	3
10. Dress:	
Dresses self without help	0
Sometimes poorly adjusted and poorly buttoned	1
Mistakes and frequent oversight in the dressing sequence	2
Incapable of dressing self alone	3
11. Sphincter control:	
Normal	0
Sometimes urinates in bed	1
Frequently urinates in bed	2
Dual incontinence	3
TOTAL II	

III. *Changes in personality and behavior*	YES	NO
12. Increased mental rigidity	1	0
13. Increased egocentricity	1	0
14. Loss of interest for the feelings of others	1	0
15. Loss of affectivity	1	0
16. Loss of emotional control, as for example excessive susceptibility and irritability	1	0
17. Inappropriate laughter	1	0
18. Decreased emotional response	1	0
19. Sexual misconduct of recent appearance	1	0
20. Abandonment of favorite pastimes	1	0
21. Loss of initiative or increasing apathy	1	0
22. Unjustified hyperactivity	1	0
TOTAL III		
TOTAL I + II + III		

The higher the score, the more pronounced the deficit

Table 2

Dementia scale by Blessed et al.

Second part: Scale B concerning interrogation of the patient

Blessed's scale B (score from 37 to 0):
Note: Circle the number corresponding to the reply obtained
B. INTERROGATION OF THE PATIENT

I. Orientation	FALSE	TRUE
Name	0	1
Age	0	1
Time (hour)	0	1
Time of day	0	1
Day of week	0	1
Date	0	1
Month	0	1
Season	0	1
Year	0	1
Personal address: street	0	1
city	0	1
postal code	0	1
Identification of place ("Where are you now?")	0	1
Identification of persons (household employees, physician, nurse, patient, parent; identification of two of these)	0	1
TOTAL I		

II. *Memory*	FALSE	±	TRUE
1. Memory for personal facts:			
Date of birth	0		1
Place of birth	0		1
School attended	0		1
Profession (or that of spouse)	0		1
Name of parents or spouse	0		1
Name of a city where the patient has worked or lived	0		1
Name of employers (or that of spouse)	0		1
2. Memory for nonpersonal facts:			
Date of beginning of the First World War	0	0.5	1
Date of beginning of the Second World War	0	0.5	1
(1/2 point if the date is exact to within three years)			
Name of the President of the Republic	0		1
Name of the Prime Minister	0		1
3. Test of short-term memory:	0		1
Mr. Jean Brun, 42, rue de l'Ouest, VESOUL			
Repeat after 5 minutes, that is:	0		1
two-minute study period, then two	0		1
test of repetition. Go on to	0		1
section III below to proceed after	0		1
repetition of the memorized text			
TOTAL II			

III. *Attention, concentration*	FALSE	±	TRUE
Count from 1 to 20	0	1	2
Count from 20 to 1	0	1	2
Months of the year backwards	0	1	2
TOTAL III			

TOTAL I + II + III	

The lower the score, the more pronounced the deficit

The average initial severity required for admission to a trial is still difficult to define. Isolated mnesic disturbance and the too advanced forms, with loss of autonomy, should probably be rejected.

Based on these principles and on significant bibliographical research, a methodology for controlled trials has been designed; it is presented here in its major outlines.

Methodology and Protocol

Objective

The study is intended to investigate whether there is a difference in the evolution of Alzheimer's disease between a group of patients treated with placebo and another group of subjects treated with a drug that has shown activity in the psychobehavioral disorders of senescence, in this case Ginkgo biloba extract (Tanakan®/Rökan®, Institut I. P. S. E. N./Intersan), according to the double-blind method versus placebo.

General study conditions

Each patient is followed for 12 months. A complete evaluation (in addition to that carried out for admission) is made at six and 12 months. The patient is also reviewed at three and nine months. This is a multicenter study, in this case involving only neurological or neuropsychiatric physicians having hospital activity, in order to assure good homgeneity of the investigators and a similar approach, in order to guarantee the neurological clinical examination and to assure easy access to the scannograph. The study is guided by a coordination committee and supervised by a monitoring committee (or by evaluation of critical events). The case history notes of the patients not included at the time of the first examination are kept and studied from the epidemiological standpoint. These are subjects presenting with an admission score outside of the preset limits for the various tests. This decision was made in order to attempt to estimate the population from which the recruited patients came.

Definitions

The disease studied is Alzheimer's type of dementia (senile dementia and Alzheimer's disease) in its mild or moderate form. The condition studied within the scope of this protocol is defined as dementia of average severity combining mnesic disorders and a deficit in intellectual capacity and/or disturbances in symbolic activities (aphasia, apraxia). The diagnosis is confirmed after the exclusion, on the basis of the history of the disease, physical examination and additional examinations (EEG, scannograph), of abnormalities originating from another cause for the dementia. The definition of patients allows for subjects of both sexes, betwen 50 and 75 years of age, French speaking, having been educated, not institutionalized, and recruited from a neurology practice.

Tools selected

In order to decide on the admission or nonadmission of the patients to the study and its conduct, a certain number of scales and tests were selected. On the basis of the difficulties mentioned above, this choice was in large part oriented towards a study by Berg et al.,(3) simplifying and reducing the number of tests in order to improve the reliability of the trial. Selection was made, retaining only the most discriminating tests. They made it possible to evaluate the following points:

- Dementia: the dementia scale of G. Blessed et al.(4) was selected, because it was the first to be correlated with the histopathological changes of the disease, and several studies have used it. The Blessed scale includes two parts: interrogation of the entourage, A; then interrogation of the patient, B. A high numerical score on scale A indicates a severe handicap, but the reverse is true for scale B (*Tables 1 and 2* give its adaptation into French, which we performed).

- Aphasia or language: the Boston aphasia battery by Goodglass and Kaplan, second edition,(9) allows quantifying the degree of aphasia and removing the patients whose impairment would be incompatible with taking other tests, and evaluating any possible exacerbation. This is a test battery simplified by Dr. Berg's group, which we have adapted for French-speaking use.

- Depression: the MADRS depression scale (Montgomery and Asberg depression rating scale) makes it possible to eliminate patients having a major depressive syndrome, whether this involves differential diagnosis (pseudodementia) or a reactive syndrome which might disturb taking the tests.(15) This scale was preferred to others (for example, those of Hamilton or Zung) because of its simplicity and its adequate metrological qualities, particularly its good sensitivity. The French adaptation by Dr. Thérèse Lempérière was selected.

- "Intelligence" (or intellectual efficiency): a single test was selected in order to avoid weighting the examination too heavily: the code test (or symbol digit test) from the Wechsler Adult Intelligence Scale (or WAIS). This test, quickly given (90 seconds), can be given without any particular competency and has already been studied in parallel with the Blessed scale. Furthermore, according to the work of Berg already cited, it appears to have significant predictive value.

- Graphic memory: a test of graphic memory, from the battery 144 of Signorct and Whitelem,(20) was selected. It is quick and easy to use, it is numerical (from 0 to 24), and although it can be "interfered with" by apraxic disturbances, it explores immediate memory and deferred memory.

These various tests* were supplemented by a neurological examination with particular investigation of the various forms of apraxia and of extrapyramidal signs which are currently suspected of being unfavorable prognostic factors. Lastly, the clinical examination was supplemented by an EEG and scannography.

Criteria

Criteria for inclusion:

Senile dementia of Alzheimer's type (senile dementia and Alzheimer's disease), early (defined by the Blessed intellectual deterioration scale, with a score on scale A ranging between 0 and 16, and a score on scale B ranging between 9.5 and 30.5), with a normal scannograph or one showing only diffuse atrophy which could possibly be asymetrical.

Criteria for exclusion:

- Age less than 50 years or more than 75 years.
- Intellectual deterioration or confused-demential syndrome of another origin: pure arteriopathic dementia (excluded by a Hachinski ischemic score >8 and the scanner), Pick's disease, alcoholic dementia, intellectual deterioration of Parkinson's disease, Huntington's chorea, amyotrophic lateral sclerosis, hydrocephalus with normal pressure, confused-demential state of metabolic, infectious or toxic origin.
- Severe depressive state (MADRS scale score more than 40).
- Severe aphasia not allowing correct evaluation of the other cognitive functions (score of more than 15 on the Boston aphasia battery).
- Dementia of advanced Alzheimer's type: institutionalization or disease requiring permanent assistance of a third person for the ordinary activities of life), score on scale A more than 16, score on scale B less than 10.
- Conditions or treatments capable of hampering evaluation of evolution: severe organic disease (renal, hepatic, cardiac, and/or decompensated respiratory insufficiency, confirmed chronic alcoholism, neoformation, regardless of site), and prolonged therapy with prohibited drugs.

Criteria for judgement and evaluation:

- essential: Blessed A. Blessed B. WAIS 4, Boston aphasia battery;
- secondary: graphic memory test according to J.L. Signoret, MADRS depression scale.

---

* The authors have available for interested readers copies of the detailed protocol and of the case-history notebook.

Epidemiological criteria

The examination of the patient comprised a certain amount of other data: personal data, level of education, living conditions, laterality, family history of dementia, investigation for apraxia, neurological evaluation. These are meant, in addition to the other criteria, to support the epidemiological data in a prompt or gradual manner, and possibly to stratify the results.

Cotherapies

The only cotherapies permitted were general drugs prescribed for more than one month, provided their prescription was indispensable. If epilepsy attacks occurred (frequency estimated at 6%), an anti-epileptic drug could be prescribed which disturbed alertness little or none: sodium valproate.** If behavioral disorders, in particular nocturnal agitation, were such that a medical supplement was indispensable, benzodiazepine was selected because of its short half-life and its frequency of use: lorazepam.*** All other psychotrophics in the broad sense (including psychotonics) and treatments which could interfere with the therapeutic evaluation were prohibited.

Possible recourse to antidepressants could create difficulties. If they are used at the beginning of the trial for a diagnostic purpose (although the depression scale should theoretically make it possible to avoid their use), or during monitoring because of aggravation or appearance of a depressive syndrome (which could be reactive), they could interfere with the evaluation of the patients and the study product. Also, it is tricky to find a product which meets all of the requirements. Consequently, abstinence is recommended, although their use is not considered as an absolute cause for exclusion during the trial. Particular attention should be paid to this point; any prescription of this type would fall under the heading of "cotherapy", without omitting the aspect "duration of treatment". All case histories in which antidepressants appear will be routinely submitted to the monitoring committee.

Conduct of the trial

An explanatory letter to the family physician is indispensable; it assumes particular importance since it can both:

  – solicit his help, useful, even indispensable, for smooth progress of the trial (cotherapy, prolongation, observance, etc.);

**   Dépakine, Laboratoires Labaz.

***   Témesta, Laboratoires Wyeth-Byla.

– assure the informed consent of the patient or of his entourage in a reasonable and realistic manner. The family general practitioner may be considered, in many cases, as guarantor in part and knowledgeable about the interests of his patient. Furthermore, he intervenes as a third party in the investigator-patient relationship, and he is a control of clarity.

Discussion

Certain limitations exist. It is obvious that this protocol does not permit studying all forms of the disease, even incipient; thus, the patients having too advanced aphasia at the outset would not be taken into consideration. On the other hand, it is possible that certain forms of rapid evolution might be too severe at the outset to be retained, even though an initial form of Alzheimer's disease might be involved.

Difficulties of a more basic type are also to be remembered. The first concerns the definition of the disease itself: Alzheimer's disease is a diagnosis of exclusion and probability. It is quite remarkable that in 1984 an American research team representing an impressive number of scientific companies sought to redefine the criteria that establish the diagnosis of Alzheimer's.(13) According to these criteria, Alzheimer's disease appears as "possible", "probable", or "confirmed" (confirmation being based on histopathological proof obtained by biopsy or autopsy). Any therapeutic trial must a priori be contented with a "probable" diagnosis, which would be even less so when the disease is more recent.

Another difficulty is the current ignorance (at least partial) concerning the natural evolution and prognostic factors. Does Alzheimer's disease constitute a single entity, or is it a heterogeneous disease? Two recent studies favor the existence of subgroups. Mayeux et al.(14) give the results of a five-year study of 121 patients; Chui et al.,(5) that of 146 patients followed for two years. It is believed(14) that there are benign forms of the disease, with little or no progression in the cognitive decline, some forms with extrapyramidal signs of more rapid exacerbation, and lastly forms with myoclonia, with a very grave prognosis.

Aside from the presence of an obvious extrapyramidal semiology, most of the other prognostic factors are debatable. In a recent study,(3) in which 43 cases of Alzheimer's disease of moderate intensity were followed for 12 months (by means of numerous tests), only the initial severity of the language disorders and the score on the code test (WAIS 4 – Weschler's adult intelligence scale) appeared to be predictive of the evolution of the demential state. The belief(1) that the evolution is more severe in younger subjects is also debatable. It is, however, quite certain that various neurotransmitter deficits are more severe when the patients are younger.(16) Furthermore, a relationship between the magnitude of the electroencephalographic abnormalities found and the severity of the disease has been reported several times, notably by Coben et al.,(6) but also not found by other authors.

In the eventuality that Alzheimer's disease does not correspond to a single and unique morbid process, the methodology used should make it possible to identify the subjects who respond to a drug, even if the overall therapeutic benefit in the entire group appears doubtful.

Finally, the fact that a diagnosis of probability is most often involved (particularly in the early stages of the disease), and the uncertainties of the evolutionary profile make selection of a homogeneous sample difficult and require the inclusion of a large group.

In practice, the strategy which has just been presented appears to be realistic and applicable. In the summer of 1986, more than 40 neurological centers accepted or adopted it; despite the difficulty in recruitment resulting from boundaries defined by the different tests (aphasia, depression, dementia), more than 230 patients have been incorporated into the study.

However, it is too soon to know whether this method is sensitive enough to demonstrate a possible difference in evolution between the two groups, whether the duration of surveillance is long enough to clarify the natural evolution of the disease, or whether the summary of the data is accurate enough to permit defining the prognostic factors.

References

1. Barclay L.L., Zemcov A., Blass J.P., Dowell F.H.M.: Factors associated with duration of survival in Alzheimer's disease. *Biol. Psychiatry*, 1985, *20*, 86-93.

2. Barclay L.L., Zemcov A., Blass J.P., Sansone J.: Survival in Alzheimer's disease and vascular dementia. *Neurology*, 1985, *35*, 834-840.

3. Berg L., Danziger W.L., Storand M., Coben L.A., Gado M., Hughes C.P., Knesevich J.W., Bojvinick S.: Predictive features in mild senile dementia of the Alzheimer type. *Neurology*, 1984, *34*, 563-569.

4. Blessed G., Tomlinson B.E., Roth M.: The association between quantitative measures of dementia and of senile change in the cerebral grey matter of elderly subjects. *Brit. J. Psychiatry*, 1968, *114*, 797-811.

5. Chui H.C., Teng E.L., Henderson V.W., Moy A.C.: Clinical subtypes of dementia of the Alzheimer type. *Neurology*, 1984, *34*, 563-569.

6. Coben L.A., Danziger W., Storandt M.: A longitudinal E.E.G. study of mild senile dementia of Alzheimer type: changes at 1 year and at 2.5 years. *Elect. Clin. Neuroph.*, 1985, *61*, 101-112.

7. Crook T.: Clinical drug trials in Alzheimer's disease. *Ann. N.Y. Acad. of Sci.*, 1985, *444*, 428-436.

8. Folstein M.F., Folstein E., Mc Hugh P.R.: Mini-Mental status: a practical method for grading the cognitive state of patients for the clinician. *J. Psychiat. Res.*, 1975, *12*, 189-198.

9. Goodglass H., Kaplan E.: The assessment of aphasia and related disorders. *Lea and Febiger, Ed.*, Philadelphia, 2ᵉ, 1983.

10. Hachinski V.C., Iliff L.E., Zilmka E. et al.: Cerebral blood flow in dementia. *Arch. Neurol.*, 1975, *32*, 632-637.

11. Israël L., Kozarevic D., Sartorius N.: Evaluation en gérontologie. *Ed. S. Karger*, 1984.

12. Kahn R.L., Goldfard A.L., Pollack M., Peck R.: Brief objective measures for the determination of mental status in the aged. *Am. J. Psychiat.*, 1960, *117*, 326-328.

13. Khann G.Mc., Drachman D., Folstein M., Katzman R., Price D., Stadlan E.M.: Clinical diagnosis of Alzheimer's disease. *Neurology*, 1984, *34*, 939-944.

14. Mayeux R., Stern Y., Spanton S.: Heterogeneity in dementia of the Alzheimer type (evidence of subgroups). *Neurology*, 1985, *35*, 453-461.

15. Montgomery S.A., Asberg M.: A new depression scale designed to be sensitive to change. *Brit. J. Psychiatry*, 1979, *134*, 382-389.

16. Mountjoy C.Q., Rossor M.N., Inversen L.L., Roth M.: correlation of cortical cholinergeric and GABA deficits with quantitative neuropathological findings in senile dementia. *Brain*, 1984, *107*, 507-518.

17. Reisberg B., Ferris S.H., Deleon M.J., Crook T.: The global deterioration scale for assessment of primary degenerative dementia. *Am. J. Psychiat.*, 1982, *139*, 1136-1139.

18. Rosen W.G., Mohs R.C., Davis K.L.: A new rating scale for Alzheimer's disease. *Am. J. Psychiat.*, 1984, *34*, 1356-1364.

19. Shader R., Harmatz J.S., Salzman C.: A new scale for clinical assessment in Geriatric Populations: Sandoz Clinical Assessment – Geriatric (SCAG). *J. Am. Geriatr. Soc.*, 1974, *22*, 107-113.

20. Signoret J.L., Whitelem A.: Memory battery scale. *I.N.S. Bulletin*, 1979, *2*, 26.

21. Soininen H., Koskinen T., Helkala E.L., Pigache R., Riekkinen P.J.: Treatment of Alzheimer's disease with a synthetic ACTH 4-9 analog. *Neurology*, 1985, *35*, 1348-1350.

Ginkgo Biloba Extract in the Treatment of Cerebral Disorders Due to Aging
Longitudinal, Multicenter, Double-Blind Study Versus Placebo

J. Taillandier[1], A. Ammar[2], J.P. Rabourdin[3], J.P. Ribeyre[3], J. Pichon[3]
S. Niddam[4], H. Pierart[5]

(1) Service de Gériatrie, Hôpital Paul Brousse. F 94800 Villejuif
(2) Centre Médical de la Caisse Nationale de Retraite des Ouvriers du Bâtiment et des travaux publics (CNRO). F 93170 Bagnolet
(3) Centre Médical de la Caisse Nationale de Retraite des Ouvriers du Bâtiment et des travaux publics (CNRO). F 77340 Pontault-Combault
(4) Centre de Gérontologie de Sarcelles. F 95200 Sarcelles
(5) Institut IPSEN, 30, rue Cambronne. F 75737 Paris Cedex 15

Summary

The efficacy of Ginkgo biloba extract in the treatment of cerebral disorders due to aging was tested in a multicenter study conducted in double-blind versus placebo, involving 166 patients.

In this study, conducted according to strict methodological conditions, a specially designed geriatric clinical evaluation scale was used. The results confirmed the efficacy of Ginkgo biloba extract in cerebral disorders due to aging. The difference between the control group and the treated group became significant by the third month and increased later on. This result was confirmed by the overall evaluation of the physician.

The disturbances characterizing cerebral aging fall under a nosological classification that is poorly defined and is constantly being modified from the standpoint of terminology and that of the diagnostic criteria or the physiopathological processes involved. Numerous more or less similar synonyms have been used to qualify the same patients or the same disturbances: chronic cerebral insufficiency, incipient primary dementia, psychobehavioral disorders of senescence. Is this a single etiopathogenic entity with forms of variable severity and evolution, or independent conditions? The question currently remains unanswered. However, even though biological, epidemiological, and clinical knowledge is still fragmentary, a certain number of methodological rules have evolved, making it possible to evaluate more accurately the

Rökan (Ginkgo Biloba). Recent Results in Pharmacology and Clinic
Edited by E.W. Fünfgeld
© Springer-Verlag Berlin Heidelberg New York 1988, pp. 291-301

influence of a therapy on the disorders, which, in view of the health requirements of each person and the demographic evolution, could pose a worrisome problem.

It is of utmost importance to rigorously select the patients recruited for a drug trial; only an initially homogenous population permits achievement of medically significant results. In particular, and although the currently available diagnostic tools still have limited efficacy, it is necessary to attempt to specify the etiology of the symptoms observed, and most particularly to differentiate degenerative syndromes from vascular syndromes.

For the same purpose, the severity and history of the disorders should be comparable, and it would be advantageous to include only recent syndromes, therefore those most accessible to therapy. Finally, in view of the slowly progressive character of the disorders studies and the existence of transitory fluctuations, the patients must also be followed for sufficiently long periods; this complicates the practical realization of such a trial, but also permits better evaluation of long-term tolerance, which is particularly important in these subjects who are so often fragile and are being treated with multiple drugs.

Methodology

General conditions

This trial brought together 166 case histories (140 women and 26 men). Admission began in November 1982, and ended in March 1984, so that the end of the study was in March 1985. Four centers participated in the study:

- The Geriatric Service, Hôpital Paul Brousse, Service of Prof. Taillandier (47 patients).
- The Medical Center, Caisse Nationale de Retraite des Ouvriers du Bâtiment (CNRO), Service of Dr. Ammar (20 patients).
- The Medical Center, Caisse Nationale de Retraite des Ouvriers du Bâtiment (CNRO), Service of Dr. Rabourdin, Dr. Ribeyre, Dr. Pichon (74 patients).
- Gerontology Center, Sarcelles (95), Service of Dr. Niddam (25 patients).

Criteria for admission

The patients admitted to the study were more than 60 years of age and had disorders related to cerebral aging (or signs of chronic cerebral insufficiency), evaluated by means of the geriatric clinical evaluation scale (GCES). They had to have been inmates of a retirement home for at least two months in order to be accustomed to their environment.

Criteria for exclusion

Excluded from the study were patients having a general decompensated disease (unbalanced diabetes, severe renal insufficiency, and more generally, any severe condition with chronic evolution), or associated pathological disorders which could hinder interpretation of the results, such as psychosis (chronic delerium, mania, depression), severe neurosis (hysterical, obsessive), any neoformation regardless of location, chronic alcoholism.

Also excluded were patients receiving necessary treatment which could bias evaluation of the results, in particular products of the same therapeutic class as the study drug.

Establishment of the diagnosis

A positive diagnosis was based on the GCES,(1) which comprises 17 items; each item is scored from 1 (absent) to 7 (severe). This scale was developed and validated for the clinical evaluation of cerebral senescence disorders and its application to therapeutic trials.

In order to be admitted, the patient had to have a score ranging between 3 and 5 for at least two of the following six items: alertness, memory for recent events, mood, vertigo, headaches, tinnitus, without the severity being maximal (coded 7) for more than two of these six items.

The total score therefore had to be between 21 for the least affected and 113 for the most serious patients.

This condition was required in order to avoid including subjects at the limit of normal or whose condition did not appear to be sufficiently severe to put them into a pathological classification, and on the other hand, patients whose deterioration was such that one could not reasonably hope for any notable improvement.

In addition to the criteria for admission, in order to better define the study population, the interrogation specified: medical and surgical history, risk factors, associated diseases, the socio-cultural class, evaluated according to the INSEE scale, and the Hachinski score,(2) which orients the etiology of senile dementias: a score less than or equal to 4 implies primary neuronal degeneration, a score above 7 is in favor of a vascular origin for the disturbances, between 4 and 7 the impairment is mixed, both cellular and vascular.

Criteria for judging efficacy

Geriatric clinical evaluation scale (GCES)

Filled in by the investigator at each quarterly consultation, this follows the evolution of each of the 17 items.

General clinical evaluation

This involves an instantaneous opinion of the patient's condition at the time of the consultation. The examining physician evaluates the severity of the impairment in the ensemble of symptoms on the basis of his clinical experience with this type of patient and the patient's score in the institutional classification previously defined. He assigns one of the following terms: impairment absent, slight, moderate, average, significant, severe.

Overall evolution

Improvement in comparison with the initial condition at the time of admission is divided into the six following categories: "much improved", "improved", "slight improvement", "no change", "slight exacerbation", and "exacerbation". This is a retrospective evaluation of the entire period as a function of the prior condition.

Criteria for clinical and laboratory tolerance

Regular monitoring of the patients during the 12 months of surveillance comprised a study of clinical tolerance. Any event occurring during the study was recorded. The laboratory tests were made at the time of admission, then at six and 12 months.

Conduct of the study

The study was randomized, in double-blind. The patient was notified of his admission to a therapeutic trial and his consent was sought. Treatments in progress were continued only if they were necessary and had been prescribed for more than three months. Their nature and dosage were recorded in the case history file.

The treatment followed consisted of the administration of Ginkgo biloba extract (EGb 761, Rökan®, Intersan), or a strictly identical placebo. Dosage was 2 mL, twice a day, or for patients having actually received EGb, 160 mg per day.

After the evaluation made at the time of admission, the patients were examined at three, six, nine, and 12 months. At each consultation, in addition to the clinical examination, the physician evaluated the degree of cerebral impairment on the basis of the judgment criteria: the geriatric clinical evaluation scale, general clinical evaluation, and overall evolution.

Compliance with the treatment did not require special surveillance, insofar as the drug was distributed daily to the patients by the supervisory personnel.

Study population and comparability of the groups

The age of the 166 patients was 82.12 ± 6.3 years (age extremes 60 and 97 years). The socio-cultutral class according to the INSEE scale was graded 2.88 on the average. The mean Hachinski score was 5.32 ± 0.21. Randomization divided the patients into two treatment groups. Eighty patients were treated with EGb and 86 with placebo. Comparison of these two groups showed a homogenous distribution of the patients; in fact, analysis of the various general parameters showed no evidence of statistically significant differences *(Table 1)*.

Table 1
Description of the population studied

Element of comparison	EGb	Placebo
Number of patients	80	86
Age (years)	82.35 ± 0.71	81.91 ± 0.69
Sex – men	13	13
– women	67	73
Chronicity of the disorders (years)	4.45 ± 0.51	5.60 ± 0.69
Tobacco	5/75	6/80
Alcohol	17/63	16/70
Social class	2.92 ± 0.186	2.83 ± 0.17
Average Hachinski	5.38 ± 0.27	5.27 ± 0.32
Hachinski less than 4	20	25
more than 7	16	16
between 4 and 7	44	45
History		
Cerebral vascular accident	6	6
Transitory ischemic accident	5	6
Cranial trauma	5	3
Infarction	8	4
Associated diseases		
Stage 1 Arteritis	16	13
Stage 2	2	4
Stage 3	1	1
Hypertension	43	33
Coronary insufficiency	8	12
Non-insulin-dependent diabetes	8	8

At the time of admission, the geriatric clinical evaluation scale revealed no differences between the two groups (EGb group 47.41 ± 1.605, minimum 23, maximum 74; and placebo group 48.425 ± 1.553, minimum 25, maximum 87. Comparison by the Student t-test: t = 0.45, 150 degrees of freedom, not significant).

At the time of admission, the classification of the patients' conditions by the physicians according to five degrees of severity showed no significantly different results (*Table 2*).

Table 2
General clinical evaluation upon admission

Impairment	Absent	Slight	Moderate	Average	Severe	Total
EGb	0	20	21	18	21	80
Placebo	0	20	15	18	30	86

χ^2 = 1.69; 3 degrees of freedom, not significant

Results

Therapeutic efficacy

The group treated with EGb presented with a significant improvement on the geriatric clinical evaluation scale as early as the third month. This improvement was continued and amplified at the time of successive evaluations (*Figure 1*). Also, the relative improvement, that is, in relation to the score at the time of admission, was significant as early as the third month, and reached 17% at one year (*Table 3*).

In the placebo group a slight improvement was noted, which became significant in comparison with admission only at the end of one year. The relative improvement for this therapeutic group is 7%.

Comparison of the group treated with EGb and the placebo group showed a statistically very significant difference (P = 0.01) by the third month, both with respect to improvement in comparison with the initial condition and comparison between the two treatments.

Examination of the distributions according to the severity of the disorders in the EGb group and the placebo group showed a significant difference beginning with the sixth month, and it was noted that the percentage of patients whose disturbances were qualified as "slight" increased from 25% to 37% in the EGb group, whereas in the placebo group it decreased from 23% to 16%.

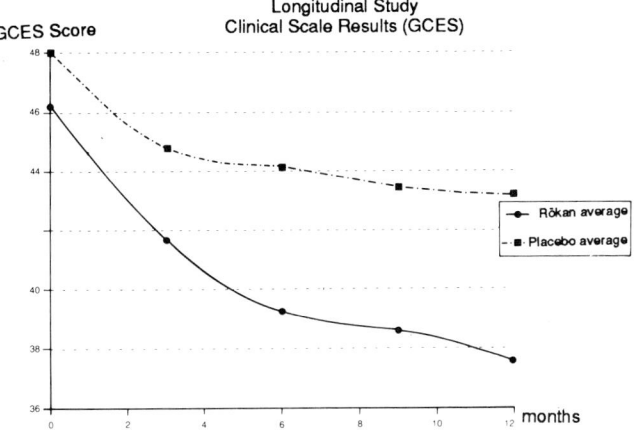

*Figure 1: Longitudinal study. Results from the geriatric clinical evaluation scale.
(Finished cases)*

Table 3
Evolution of the GCES scores

Evolution	Admission		3 months	6 months	9 months	12 months
Absolute score	EGb	47.41	42.36	36.92	39.46	37.57
	placebo	48.42	46.05	46.00	43.95	43.18
	Intergroup significance	NS	P < 0.05	P = 0.01	P = 0.02	P = 0.01
Relative improvement	EGb		9.89%	14.5 %	15.12%	17.10%
	placebo		3.89%	4.29%	7.59%	7.8 %
	Intergroup significance		P = 0.02	P = 0.003	P = 0.03	P = 0.05

For overall evolution graded by the clinician, a significant difference was noted in the distributiion of the two therapy groups beginning with the ninth month. In particular, at the end of treatment, 58% of the patients in the EGb group were improved in comparison with 43% in the placebo group. Furthermore, no center effect was noted.

Thus an improvement was noted on all of the evaluation criteria, which increased in the course of successive tests. The placebo group presented a slight improvement, but of mild intensity and rapidly plateauing.

Detailed analysis by groups

Without its being possible to draw statistically interpretable conclusions, it was worthwhile to attempt to determine whether, among the 166 patients examined for one year, it was possible to establish subgroups whose characteristics known at the time of admission to the study would make it possible to predict a difference in evolution.

It was found that the patients treated with EGb with a history of disorders for longer than two years improved more than the patients more recently afflicted, despite identical severity at the start (*Table 4*). This difference was even more marked for the placebo group, which presented a relative improvement for only 1.6% of the patients whose disorders dated back at least two years.

As a function of the admission score, analysis of the results shows (*Table 4*) that the improvement obtained was greater when the patients were severely affected initially.

According to the Hachinski score, it appears that the higher the score, the greater the improvement in the patients (*Table 4*), that is, implying vascular participation.

Tolerance and dropouts from the study

The causes for dropping out in the course of the study were not statistically different in the two groups. In the EGb group there were 11 suspensions, one cerebral vascular accident less than one month after inclusion in the study, eight deaths, and one problem with tolerance. In the placebo group there were eight suspensions, 13 deaths, and two problems of tolerance. The suspensions corresponded to dropouts during the study unrelated to the treatment or to the evolution of the disease. These were usually a change in retirement home or return to the family. Three patients (two of whom were receiving placebo) who stopped treatment because of intolerance were complaining of gastric disturbances. The distribution of the deaths, more numerous in the placebo group, was not statistically significant and does not permit drawing any conclusions.

Table 4

Relative improvement according to chronicity, initial GCES score, and Hachinski score

Element of comparison	EGb	Placebo
Time disease present less than or equal to two years	15.4% n = 26	1.6% n = 26
Chronicity more than two years	18% n = 46	10.4% n = 54
Score less than 35	9.8% n = 18	− 7.7% n = 16
Score from 35 to 46	17.82% n = 15	13.13% n = 20
Score from 47 to 59	18.67% n = 22	5.13% n = 24
Score more than 59	24.51% n = 17	20.25% n = 20
Hachinski less than or equal to 4	11.5% n = 17	1.2% n = 23
Hachinski more than 4, less than 7	15.48% n = 40	7.1% n = 42
Hachinski more than 7	27.18% n = 15	21.71% n = 10

Biological surveillance

During the 12 months of monitoring of the 86 patients treated with EGb, the following parameters were followed: prothrombin rate, uricemia, total lipids, total cholesterolemia, triglyceridemia, fasting glycemia, transaminases, creatininemia, complete blood count, sedimentation rate, glycosuria, proteinuria. No laboratory test showed any significant variations between the initial values and those recorded at six months and 12 months. The same procedure was followed for the placebo group, which also had no differences.

Discussion and Conclusion

The patients included in this study form a group whose homogeneity could be qualified satisfactorily, whether from the standpoint of age, social class, history, or associated diseases. We should also stress that it was the great uniformity of their lifestyle, that of retirement homes and not a long hospital stay, which assured them of both their protected space and a good degree of autonomy.

Even more important, the conditions fro admission excluded subjects who were too deteriorated, but also subjects who were too "normal". Certainly, despite this precaution, their degree of handicap was situated within a relatively broad bracket, but more severe criteria would have rendered the testing impossible from the practical standpoint by reducing the population too much.

The geriatric clinical evaluation scale used (GCES) was designed to evaluate the elderly subjects in an overall manner: intellectual functions (memory, alertness, attention), mood, social insertion, neurosensorial disturbances. It was particularly well adapted to monitoring of moderately deteriorated subjects rather than for the evaluation of confirmed dementias or depressions.

Most of the patients in this multicenter therapeutic trial could be classified in "moderate cognitive deficit" categories (annoying memory disturbances, definite decrease in attention and concentration), or even "deficit of moderate severity" (help by a third person necessary, major memory disorders, difficulties in calculating, beginning temporospatial disorientation).

It is remarkable that the most affected subjects seem to be those who benefited most from the treatment (*Table 4*). The same is true for those whose disorders were the oldest; but in fact, it was probably usually the same subjects. The finding is perhaps paradoxical only in appearance: it is easier to quantify an improvement when the deficit is distinct at the beginning.

In the two therapeutic groups, the patients whose Hachinski score was highest, that is to say, the "vasculars", were those whose relative gain at one year was highest.

Among the 17 factors studied by the GCES, those who had the most "movement" were those who corresponded to dynamism and social openness; this seemed to be particularly worthwhile for subjects for whom it was desired to maintain an active life as long as possible, whether they were pensioners in a retirement home or whether they lived alone or with families.

The ten-point gain on the behavioral scale, the average for subjects treated with EGb, might seem modest. It is, however, more than double that recorded for the patients on placebo; such a gain is often enough to move a patient out of a "semi-invalid" category to the "semi-valid" category, which could change everything for their relatives, for the nursing personnel, and also for themselves, delaying "institutionalization".

The apparent efficacy of the placebo should not be surprising: a senescent subject to whom attention is paid does better; this is a well-established fact. *Table 4* is interesting however, since it shows, as to the difference in the other categories, that the patients little affected grew worse under placebo. At one year, the difference between the two treatment groups was particularly significant. It therefore seems that there is value in treating as soon as possible and that then one might hope to delay or amend the degenerative processes.

Study of *Figure 1* is instructive: not only did the subjects treated with EGb see the gap between them and the patients in the placebo group gradually widen, but their condition continued to improve, whereas that of the patients on placebo tended toward a plateau. In other words, the patients treated with EGb continued to draw obvious benefit from the treatment after one year, contrary to what was observed with placebo.

Finally, we should stress the innocuousness of the drug, which appeared to us to be practically complete.

In conclusion, the use of a geriatric clinical evaluation scale (GCES) confirmed the effectiveness of Ginkgo biloba extract in disorders due to cerebral aging at the end of a multicenter study conducted according to a rigorous methodology (double-blind, randomization), meeting the criteria currently required to evaluate the therapeutic efficacy of drugs.

The patients receiving placebo recorded a slight improvement at the beginning of the study (which is customary), then stagnation. In summary, in the EGb group, the improvement which appeared during the first few weeks progressed throughout the successive control evaluations, and the difference between the two groups became significant by the third month and increased over the course of time.

The results according to the clinical evaluation scale agree with the subjective evaluation by the physician, who made an overall judgment on the evolution of his patients and concluded at each control and at the end of the treatment that there was obvious improvement in all of the patients treated with EGb.

References

1. Georges D., Lallemand A., Constenoble I., Loria Y.: Validation par l'analyse factorielle d'une échelle d'évaluation clinique des troubles de la sénescence cérébrale. Application à l'essai thérapeutique. *Thérapie,* 1977, *32*, 173-180.

2. Rosen W.G., Terry R.D., Fuld P.A. et al.: Pathological verification of ischemic score in differentiation of dementias. *Ann. Neurol.,* 1980, *7*, 486-488.

The Clinical Effect of Ginkgo Biloba Extract in the Case of Cerebral Insufficiency Documented by Dynamic-Brain-Mapping – A Computerized EEG Evaluation.

E.W. Fünfgeld[1], D. Stalleicken[2]

(1) Schloßbergklinik Wittgenstein, Bad Laasphe (West Germany)
(2) Intersan GmbH, Ettlingen (West Germany)

Summary

The advantages of the Computer EEG, its applications, and the easily readable equipment used (dynamic brain mapping according to Itil) are described on the basis of the reaction to Ginkgo biloba extract. Without a doubt, a cerebral dysfunction can so be detected in 90% of the cases before any essential clinical failures are observed. Ginkgo biloba (Rökan®), clinically tested in a multicenter study with more than 8000 patients, promises to be successful in the treatment of cerebral dysfunction with combined impairment of intellectual abilities and vigilance.

In the industrialized countries a far-reaching change in the demographic profile can be observed. Whereas in the fifties the percentage of those aged over 65 was about 8% of the population, it has already risen to 15% in the eighties and will go beyond the 20% mark in 2025.(1) Accordingly, the age pyramid is changing its form; it is getting narrow at the base and approaching a square. The rise in the average life-age has changed the age structure of the population and is accompanied by a considerable increase in demential diseases. Depending on the author, the incidence in those between 65 and 70 years varies from 2 to 5%, in those between 80 and 90 from 20 to 25%.

Today, cerebral insufficiency, states of confusion and other symptoms of the cerebro-organic psychosyndrome are considered to be serious enough for medical treatment. Undoubtedly, one of the best established preparations for medical therapy is Ginkgo biloba extract (Rökan®) whose therapeutic efficacy can be documented casuistically – in the sense of a representative case from a study still in progress which will be reported on in another publication – by a new method of EEG evaluation.

Rökan (Ginkgo Biloba). Recent Results in Pharmacology and Clinic
Edited by E.W. Fünfgeld
© Springer-Verlag Berlin Heidelberg New York 1988, pp. 302-313

The Ginkgo biloba extract, according to Tea and Colleagues (25), positively influences the cerebral metabolism, the absorption of oxygen and glucose and also – through the terpenoid Ginkgolid B (an antagonist of the thrombocyte-activizing factor) present above all in the infusion – causes the inhibition of the aggregation of thrombocytes.[27]

In the Ginkgo biloba infusion therapy a standardized extract (Rökan® Amp., not marketed) in ampules with 50 mg of the active substance per ampule is applied.

This substance is gained from the dried leaves of the Ginkgo biloba tree in an extraction procedure by using an acetone-water-mixture and removing the acetone afterwards. The extract is standardized on 24% of Ginkgo flavonglucosides (heterosides) which serve as a guiding substance. Apart from that the extract contains ginkgolides, bilobalides, proantocyanides with the prototypes delphinidin and cyanidin [6].

At present the following pharmacological properties of Ginkgo biloba are the main items of research and contribute to the understanding of its clinical efficacy:

1. the effect of the hemodynamics, verified by blood flow measurements in various vessel regions and by the positive influence on the capillary permeability and the vein tone [2, 17, 18].

2. the effect on the metabolism, proved both by a rise of ATP and glucose level, especially in infused brain regions, and by the protective action against the triethyltin edema.[20]

3. the effect on the rheology by stopping the exceeding aggregation of thrombocytes [4, 18]

4. the effect on the rarefication of the receptor conjunctions for neurotransmitters of the acetylcholinergic system due to aging [24]

Rökan®, clinically tested and documented in literature, has also recently been permitted by the West German Federal Health Agency for the treatment of cerebral dysfunction with combined decline of intellectual abilities and vigilance as well as cerebral symptoms such as dizziness, headache, ringing of the ears, impairment of memory and concentration, mood lability. [3, 5, 9, 10, 11, 19, 23, 26]

The outstanding success of therapy with Ginkgo biloba with its excellent compatibility in cases of demential phenomena were shown in a multicenter study with more than 8000 patients [22].

For over 40 years considerable effort has been made to objectify and standardize the EEG evaluation. Due to the advanced computer techniques it is now possible – within reasonable terms of expenditure – to get hold of objective test data by means of the Fast-Fourier-analysis. Moreover, this method brings about a greater information density, since on the conventional paper registration low waves repeatedly overlap and thus do not show up; they rather merge in higher tension waves.

Adequate apparatuses have been developed mainly in the USA, eg. Cadwell, Nicolet etc. The system of Dynamic-Brain-Mapping developed by Itil in Tarrytown (New York) is particularly easy to read, because differences in progress can clearly be seen.

The usual four frequency zones appear on the monitor in colour: various shades of red for the Delta-area, of violet for the Theta, of blue for the Alpha and of green for the Beta area. Beyond that – and this is the essential advantage of the Itil method – the percentage of the four frequency zones can immediately be read from the points of derivation, so that intra-individual and inter-individual comparison can easily be made. Arising from the demand for practicability, there are 9 different computer programs available for each EEG fitting and they can be displayed on monitors: 4 programs refer to the four different frequency zones, the percentage of the delta, theta, beta, and alpha waves are depicted separately as to distribution and frequency; five programs were developed according to the clinically most relevant aspects, which are defined as follows: first the "Absolute Highest" activity in the brain area concerned or the "Second High" respectively. In the programs 'primary (or secondary) clinical activities' the low frequencies are given priority because of their clinical relevance. In the program 'topographical distribution' all four frequency zones are represented, as far as they occur repeatedly in certain brain areas [13-16].

During an application on over 500 patients which lasted more than a year with progress controls during the therapy (more than 10 derivations in a number of patients, even more than 15 in some), the clinical relevance of these five standard programs – apart from the separate display of the four frequency zones – could always be considered as very positive when immediate evaluation of the individual success of the therapy was asked for.

Normal values and border case findings

Figures 1 and 2 show computer EEG findings of patients whose EEG looked completely normal in the conventional derivation (*fig. 1* – here in profile only alpha waves) or could at least be considered as ranging within standard (*fig. 2* – top view). *Figure 2*, however, reveals additional information by means of the computer EEG: the alpha production being normal occipital and equilateral, we can discern a precentral theta-activity predominating in the left front whereas in the right front beta-activity is clearly prevailing. Artefacts could be excluded. Thus according to the computer EEG the finding is not normal, but at least a border case with asymmetry in disfavour of the left front of the brain half (even after an overcheck of the conventionally registered EEG the above finding could not be detected!).

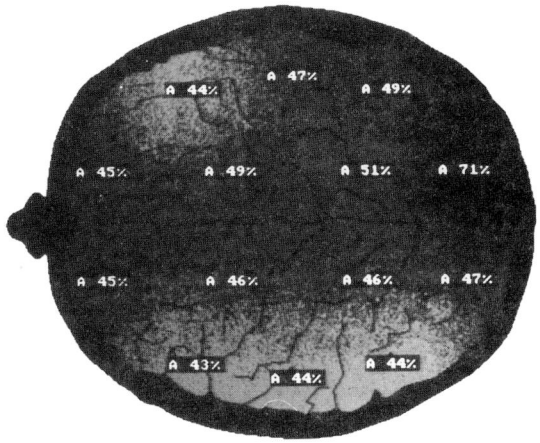

Figure 1: Normal alpha-EEG

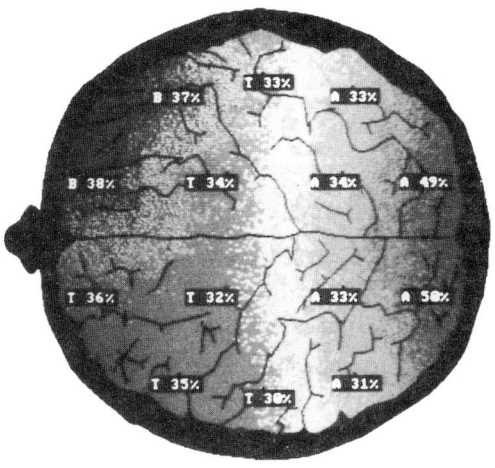

Figure 2: Borderline state with slight theta interspersing (not visible on conventional EEG)

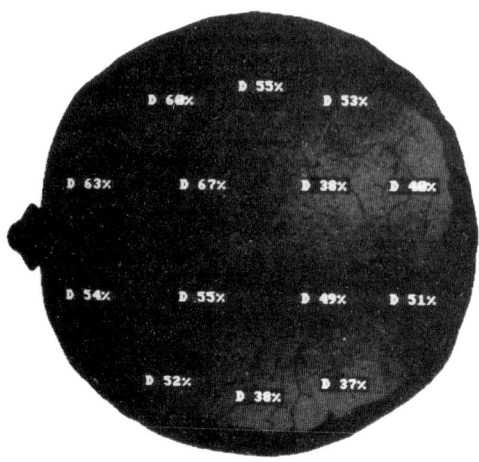

Figure 3: Severe general change, pure delta activity. Severe presenile Alzheimer illness

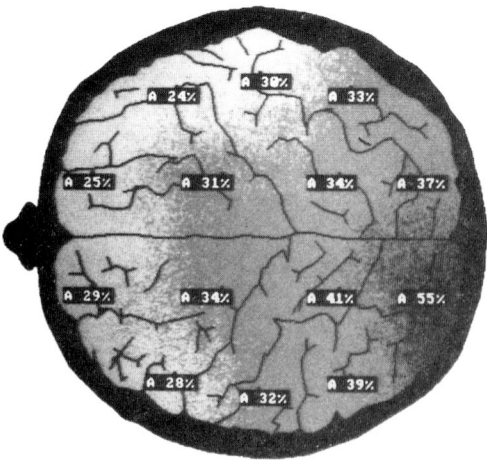

Figure 4: Alpha activity in recidive of a right-brain insult 3 months before

Figure 3 shows in the program "Absolute Highest" exclusively delta activity and this mainly in the front.

Figure 4 shows the EEG of a 81 year old patient who, 3 months before his first derivation of a C-EEG, had been taken to a different hospital with a relapse into a left side hemiparese. In the C-EEG exmaination on 22/4/87 a (relative) steady state with complete pares of the left arm and a partial parese of the left leg had already been a matter-of-fact. Accordingly delta- and theta activities could be found in the right hemisphere.

In what follows we want to introduce a representative casuistic of a Ginkgo biloba study still in progress. It concerns geriatric patients with symptoms of cerebral insufficiency who partly suffer from additional neurological diseases such as M. Parkinson.

In July 1987, 74 year old Willi W. was brought to the hospital for the second time for the treatment of his parkinson-syndrome which he had had for several years. Earlier, in connection with a rather high anti-parkinson-medication, considerable states of delerium had already occurred. On the first as well as on the second recording the conventional EEG showed a distinct general change.

Figure 5 shows the program "Absolute Highest" before the therapy started. *Figure 8* shows the program "second high" at the same point of time. Whereas in *Figure 5* a very clear difference between the two hemispheres can be observed – on the right side exclusively theta waves, on the left side exclusively beta waves – in *Figure 8* we find only alpha activity which predominates on the left side. *Figure 6* and *Figure 9* show the changes in both programs 2 hours after the first injection of 200 ml of a parenteral preparation of Ginkgo biloba. In the program "Absolut highest" (*Figure 6*) the theta activity in the right hemisphere has slightly increased in front and occipitally, but has also spread over the left hemisphere with the exception of an area of alpha-waves in the precentral, central and temporal zone. In the program "Second High" (*Figure 9*) a distinct change has occured in the left hemisphere too: instead of alpha and a narrow strip in the precentral, central and temporal zone, on the right side a slight general regression of alpha activity. *Figures 7 and 10* show the findings after 10 infusions of 200 ml Ginkgo biloba each: In *figure 7* we now find a rather even, on the right slightly predominating theta activity; *figure 10* shows a regression of alpha activity in the right hemisphere and on the left a shift of alpha activity which is now encircled by beta waves in front and occipitally; in *Figure 5* (before the therapy started) this hemisphere shows a very strong beta activity.

The findings under the infusion therapy with Ginkgo biloba extract can be interpreted to the effect that a balance between both hemispheres can be established, since the distinct differences on both sides at the beginning are hardly or only residually traceable after 10 infusions. The clinical picture has conisderably impro-ved, too: visible intensification of impulse, good compatibility of the gradually increased antiparkinson medication, no new states of delerium. (When asked 2 months

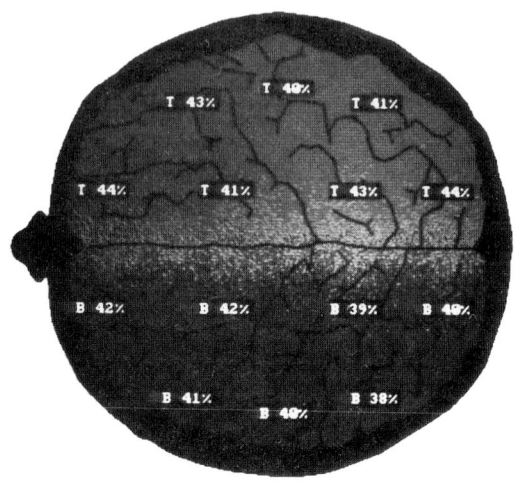

Figure 5: Before therapy begin

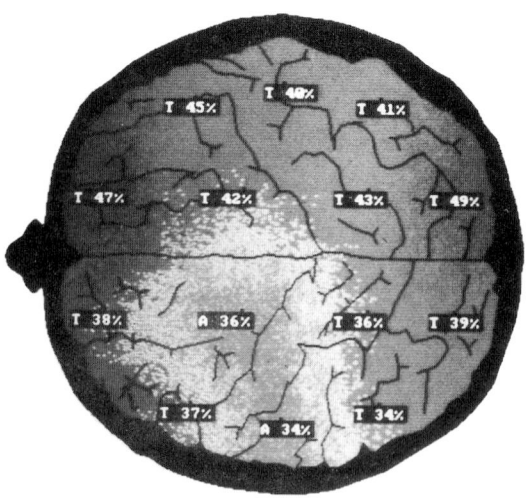

Figure 6: 2 hours after the first infusion

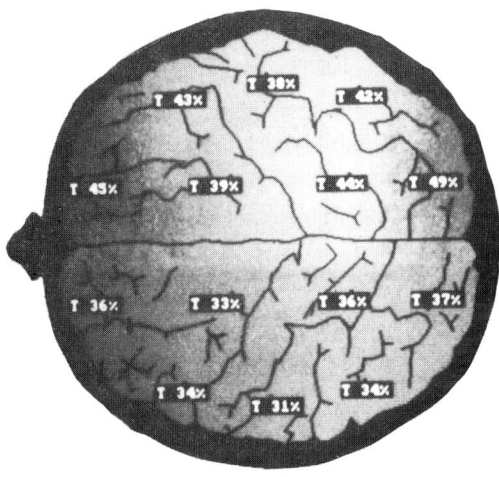

Figure 7: Patient as in figure 5 after ten infusions of 200 mg Ginkgo biloba

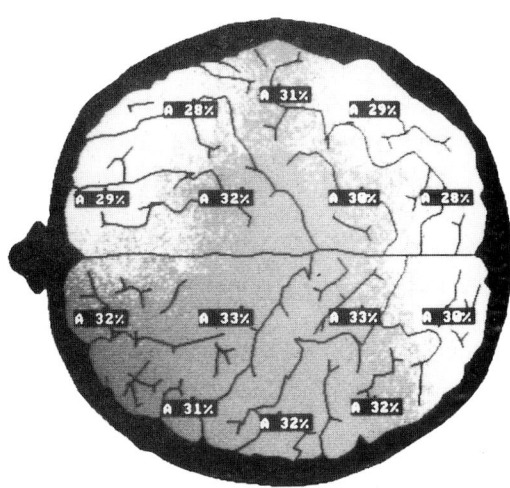

Figure 8: Before therapy begin

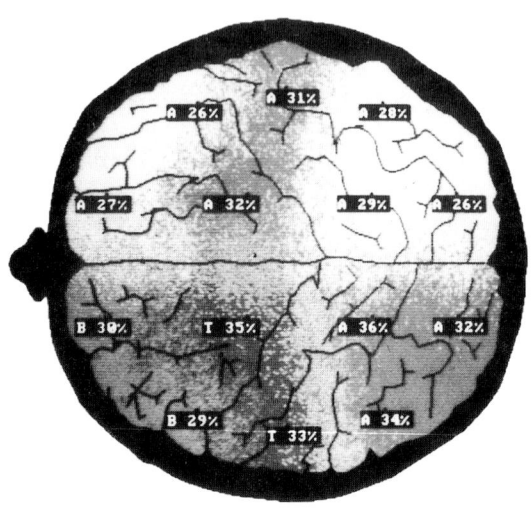

Figure 9: 2 hours after the first infusion

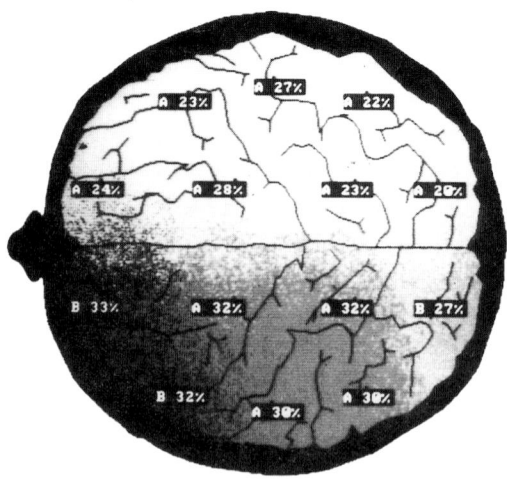

Figure 10: Findings after 10 infusions of 200 mg Ginkgo biloba daily

after his discharge the patient reported that he was quite content and his health was still good and steady.)

Although quite a number of highly technicalized and very differentiated methods have been available lately (positron-emission-tomography, nuclear magnetic resonance technique etc.) we are far from knowing the actual cause or the base disturbances of senile dementia of the Alzheimer type. Various authors report that in such cases they found a reduced absoprtion of glucose, changes of the transmitter, membrane rigidity, calcium overloading and much more. If one wants to relate the possible variations of disturbances to the clinical pictures, the information gained by different technical approaches is still relatively uniform, it is reduced to a few clinical syndromes, or symptoms. But for the time being the following indirect approach to retrospective diagnostics of certain degrees of disturbance seems practicable: the observation of neurophysiological reactions to medications by means of the computer EEG with regards to quality, quantity and localization of the various frequencies. Along with that, the dimension of 'time' should be taken into consideration moreso than before: the reaction to a single dose and the development of the computer EEG under permanent treatment.

The reactions which can be observed during the individual treatment of one patient can surely be taken as a sign of his own brain physiology and physiopathology.

CEEG findings under the influence of Ginkgo biloba extract are not yet at hand. The publication of Tea et al. emphasizes the positive effect in some metabolism parameters. The recently published study by Hofferberth reports – similar to earlier studies – on a statistically significant clinical effect of an oral dose of Ginkgo.

Without a doubt EEG-findings represent objective results, and carrying out blind, double-blind or double-blind cross-over studies could become unnecessary or at least be reduced.

References

1. Allard M., J.L. Signoret, D. Stalleicken: Alzheimer Demenz, *Springer,* Berlin-Heidelberg-New York-Paris-Tokyo 1988

2. Auguet M. et al.: Bases pharmacologiques de l'impact vasculaire de l'extrait de Ginkgo biloba. *Presse ined. 16,* 1524-1528 (1986)

3. Aust G.: Therapie mit Rökan bei vertebro-basilärer Insuffizienz. *In:* Schlitter K. (Hrsg.): Vertigo-Interdisziplinäres Symposium, Berlin 1986, S. 64-74. *Harsch, Karslruhe*

4. Borzeix M.G. et al.: Recherches sur l'action antiagrégante de l'extrait de Ginkgo

biloba. Activité au niveau des artères et des veines de la pie-mère chez le lapin. *Sem. Hôp. Paris 56,* 393-398 (1980)

5. Claussen C.-F., M.V. Kirtane: Randomisierte Doppelblindstudie zur Wirkung von Extractum Ginkgo biloba bei Schwindel und Gangunsicherheit des älteren Menschen. *In:* C.-F. Claussen (Hrsg.): Presbyvertigo, Presbyataxie. Presbytinnitus, Gleichgewichtsstörungen im Alter, S. 103-115. *Springer,* Berlin-Heidelberg-New York-Tokio 1985

6. Drieu K.: Préparation et définition de l'extrait de Ginkgo biloba. *Presse méd. 15,* 1455-1457 (1986).

7. Fünfgeld, E.W.: Spectral and Frequence Analysis of the Central EEG Activity in Alzheimer's Disease: The development during nootropic therapy. Conference at International Symposium and Workshop on Topographic Brain Mapping of EEG and Evoked Potentials, Würzburg 1987. *Springer* (in Press)

8. Fünfgeld E.W., M. Baggen, P. Nedwidek, R. Speck: New nootropic drugs in SDAT-Ratings and objective Results with a Brain Mapping and Imaging System. *In:* Conference at The Third Congress of the International Psychogeriatric Association, Chicago, August 1987

9. Geßner B., A. Voelp, M. Klasser: Study of the long-term action of a Ginkgo biloba Extract on vigilance and mental performance as determined by means of quantitative pharmaco-EEG and psychometric measurements. *Arzneimittel-Forsch. 35,* 1459-1465 (1985)

10. Hagenauer J.P., F. Cantenot, H. Koskas, H. Pierart: Traitement des troubles de l'équilibre par l'extrait de Ginkgo biloba. Etude multicentrique à double insu face au placebo. *Presse méd. 15,* 1969-1572 (1986)

11. Hofferberth B.: Die Therapie neurologischer Vertigo-Fälle mit Ginkgo biloba (Rökan®) bei hirnorganischem Psychosyndrom. In: Schlitter K. (Hrsg.): Vertigo – Interdisziplinäres Symposium, Berlin 1986, S. 47-63. *Harsch,* Karlsruhe

12. Hofferberth, B.: The influence of Ginkgo Biloba Extract (GBE) on the Neurophysiological and Psychometrical Test results in patients suffering from organic cerebral Psychosyndrome: A Double-Blind Study Versus Placebo. Conference at The Third Congress of the International Psychogeriatric Association, Chicago, August 1987

13. Itil T.M., D.M. Shapiro, E. Eralp, A.Akman, K.Z. Itil, C. Garbizu: A new Brain function function diagnostic unit, including the Dynamic Brain Mapping of computer analyzed EEG, evoked potential and sleep (a new Hardware/Software System and its application in Psychiatry and Psychopharmacology) – grundlegende Arbeit. *New trends exp. clin. Psychiat. 1,* 107-177 (1965)

14. Itil T.: CEEG Brain Mapping in Psychiatry, Conference in : Computer Analyzed EEG (CEEG) and evoked potential in Clinical PSychiatry and Research. 140th Annual Meeting of the American Psychiatric Association Chicago May 1987

15. Itil T.M., K. Itil, E. Eralp, A. Kunitz: CEEG Dynamic Brain Mapping of aging Brain and a theory to reverse Physiological aging. Conference at The Third Congress of the International Psychogeriatric Association, Chicago, August 1987.

16. Itil T.M., E. Eralp, K. Itil, A. Manco, P. Mehta: Brain Function Monitoring (BFM) System in Geriatric Psychopharmacology. *Conference at The Third Congress of the International Psychogeriatric Association.* Chicago, August 1987

17. Lagrue G., J. Baillet, A. Behar: Activité d'un extrait végétal complexe dans les oedèmes idiopathiques orthostatiques. *Sem. Hôp. Paris 54,* 214-217 (1978)

18. Marcy R.: Pharmakologisches Gutachten. Pharmacological Report (1986)

19. Pidoux B.: Clinical and Quantitaive EEG Double-Blind Study of Ginkgo Biloba Extract (GBE). *J. Cerebral Blood Flow Metab. 3 (Suppl. 1)* (1983)

20. Rapin J.R., M. Le Poncin Lafitte: Modèle expérimental d'ischémie cérébrale – Action préventive de l'extrait de Ginkgo. *Sem. Hôp. Paris 55,* 2047-2050 (1979)

21. Rotrosen J.: Membrane Lipids: Can Modification Reduce Symptoms or Halt Pregression in Alzheimer's Disease? Crook T., R.T. Bartus, S. Ferries, S. Gershon (eds): Treatment Development Strategies for Alzheimer's Disease, *Powley Ass.,* Madison/Con. 1986

22. Stalleicken D., P. Ihm: Rökan® flüssig bei zerebraler Insuffizienz – Daten einer multizentrischen Studie mit mehr als 8000 Patienten. Symposium Zerebrale Insuffizienz, Berlin, September 1987

23. J.P. Ribeyre, J. Pichon, S. Niddam, H. Pierart: Traitement des troubles du viellissement cérébral par l'extrait de Ginkgo biloba. *Presse méd. 15,* 1583-1587 (1986)

24. Taylor J.E.: Liaison des neuromédiateurs à leurs récepteurs dans le cerveau de rats. *Presse méd. 15,* 1491-1493 (1986)

25. Tea S., P. Celsis, M. Clanet, J.-P. Marc-Vergnes, U. Boeters: Quantifizierte Parameter zum Nachweis von zerebraler Durchblutungs- und Stoffwechselsteigerung unter Ginkgo-biloba-Therapie, *Therapiewoche 37,* 2655-2657 (1987)

26. Vorberg G.: Ginkgo biloba extract: a longterm study of chronic cerebral insufficiency in geriatric patients. *Clin. Trial J. 22,* 149-157 (1985)

27. Weber N.: Platelet Activating Factor – ein physiologisch aktives Etherlipid. *Pharmazie uns. Zeit 15,* 107 (1986)

Effects of Ginkgo Biloba Extract on Cerebral Functional Activity
Results of Clinical and Experimental Studies

B. Pidoux

Laboratoire de Physiologie. 91, boulevard de l'Hôpital. F 75634 Paris Cedex 13

Summary

Electroencephalography is the only convenient method for functional exploration of the brain. The recent introduction of signal analysis techniques has given it a quantitative dimension and has resulted in pharmacological studies of electroencephalograms. In four studies of this kind the effects of Ginkgo biloba extract were investigated on three pathological animal models, in young healthy volunteers, and in elderly people with demential disorders. In man, the EEG tracings could be analyzed in relation to different psychometric tests. The results obtained confirm those of clinical trials, and notably the activity of Ginkgo biloba extract on alertness.

The only practical method for functional investigation of the brain, electroencephalography (EEG) has been enriched during the past few years with signal (power spectrum) analysis techniques that have given it a quantitative dimension. This advance in EEG not only allows us to draw functional maps of cortical activity, but also to increase the objectivity of the examinations and to make longitudinal comparative studies of patients and healthy volunteers. The EEG reflects in an extremely sensitive manner all of the metabolic circulatory changes that affect the life of the neurons. It also reflects the state of alertness and the responses of the nervous system to psychotropic substances. Thus a veritable pharmaco-EEG was created, the purposes of which are to identify new drugs, to compare two or more substances, to follow the kinetics of the central activity of a medication, and to evaluate tolerance to treatment.

A certain number of studies have been devoted to Ginkgo biloba extract (EGb 761, Rökan®, Intersan), in elderly adults with senile dementia, in young healthy volunteers, and in animals. We are presenting here a review of these studies.

Rökan (Ginkgo Biloba). Recent Results in Pharmacology and Clinic
Edited by E.W. Fünfgeld
© Springer-Verlag Berlin Heidelberg New York 1988, pp. 314-320

Alertness and intellectual performance of the elderly subject

The purpose of the study by B. Gessner et al.(2) was to measure the action of EGb in patients from 57 to 77 years of age. They were not suffering with any special neurological condition, other than disturbances related to their age.

Sixty volunteers were divided at random into three groups of 20 subjects each. Some received 40 mg/day EGb three times a day, others 5 mg nicergoline, and the last, a placebo identical in appearance. All were submitted to a battery of tests and examinations before the study began and at the end of 4, 8, and 12 weeks of treatment. The EEG was recorded from four bipolar leads 01–C1, C1–F1, 02–C2, C2–F2. The patients were comfortably settled in an easy chair with their eyes closed. Two sequences were recorded each time: an awake EEG in the course of which alertness was verified by asking the subject to press a button in order to differentiate between two sounds of different frequency (500 and 1000 Hz); a resting EEG without verifying alertness. Quantification of the EEG was done by spectral analysis and the results as energy in the delta, theta, alpha-1, alpha-2, beta-1, and beta-2 bands, or as relative intensity in comparison with the total energy of the EEG spectrum. The dominant frequency was calculated at the place on the spectral density with maximal power.

The psychometric tests included, among other things, simple reaction tests and multiple-choice reaction times, search tests which evaluate the faculties of concentration and motor control. The subjects also filled out a self-evaluation questionnaire.

The results from analysis of the EEG showed that, in comparison with the initial measurements before treatment, there was observed only in the EGb group a distinct increase in alpha-1 in the course of the awake EEG (*Figure 1*). Subdivision of the subjects into subgroups on the basis of initial EEG values yielded some interesting information. In the subjects with a dominant low frequency on the resting EEG, an increase of 2 Hz in alpha-1 was found only in the EGb group. There was also found, in patients who initially showed a high value in theta/alpha ratio, a distinct diminution in this ratio in EGb group. This corresponds to an increase in vigilance.

The psychometric results also showed the superiority of EGb over the other two products. Thus, in the EGb group, simple reaction time was shorter at time M2 than at the beginning of the test.

To conclude, no manifest psychostimulant effect of the two drugs in comparison with placebo was found in the entire population studied. However, in the subgroup in which the theta/alpha ratio indicated low alertness at the beginning of the trial, a distinct elevation was noted in alertness on the resting EEG under EGb treatment and not in the other subgroups.

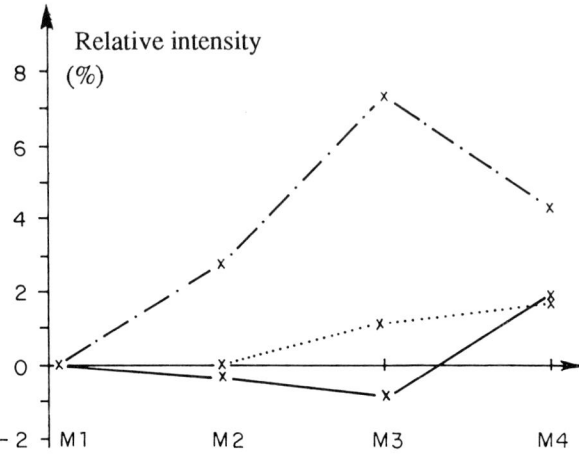

Figure 1: Change in alpha-1 proportion in the EEg power spectrum of three groups of 20 subjects. Placebo (—), EGb (–.–.–), and nicergoline (....) at times M2 (1month), M3 (2 months), M4 (3 months) after the initial M1 recording. Ordinate: relative intensity; abscissa: time. EEG under controlled vigilance, lead 01-C2. (B. Gessner et al.(2)).

Senile dementia

The study by Pidoux et al.(4) involved a group of senile dementia patients. The average age of the 14 patients was 85 years. The initial EEGs were disturbed, as might be expected. However, the only subjects retained were those who were presenting no focalized abnormalities on the EEG, but a slowed baseline rhythm. Patients were rated by evaluation scales (GCES and SGRS) and EEG examinations were performed twice before initiation of treatment with EGb at the rate of 160 mg/day or with placebo in identical packaging. The recordings were repeated after 3, 6, and 12 weeks of treatment. The EEGs were recorded from four leads, T4-C4, P4-02, T3-C3, P3-01. The subjects were recorded for five minutes with eyes closed.

Spectral analysis of the EEG was done in order to calculate the spectral parameters in the delta, theta, alpha, and beta bands. The EGb and placebo groups were compared by means of parametric and non-parametric statistical tests. The results show a clinical improvement indicated by reduction of the evaluation scales score by 29% (P<0.05) for the EGb groups, and non-significant reduction for the placebo group (13%). The EEG changes (*Figure 2*) are indicated by restructuring of the EEG, with an increase

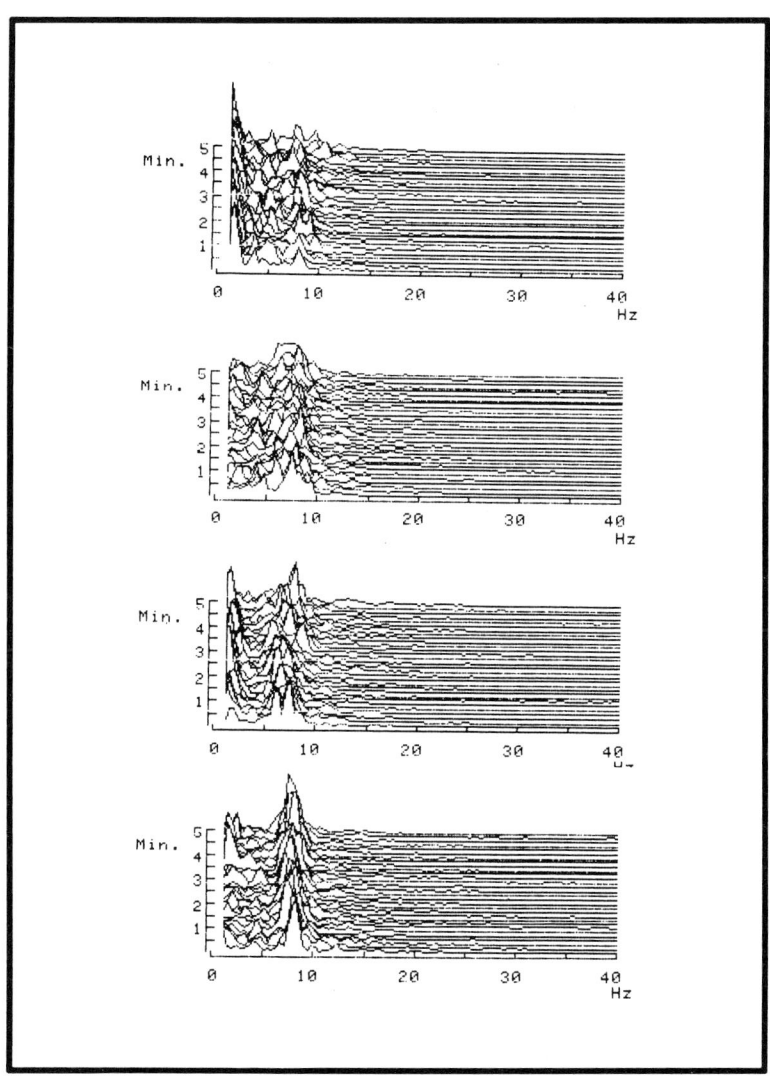

Figure 2: Evolution of the EEG power spectra in a 96-year-old dementia patient before (A) and after three weeks (B), six weeks (C), and 12 weeks (D) of treatment at the rate of 120 mg/day EGb. A distinct improvement was found in the EEG, with a gradual diminution in the delta activity ratio (0 to 4 Hz), and an increase in the alpha (8-9 Hz) which became more stable during treatment. Temporo-Rolandique T4-C4 lead. (Pidoux et al.(4)).

in the spectral intensity of alpha and reduction in the slow frequencies (P<0.05), shown by the reduction in the theta/alpha ratio. The EEG changes for the placebo group were not significant.

In the young healthy subject

The study by Krauskopf et al.(3) investigated the short-term pharmacodynamic effects of EGb in six healthy young volunteers from 18 to 31 years of age (average age 23.4 years). These volunteers took no medication in a habitual manner, and their EEGs were normal. This double-blind study was carried out with increasing doses of 120, 240, and 600 mg EGb or placebo, at intervals of several days and at the same times. The EEG was recorded from eight leads Fp1, F3, C3, 01 and Fp2, F4, C4, P4, 02. At each examination, the baseline EEG was recorded for 15 minutes before and 30 minutes after administration of the product, for 240 minutes. The alertness of the subjects was not tested. The EEG spectral analysis was made over 27-second periods. At the end of the study this analysis supplied the dominant frequency, the absolute and relative spectral power of the dominant frequency, and the various frequency bands. Intra-individual changes in the EEG were calculated by comparison with the mean of the first five periods. In the course of these, it could reasonably be estimated that the subjects were indeed awake and their level of vigilance was high. A distance index based on a noneuclidian distance between values of the spectral energies made it possible to calculate a vigilance index.

The results were the following: evolution of the dominant frequency in the baseline EEG showed a relaxation effect which indicated good adaptation of the subjects to the experimental conditions. The frequency of alpha dropped from 10 Hz to 9.5 Hz.

After placebo, a chronic fluctuation was observed in spectral energy and in frequency on all leads, which reflects fluctuation of the level of vigilance.

At the dosage of 120 mg EGb, alpha power was increased on all leads, except for the frontal regions. On the contrary, beta-1 activity was diminished fro the occipital regions. The fluctuations in spectral energy were diminished. At the dosage of 140 mg EGb, the alpha power spectral was increased in comparison with the values under placebo treatment and with 120 mg, except for the frontal regions. Beta-1 power was weaker than in the placebo group, but higher than with 120 mg. Stabilization of spectral energy was again observed in all frequency bands. At the dosage of 600 mg EGb, an increase was noted in alpha spectral power in both the frontal and occipital regions of both hemispheres. This effect was observed 100 to 120 minutes after administration of the product. An increase was also noted in beta-1 throughout the duration of the recording for the fronto-central regions.

With respect to the dominant frequency, on placebo the mean frequency was around 9 Hz and presented fluctuations. With 120 mg EGb, a diminution of 8.5 Hz was recorded after 120 to 140 minutes, then a return of 10.5 Hz after several minutes. With

250 mg, the frequency was stable on all leads, other than a slight slowing for five minutes, less marked than with placebo. With 600 mg, the most important changes occurred after 120 minutes. The dominant frequency increased to 12 Hz on all leads. This increase lasted throughout the recording. In young subjects, the EEG changes induced by EGb were therefore in favor of stabilization of spontaneous vigilance, which is perceptible with the usual dosage and reaches statistical significance with a double dosage. The effect begins less than 30 minutes after administration of the product, is proportional to the dose prescribed, and lasts longer with the high doses (more than four hours). With 600 mg, the occurrence of a state of hyperalertness could even be detected.

In acute cerebral afflictions

The study by M.G. Borzeix et al.(1) is based on experimental models of acute cerebral damage. Three models were used. The first is a model of cerebral edema of traumatic origin. The second, lithium poisoning, and the third, total but transitory ischemia. These preparations were made in the awake rabbit. The EEG spectrum of activities was calculated in the usual four EEG bands: delta, theta, alpha, beta. The theta+beta/delta+alpha ratio, which gives an index of the proportion between the arousal rhythms (numerator) and the pathological rhythms (denominator) was eva- luated. The evolution of this ratio was determined over 30-second periods. In the case of traumatic edema, the latter showed a significant fall 18 hours after creation of the edema and in the course of the six hours of continuous recording. After intoxication with lithium chloride, a rather similar evolution was observed. However, in this latter case, the decrease in the ratio is due to an increase in delta activity, whereas in post-traumatic edema it is the arousal theta rhythm which is reduced. The authors compared the evolution of the index after administration of four substances: vinca- mine base, depot-effect vincamine, codergocrine, and EGb, in traumatic edema. The results show a significant increase ($P<0.05$) in the index in comparison with the control animals for the last three substances. The efficacy of EGb was better than for the other preparations. *Figure 3* shows the evolution of the EEG power spectrum in the delta band under the same conditions. It was found that EGb is responsible for a greater decrease in pathological delta in the course of the six hours of observation.

Conclusion

The studies which we have just reported show the value of the quantitative analysis of the EEG for studying the cerebral effects of Ginkgo biloba extract. The EEG confirms the clinical results supported by the various performance tests and de- monstrates activity of the product at therapeutic doses in a population of subjects without major cognitive disorders, as well as in elderly persons suffering with senile dementia. At the highest doses, the quantitative EEG revealed a stabilizing effect of Ginkgo biloba extract on spontaneous vigilance in young subjects. The experimental animal studies demonstrated the existence of beneficial effects on the sequelae of accidents which destroy cellular biological equilibrium. This approach should also make it possible for us to better understand the mechanisms of activity of the complex substances which compose Ginkgo biloba extract.

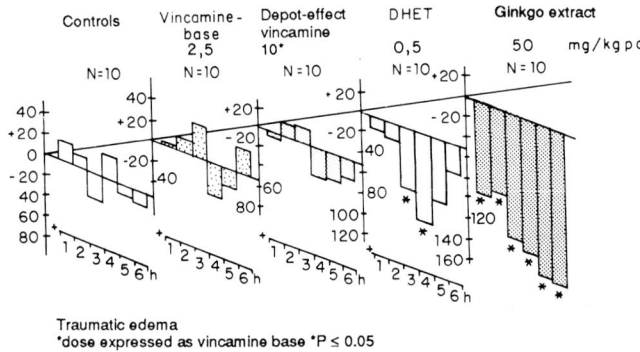

Figure 3: Evolution of the power spectrum in the delta frequency (Borzeix et al.(1)).

References

1. Borzeix M.G., Labos M., Hartl C.: Perméabilité membranaire et EEG. Etude comparative de l'EEG quantifiée dans les atteintes cérébrales aiguës d'origine ischémique ou toxique chez le lapin vigile. *In*: Pathogénie des maladies cérébro-vasculaires. Symposium international, Paris, 13 décembre 1978, *G.G. Editeur.*

2. Gessner B., Vœlp A., Klasser M.: Study of the long-term action of Ginkgo biloba extract on vigilance and mental performance as determined by means of quantitative pharmaco-EEG and psychometric measurements. *Arzneim. Forsch./Drug Res.*, 1985, *35*, 1459-1465.

3. Krauskopf R., Guinot Ph., Peetz H.G.: Long term on line EEG analyses demonstrating the pharmaco-dynamic effect of a defined Ginkgo biloba extract. *Beaufour-Schwabe Internat. Report*, 1983.

4. Pidoux B., Bastien Cl., Niddam S.: Etude à double insu, face au placebo, des effets de l'extrait de Ginkgo biloba sur l'état clinique et l'EGG quantifié. *Cerebr. Blood Flow Metabol.* 1983, *3*, suppl. 1, 5556-5557.

Activity of Ginkgo Biloba Extract on Short-Term Memory

I. Hindmarch

Department of Psychology. Human Psychopharmacology Research Unit. University of Leeds. Leeds, United Kingdom

Summary

Eight healthy female volunteers were included in a double-blind, cross-over trial comparing Ginkgo biloba extract in acute and ascending doses (120, 240, 600 mg) with a placebo. One hour after treatment they were subjected to a battery of tests, including: critical flicker fusion, choice reaction time, subjective rating scale and Sternberg memory scanning test. No statistically significant differences with the placebo were observed in the first three tests. In contrast, short-term memory, as assessed by the Sternberg technique, was very significantly improved following 600 mg of Ginkgo biloba extract, as compared with the placebo. These results differentiate Ginkgo biloba extract from sedative and stimulant drugs and suggest a specific effect on memory processes.

We studied in healthy volunteers the effects of the acute oral administration of increasing doses of Ginkgo biloba extract (EGb 761, Rökan®, Intersan) on cognitive function and the information process. The battery of tests used was selected so as to evaluate the subjective effects of the product and to measure objectively alertness, psychomotor performances, and short-term memory.

Methodology

The eight females recruited, from 25 to 40 years of age (average age 32 years), were in good physical health and without pathological history (cardiovascular, gastric, hepatic, renal, psychiatric). The criteria for exclusion included any drug treatment (except contraceptives) and confirmed or suspected pregnancy. On test days, standard meals were served, and all drinks containing caffeine or alcohol were excluded.

The test was conducted according to the crossover double-blind method. The treatments consisted of 120, 240, and 600 mg EGb, or the corresponding placebo. The order of administration was established by prior randomization. Two Latin squares

Rökan (Ginkgo Biloba). Recent Results in Pharmacology and Clinic
Edited by E.W. Fünfgeld
© Springer-Verlag Berlin Heidelberg New York 1988, pp. 321-326

were used in order to determine the sequence of the different treatments. Each subject received the four treatments while observing a free interval of one week between treatments in order to avoid any residual effect.

Before the beginning of the trial, all of the subjects were intrstructed and familiarized with the test procedures in order to avoid a learning effect. Each test day began with a training exercise. The effects of treatment were tested one hour after administration.

Tests and Scale

Critical flicker-fusion test (CFF)

The critical flicker-fusion test(4),(7) measures the activity of the entire central nervous system and more precisely explores sensory capability. The subject is asked to recognize the light which flickers in a battery of four luminous diodes placed one meter away within the perimeter of central vision. The threshold of frequency at which the light appears continuous is determined by using an ascending and descending scale according to the method of the Leeds Psychomotor Tester.

Choice -reaction time (CRT)

Sensorimotor performances were evaluated by the choice-reaction time from the Leeds Psychomotor Tester. It measures both motor response (MR) and stimulus-reaction time (SRT). The subject is asked to extinguish a lamp, among six colored lamps which light at random, by pressing the corresponding key. The reaction time recorded is the average of the response times in 20 successive tests.

Memory

In order to measure rapid discriminant memory and short-term memory (STM), the procedure described by Sternberg(9),(10) was used. A microcomputer and a video monitor used together with a computer program facilitates giving the test, measuring reaction time, and recording the results.

The subject had to memorize series of four, five, or six numerals presented sequentially at intervals of 1.2 seconds. Two seconds after the appearance of the last numeral, a sound signal (750 ms in duration) was followed by the appearance of the test. The subjects had to answer by pressing one of two keys: "yes" if the numeral shown was part of the list to be memorized, or "no" in the opposite case. A variation comprised four to six numerals alternated at random during successive tests. Each subject had to respond as quickly as possible and take 20 successive tests at three-second intervals. In 40 tests, the reply should be "yes" in half of the cases and "no" in the other half. The proportion of incorrect replies being low, only the correct responses were taken into consideration for the final analysis.

Analog visual scale

A 10-cm analog visual scale(7) was used in order to judge the subjective effects. The average evaluation score for asthenia, sensations of loss of balance, and decrease in alertness (appearing among several scales measuring concentration) was used to evaluate the subjective level of mood and drowsiness.

Results

All of the results from these various tests were submitted to analysis of variance by randomized groups. Later the means were compared, using a confidence interval of 95%.

Analysis of the discriminant memory test showed a significant decrease in overall response time (*Figure 1*), one hour after administration of 600 mg EGb (F = 13.4, degrees of freedom = 3-21, P < 0.0001, for the principal effect of the drug).

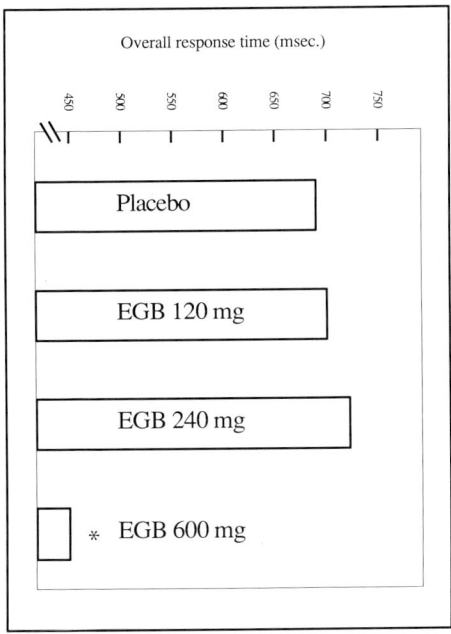

Figure 1: Discriminant memory test. A significant decrease was observed in overall response time after administration of 600 mg Ginkgo biloba extract.

Figure 2 shows the mean reaction times from combined positive and negative test data, as a function of test difficulty (larger or smaller number of figures to memorize). The slopes of the lines were obtained by the least-squares method. Later analysis (Z-test) of the slopes and intersections (*Figure 2*) shows significant differences (P < 0.05) between placebo and EGb.

No significant difference appeared for the critical flicker-fusion frequency test and the choice-reaction time.

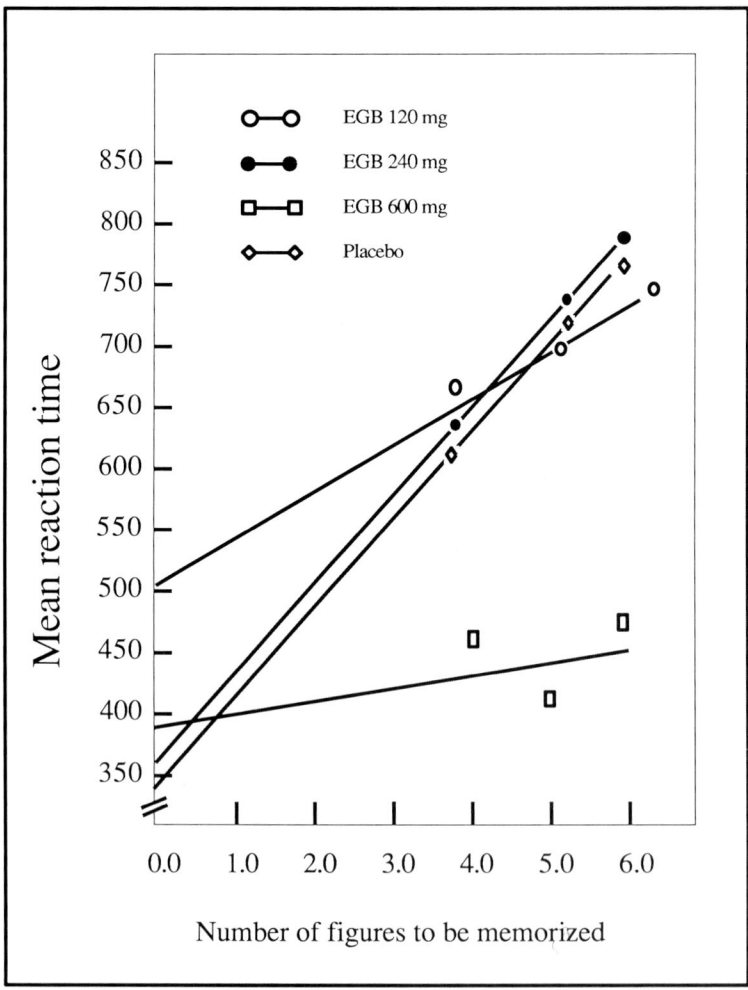

Figure 2: Mean reaction time from combined positive and negative test data as a function of test difficulty.

Discussion

With respect to memorizing, the effects of EGb on overall reaction time are obvious; one hour after administration of 600 mg EGb, a decrease in reaction time was found.

According to Sternberg,(9) in the course of such a task, the process of reaction to a stimulus takes place according to a sequence comprising at least three successive stages. While acknowledging that the subject has stored the test series in his short-term memory (STM), he must first perceive and record the stimulus (stimulus recording) which is then compared to the elements in the memorized series (serial discriminative or comparison memory); finally, an answer is given, based on these comparisons (formation of a selective response). The reaction time observed may also be represented by a straight line:(1) the slope of this line is an estimate of the serial comparison time, and the intersection is an estimate of both stimulus-recording time and time taken to formulate a selective response.

In the subjects on placebo, the increase in number of figures offered in the series is reflected by an average increase in reaction time of 48.8 ms for each figure added. In the EGb group at dosages of 120 mg and 240 mg, the reaction times increased only by 26.3 ms and 48.8 ms and only by 22.6 ms for 600 mg. These data are indicated by the significant differences in slopes (*Figure 2*).

Although we cannot spell out in detail what process – recording or response – is influenced, the system of analysis not allowing us to separate them, the effects of EGb on the serial comparison stage of reaction to stimulus are obvious.

It will be noted with interest that no significant change appeared in subjective evaluation of the effects of the product, or in CFF and CRT. The CFF threshold has been used by numerous investigators in orer to situate psychotropic drugs on an activity scale ranging from sedation to stimulation.(5),(6),(8),(11) The result is that three categories of drugs may be distinguished which affect CFF differently.(4) In general, sedatives such as barbiturates and benzodiazepines lower the CFF threshold, whereas psychostimulants (for example, amphetamines) raise it. A third group of products (codergocrine, nomifensine) may have positive effects on mood and activity and also raise the CFF threshold.

Some simple tests and the CRT have been widely used in order to measure the changes in sensorimotor functions induced by drugs.(3) Sedatives(2) generally bring about a decrease in performance (lengthening of response time), whereas stimulants such as nicotine and amphetamine(11) improve it (decrease in response time).

Curiously, only the Sternberg test was modified significantly by administration of EGb, indicating the specific activity on the central cognitive processes. Such results lead us to propose treatment with Ginkgo biloba extract of subjects suffering with senile dementia or pre-senile dementia in whom memory disorders are in the foreground of the clinical picture.

References

1. Darley C.F., Tinklenberg J.R., Hollister T.E., Atkinson R.C.: Marihuana and retrieval from short-term memory. *Psychopharmacologie*, (Berlin), 1973, *29*, 231-238.

2. Hindmarch I.: Effects of hypnotic and sleep inducing drugs on objective assessments of human psychomotor performance and subjective appraisals of sleep and early morning behaviour. *Br. Clin. Pharmacol.*, 1979, *8*, 43S-46S.

3. Hindmarch I.: Psychomotor function and psychoactive drugs. *Br. J. Clin. Pharmacol.*, 1980, *10*, 189-209.

4. Hindmarch I.: Critical flicker fusion frequency (CFF): the effects of psychotropic compounds. *Pharmacopsychiatra*, 1982, *15*, (suppl. 1) 44-48.

5. Hindmarch I., Clyde C.A.: The effects of triazolam and nitrazepam on sleep quality, morning vigilance and psychomotor performance. *Arzneim. Forsch.*, 1980, *30*, 1163-1166.

6. Hindmarch I., Gudgeon A.C.: The effects of clobazam and lorazepam on aspects of psychomotor performance and carhandling ability. *Br. J. Clin. Pharmacol.*, 1980, *10*, 145-150.

7. Hindmarch I., Parrott A.C.: A repeated dose comparison of the side effects of five anti-histamines on objective assessments of psychomotor performance, central nervous system arousal and subject's appraisals of sleep and early morning behaviour. *Arzneim. Forsch.*, 1978, *28*, 483-486.

8. Parrott A.C., Hindmarch I.: Haloperidol and chlorpromazine comparative effects upon arousal. *IRCS Medical Science*, 1973, *3*, 562.

9. Sternberg S.: Memory scanning: Mental processes revealed by reaction time experiments. *American Scientist*, 1969, *57*, 421

10. Sternberg S.: Memory scanning: news findings and current controversies. *Quarterly J. Experiment. Psychol.*, 1975, *27*, 1-32.

11. Taeuber K., Zapt R., Rupp W., Badian M.: Pharmacodynamic comparison of the acute effects of nomifensine, amphetamine and placebo in healthy volunteers. *Int. Pharm. Biopharma.*, 1979, *17*, 32.

Clinical Psychopharmacology of Ginkgo Biloba Extract

D.M. Warburton

Department of Psychology, University of Reading. United Kingdom

Summary

From this general review of the pharmacological, psychopharmacological and clinical studies performed with Ginkgo biloba extract, the following conclusions can be drawn: the drug seems to be effective in patients with vascular disorders, in all types of dementia and even in patients suffering from cognitive disorders secondary to depression, because of its beneficial effects on mood. Of special concern are people who are just beginning to experience deterioration in their cognitive function. Ginkgo biloba extract might delay deterioration and enable these subjects to maintain a normal life and escape institutionalization. In addition, Ginkgo biloba extract appears to be a safe drug, being well tolerated, even in doses many times higher than those usually recommended.

Aging is accompanied by an ensemble of symptoms involving the cognitive, affective, and behavioral spheres that reflect an organic deficiency in the brain. Aside from this organic deficiency related to age, dementia can result from degeneration of the cortex, as in senile dementia (29% of cases) and Alzheimer-type dementia (19% of cases), or vascular lesions as in athero-sclerosis and multiple infarctions (19% of cases), or even a combination of these two conditions (18% of cases). The differential diagnosis is difficult, but vascular dementia progresses in spurts and degenerative dementia tends to become gradually exacerbated with age, while the mixed pathology combines both patterns of evolution. The first symptoms of organic deficiency of the brain during normal aging are the same as in dementia. The underlying mechanisms have not been elucidated, and the distinction is still arbitrary. That is why it seems that it would be better to take both of these syndromes into account at the same time, when considering the therapeutic problem.

The study of the changes related to age, and that of their treatments, is becoming increasingly crucial because the average age of the American and European population is rising. That is why extensive research has been devoted to studying the nature of the neurochemical changes related to age for the purpose of discovering drugs that

Rökan (Ginkgo Biloba). **Recent Results in Pharmacology and Clinic**
Edited by E.W. Fünfgeld
© Springer-Verlag Berlin Heidelberg New York 1988, pp. 327-345

could improve the psychological infirmities resulting from it. Thus the concentration of various metabolites in the urine, blood, or cerebrospinal fluid can be measured for the purpose of establishing the diagnosis, selecting the adequate drug, and following the treatment. Computerized scanography and nuclear magnetic resonance may be found useful, but have been mainly research tools up to the present.

An exhaustive analysis of behavior in order to classify the patients and give them the appropriate medication is difficult. Many variables make a precise evaluation arduous, and not all deficits are related to cerebral lesions. They can simply result from poor physical and mental health, which is frequent in elderly persons; in particular, patients who are suffering with a psychiatric disorder, such as the memory disorders so frequently encountered in depressive states must be set aside.

It is obvious that there is a need for drugs to prevent cognitive disorders in the course of dementia, but the primary purpose of this therapy should be mainly pragmatic: to improve the symptoms until the difficult problem of the etiology of the cognitive deficit of aging is elucidated. Although a certain number of products may be suggested for the treatment of these disturbances, doubts have been expressed about the efficacy of most of them.(30)

Not only is it necessary to accept with caution information concerning the possible therapeutic role of the suggested medications, but also to emphasize that there is not always a consensus as to the methods for gauging therapeutic efficacy.

In an attempt to clarify the problem, this article will discuss clinical evaluation scales and psychometric tests appropriate for the study of these medications. Clinical and psychopharmacological studies on Ginkgo biloba extract (EGb) will be used as an example of therapeutic tests suitable for this use. EGb is marketed under the names Tanakan, Rökan, Tanakène, Tanacaïn, Gincoben, etc., in several European and American countries. It has been used since the mid-1970s.

Pharmacology

A concentrated solution of an extract of Ginkgo biloba leaves, EGb 761, was used. The pharmacologically active fractions are flavonoids, proanthocyanidines, ginkgolids, and bilobalid. The pharmacological studies were directed towards its effects on cerebral circulation, neuronal metabolism, and cerebral neurochemistry.

Cerebral circulation

The preliminary studies were focused on the possible effects of EGb on cerebral circulation. One of the first elements was a study using rheoencephalography, which measures the electrical resistance of the tissues. This resistance is proportional to the quantity of blood contained in the tissue studied. Boismare(4) measured the variations in resistance after an i.v. injection of 17.5 mg EGb in both young subjets (average age 30 years) and elderly subjects (average age 77 years). The increase recorded was identical in the two groups, with an average increase of 9% ($\pm$6%).

An increase in cerebral flow under the influence of EGb has also been recorded by means of radiocirculography, which measures the variations in radioactivity at the base of the skull after injection of a radioactive isotope.(22) In radiocirculography, the variations in radioactivity as a function of time show an arterial peak, a corresponding drop in capillary passage, and a venous peak. Twenty patients suffering with cerebrovascular insufficiency were treated with 160 mg EGb per day for 15 days; 15 patients had a distinct increase in cerebral circulation, with an increase in amplitude of the aterial peak and the capillary drop, and doubling of the venous peak. The activity on cerebral circulation and particulary on venous return is distinct. These hemodynamic changes were accompanied by a distinct clinical improvement in seven patients.

In a comparative study involving 29 products, one of which was EGb, Heiss and Zeiler(14) measured the effects of these drugs on regional cerebral blood flow, using the technique of radioactive Xenon injected into the carotid. In 12 cases of cerbral vascular accidents who had received a dose of 35 mg EGb intravenously, an increase of 8.4% was obtained in total cerebral blood flow, and the same increase in blood flow in the ischemic zone, thus excluding the hypothesis of a blood diversion. This was the most distinctly active agent among the 30 products tested. In another study using radioactivity, 19 patients who had presented with a cerebral ischemic accident received 160 mg EGb for two months.(26) Cerebral transit time decreased from 14.48 seconds (that is, 161% of the normal mean value, which is nine seconds) to 12.08 seconds (134% of normal and at the upper limit of normality).

Neuronal metabolism

The last study mentioned above also measured consumption of glucose and oxygen by the brain, using complex biochemical techniques. For oxygen, the departure level was 2.76 mL/min/100 mg cerebral tissue, that is, 84% of normal (approximately 3.25 mL). After two months of treatment with EGb, consumption had increased to 3.37 mL/min/100 g, that is, normal. Glucose consumption also increased by 40% during the two months, but without reaching normal. As the level of lactates showed no variation, it seems that cellular energy metabolism of the cerebral neurons had been improved, in view of the better uptake of oxygen and glucose by the tissues.(26) A similar result was recorded in an animal model of cerebral ischemia: increased cerebral blood flow, increased uptake of glucose, and increase in ATP concentration at the end of three weeks of EGb treatment.(21) Parallel with this improvement in energy metabolism, a decrease was found in cerebral edema.(7)

The studies pursued in animals under conditions of normal oxygenation or hypoxia could not explain these changes by the simple increase in blood flow. The accumulated data show that deoxyglucose uptake is notably increased under the influence of EGb, whether in animals maintained under normal conditions or in hypoxia, whereas cerebral blood flow varied very little, particularly in hypoxia. These results are significant, since they suggest a direct action of EGb on cellular metabolism, which is independent or partially independent of the improvement in cerebral flow. It is interesting to note that this protective effect on cellular metabolism is found as much in normal neuronal tissue as when an improvement is involved in functional deficit after neurotoxic damages in rats and after a vascular accident.

Ginkgo biloba extract and neuromediators

One of the most important discoveries from a neurochemical standpoint concerns the binding capacity of the musarinic acethylcholine receptors.(25)

Investigations into catecholaminergic functions also show facilitation of this transmission system. EGb opposes the catalepsy generally produced by haloperidol, as well as the peripheral effects of reserpine. This fact constitutes a significant argument in favor of an activity of EGb on the catecholaminergic system.

Electrophysiology

Electroencephalography has given physiological indications relative to improvement in cortical function. The effects of EGb on electroencephalographic activity (12, 19) were studied in two investigations. There are two possible strategies for evaluating psychotropic drugs. The most obvious consists of attempting to reduce the deficit in patients presenting with cerebral deterioration, while the other method uses a homogeneous population of healthy volunteers in whom an attempt is made to improve cerebral function. In an experiment conducted in healthy subjects,(16) the effects of acute doses of 120, 240, and 360 mg EGb were tested in a randomized double-blind cross-over study. A dose of 400 mg was also tested in an open study in order to obtain additional information on the active dosage. A four-hour recording period made it possible to study the response over time. Under placebo, fluctuations were recorded in power and vigilance, and a transitory decrease in the arousal state. Instability of frequency was observed, mainly in the 2-5 Hz and 5-8 Hz bands in the parieto-occipital region. The power fluctuations were reduced by the lowest dose of EGb, and even more by the highest doses. The dominant frequency showed a dose-dependent increase of 9 Hz after placebo and up to 12 Hz after 600 mg EGb; the maximal effects were manifested 120 minutes after administration. A dose-dependent increase in power was also found in the dominant frequency. These results suggest that EGb improves cortical function in healthy volunteers and allow us to hope that it may also improve cognitive function in elderly persons.

Psychopharmacology

Another psychopharmacology study in healthy volunteers supports the hope of obtaining such activity in elderly persons.(24)

A summary of the psychopharmacology studies is presented in *Table 1*; it can be seen that all of these studies have been published since 1975. Eleven of them were conducted in double-blind, and the other nine were open studies. The clinical studies include four comparative double-blind studies and one comparative open study, the comparison products being ergot derivatives. No behavioral therapy such as conditioning or practice in cognitive ability, sensorial stimulation, or socialization methods was combined with the treatment.

In all, 758 patients were tested with EGb, 263 with placebo, 59 with ergot derivatives, 24 with raubasin combined with ergot derivatives, and 19 with nicergoline. The inclusion diagnoses included chronic cerebrovascular disorders, sequelae of cerebral vascular accidents, senile dementias (organic change in the brain). The characteristic symptoms comprise cognitive disturbances, mood lability, and decreased sociability. The duration of these studies varied from one week to 18 months (five weeks or more, for the majority); dosage was 120, 240, or 360 mg EGb per day in the form of drops, except for certain patients to whom 17.5 g were administered intramuscularly(27) and 35 mg intravenously.(22)

Evaluation methods

The efficacy of EGb was evaluated by various methods, sometimes according to an overall clinical evaluation, but generally by means of a clinical evaluation scale, to which a battery of psychometric tests was added in some cases. Evaluation scales and psychometric tests correspond to well-known tests, described and explained in various publications by Israel, Kozarevic, and Sartorius.

Clinical evaluation scales

These are multidimensional evaluation instruments conceived to explore a variety of functions, including symptoms of mental deterioration, social activities, and activities of daily life.

They give the inventory of the various criteria comprising self-evaluation by the subject, or those which demonstrate psychiatric, medical, and social problems. They

Table 1
Synoptic table of clinical studies

Author	Year	Number of patients	Age (years)	Average duration of treatment (weeks)	Dosage (mg/day)	Type	Comparison product
Agnoli(1)	1984	30	60	4	120	DBCS	Placebo (n=30)
Arrigo and Cattaneo(2)	1984	80	40-80	7	120	DBCS	Placebo (n=40)
Augustin(3)	1976	99	77	24	120	DB	Placebo (n=90)
Bono and Mouren(5)	1975	14 40	65 67	5 5	120 120	DB O	Placebo (n=14) ED (n=19)
Boudouresques et al.(6)	1975	47	35-80	3	120	O	
Choussat et al.(8)	1977	48	65-95	8	360	O	
Dieli et al.(10)	1981	20	62	5	160	DB	Placebo (n=20)
Eckman and Schlag(11)	1982	25	60	4	120	DB	Placebo (n=20)
Gessner et al.(12)	1983	19	57-88	12	120	DB	Placebo (n=19) Nicergoline (n=19)
Israel et al.(15)	1977	48	72	8	240	O	
Kugler et al.(16)	1982	10	59	9	120	DB	ED (n=10)
Leroy et al.(17)	1978	27	78	8	120	DB	Raubasine + ED (n=24)
Moreau(18)	1975	30	84	12	120	DB	Placebo (n=30) ED (n=30)
Pidoux(19)	1983	12	87	12	160	DB	Placebo
Safi and Galley(22)	1977	20	47-86	2	35 (i.v.)	O	
Tea et al.(26)	1979	19	67	8	160	O	
Terrasse and Morin(27)	1976	20	59-84	1-3	17.5 (i.v.)	O	
Vorberg(28)	1985	112	55-94	52	120	OM	
Wackenheim(29)	1977	50	50	27	160	O	

DB = double-blind; CS = crossover study; O = open; M = multicenter; ED = ergot derivatives make it possible to describe precisely the levels of the initial deficit and to follow the evolution during treatment.

Crichton's geriatric evaluation scale is a scale specifically conceived to evaluate the effects of a treatment. It covers 11 aspects of behavior including mood, orientation, autonomy, and communication. It is applicable to elderly psychiatric patients and uses a five-degree score. A simplified version of this scale was used in the long-term multicenter study by Vorberg.(28)

The Parkside behavior evaluation scale was conceived to measure the degree of impairment of elderly hospitalized subjects. It has been modified for the evaluation of chronic insuffiency. It includes 16 items subdivided into eight groups; it is scored according to a five-point scale by the nurses. It was used in a study of EGb by Agnoli.(1)

Stockton's geriatric behavior scale has been used frequently in studies of elderly persons; it is therefore well validated. Designed to evaluate the behavior of hospitalized patients, most of the time seriously afflicted, it includes 33 items which were evaluated by the nursing personnel according to a three-point score. Stockton's scale was used in the EGb study by Leroy et al.(17)

Plutchik's geriatric evaluation scale was derived from Stockton's scale. It contains 31 items, some of which reflect behvioral disturbances; this score is also based on a three-point scale. Considered as reliable and useful for evaluating the effects of a therapy in elderly persons, it was used by Dieli et al.(11) and by Agnoli(1) in addition to the Parkside scale.

The Sandoz geriatric clinical evaluation sclae was especially designed to constitute a simple, reliable, and polyvalent tool to measure the efficacy of a therapy. It covers 18 specific symptoms of senile dementia and depressive states; it uses a seven-point grading scale and has been standardized as a result of numerous therapeutic studies. Pidoux evaluated the improvement in cognitive functions under the influence of EGb by means of this scale.(19),(20)

Psychometric tests

In several studies with EGb, a battery of psychometric tests was used in order to obtain more precise and more objective data on patient cognitive capacities than that supplied by clinical evaluation scales. The psychometric tests used in the EGb studies measure memory (Benton's visual retention test, the U.C. memory table, Rey's verbal memory test, and the numeral test derived from Wechsler's adult intelligence scale), conceptual exploration (progressive matrices, addition, crossing out letters, the digit symbol substitution test, and similar tests derived from the Wechsler adult intelligence scale, the series completion tests), orientation (trail marking test, labyrinth test), and visuomotor coordination (rotor following).

Benton's visual retention test, the test of verbal memory, distance between figures, progressive matrices, addition, crossing out letters, the digit symbol substitution test, series completion, the labyrinth test, and the rotor pursuit test are standard psychometric tests which have been used extensively to evaluate cognitive functions in neuropsychology and psychopharmacology.

Electroencephalography

A therapeutic study using the EEG power spectral analysis(19),(20) as criterion analyzes the electroencephalograhic changes which appear during treatment with EGb and which are correlated with the clinical condition. It is known that senile deterioration is accompanied by electroencephalographic abnormalities, with the magnitude of the abnomalities being correlated with the severity.

In the study by Pidoux et al.,(19) the patients were incorporated into an EGb group or a placebo group; the EGb group was treated for 12 weeks at the rate of 160 mg per day. At the beginning of the test both groups were comparable as to their cerebral activity, but the tracing of their EEG activity began to change shortly after treatment began.

With an average age of 87 years, the patients in the EGb group quickly presented an increase in amplitude of alpha rhythm with a relative increase of the latter, to the detriment of theta rhythm. The significant reduction in slow frequencies and the coefficient of variation of the rhythm frequency (statistically significant from the third week) persisted throughout the duration of treatment. In the placebo group, only nonspecific changes were observed on the EEG.(19)

The EEG improvement was correlated with a clinical improvement: 29% reduction in the overall clinical deterioration score at the end of 12 weeks of treatment; on the contrary, the overall clinical score for the placebo group showed only a nonsignificant reduction of 13%. It is therefore obvious that the EEG changes were reflected clinically.

These results were corroborated by a nine-week double-blind EEG study comparing EGb with codergocrine. It included patients suffering with cerebro-vascular insufficiency; they were treated with 120 mg of one or the other product.(12)

The power spectral analysis showed that both compounds increased alpha activity and decreased rapid beta activity a little. The increase was significant in the 6-15 Hz band. The improvement in cerebral vigilance was reflected by an improvement in cognitive functions in both treated groups, with the better percentage of improvement being obtained on the arithmetic test and the general knowledge test, general comprehension, object assembly, drawing completion, and the digit symbol test, derived from the Wechsler adult intelligence test.

Results from the pharmacoclinical evaluation

Global results

The double-blind clinical trials are reported in *Table 2*. It may be seen that the overall estimates conclude to the efficacy of EGb in 56% of 394 patients of various ages suffering with varied conditions. *Table 3* gives the results of the open studies; the overall success rate (63%) is essentially comparable to that for the double-blind trials.

Table 2

Summary of the Results from the Double-Blind Studies

Principal author	Diagnosis	Number of patients	Mean duration of treatment (weeks)	Dosage (mg/day)	Comparison product	Overall efficacy
Agnoli(1)	CCI	30	4	120	Placebo	76%
Arrigo and Cattaneo(2)	CCI	80	7	120	Placebo	65%
Augustin(3)	misc.	99	24	120	Placebo	44%
Bono and Mouren(5)	CCI	14	5	120	Placebo	65%
Dieli et al.(10)	CCI	20	5	160	Placebo	80%
Eckmann and Schlag(11)	CVA	25	4	120	Placebo	92%
Gessner et al.(12)	senescence	57	12	120	Nicergoline-placebo	69%
Kugler et al.(16)	CCI	10	9	120	Ergot derivatives	NS
Leroy et al.(17)	CVA	27	8	120	Raubasine	74%
Moreau(18)	CCI	30	12	120	Placebo	79%
Pidoux et al.(19)	CCI	12	12	160	Placebo	85%

CCI = chronic cerebral insufficiency; CVA = cerebral vascular accidents; NS = not specified

Table 3
Summary of the results from open studies

Principal author	Diagnosis	Number of patients	Mean duration of treatment (weeks)	Dosage (mg/day)	Comparison product	Overall efficacy
Bono(5)	CCI	40	5	120	Ergot derivatives	90%
Boudouresques(6)	CCI+CVA	47	3	120-360	no	80%
Choussat(8)	CCI	48	8	360	no	60%
Israel(15)	D	48	8	240	no	NS
Safi(22)	CCI	20	2	35 (i.v.)	no	76%
Tea(26)	CVA	19	8	160	no	
Terrasse(27)	misc.	20	1-3	17,5 (i.v.)	no	55%
Vorberg(28)	CCI	112	52	120	no	68%
Wackenheim(29)	CCI CCT	25 25	27 27	160 160	no no	76% 72%

CCI = chronic cerebral insufficiency; CVA = cerebral vascular accidents; NS = not specified; D = dementia

Clinical evaluation scales

The following scales were used during EGb studies: the Crichton geriatric behavioral scale,(28) Parkside's scale,(1) Plutchik's scale,(1),(10) the Sandoz scale,(19),(20) and Stockton's scale.(17) *Table 4* shows that EGb caused significant improvements in the seven studies in which it was used. Five different scales supplied proof of the efficacy of EGb. However, we must take into consideration the fact that these different instruments are more or less correlated with each other; for example, Plutchik's scale is derived from Stockton's scale. The evaluation criteria which correspond best to EGb are summarized in *Table 5*; the cognitive functions are unquestionably inproved, in particular memory, vigilance, and disorientation. The same is true for mood, which is important in view of the frequency of this symptom in demential states, whether these are of organic origin or not.

Another way of presenting the data is to classify the results according to the Sandoz geriatric scale. The pertinent factors are cognitive dysfunction (vigilance, confusion,

Table 4

Results of Ginkgo biloba extract on clinical evaluation scales

Clinical evaluation scales	Criteria	(1)	(10)	(17)	(20)	(28)
Plutchik's scale		+*	+*			
Stockton's scale				+*		
Crichton's scale	Symptoms					+*
Sandoz scale					+*	
Parkside's behavior scale		+*				

+ = test used; * = statistically significant results;
(1) = Agnoli; (10) = Dieli; (17) = Leroy; (20) = Pidoux; (28) = Vorberg.

recent memory, and disorientation), somatic function (appetite, vertigo, and fatigue), autonomy, affectivity (emotional lability, depression, and anxiety), apathy (lack of motivation, indifference to surroundings, and withdrawl), and social behavior (lack of cooperation, agitation, aggression, hostility).

Table 5

Criteria having responded best to treatment with Ginkgo biloba extract

Study	Agnoli	Dieli	Leroy	Vorberg
Scale	Parkside (modified)	Plutchik	Stockton	Crichton (modified)
Item	Autonomy	Eating	Attention	Mood
	Vigilance	Grooming-Dressing	Intellect disturbances	Vigilance
	Recent memory	Personal care	Sociability memory	Short-term
	Mood	Disorientation	Mood	
		Nocturnal agitation		
		Sociability		
		Initiative		

Table 6 presents the various items on the Sandoz scale and the percentage of patients whose improvement was evaluated as good or very good, regardless of the initial diagnosis. The same general picture emerges; we see that memory, vivacity, intellectual capacities, and mood are distinctly more improved than social behavior. It is clear that EGb has favorable effects on cognitive and affective dysfunction; as to efficacy on mood, it is closely correlated with the improvement in memory and intellectual efficacy.

Table 6
Percent improvement in the various items

Cognitive disorders	Disturbed vigilance	41%
	Recent memory	48%
	Intellectual deterioration	48%
Mood disturbance	Including emotional lability depression, and anxiety	41%
Social behavior	Cooperation, instability, agitation, hostility, withdrawn attitude	26%
Somatic disturbances	Appetite	0%
	Equilibrium disturbance	81%

Psychometric tests

The studies which used psychometric tests corroborate the evaluations according to the clinical scales. *Table 7* summarizes the results that are significant or close to significance from ten studies conducted in double-blind in patients or healthy volunteers. The distinct improvements concern essentially memory, intellect, orientation, and psychomotor performances. *Table 7* shows the improvements demonstrated by the Benton visual retention test, Rey's verbal memory test, and the trail-marking test, in more than half of the patients tested, regardless of clinical context. These data objectively corroborate the observations of clinicians who conclude to an improvement in cognitive functions.

Other beneficial effects

In addition to evaluation of the so-called intellectual capacities, certain studies mentioned above studied other aspects of sensorimotor behavior such as visual and auditory disturbances, tinnitus, headaches, vertigo, and dizzy sensations which are often associated with cognitive dysfunction.

Table 7

Results from the psychometric test and the electroencephalographic examinations (EEG), after treatment with Ginkgo biloba extract

Psychometric tests	Function	(2)	(3)	(10)	(12)	(16)	(17)	(20)	(24)
Benton (visual retention)	Memory		+*				+*		
Rey (word memory)			+*				+*		
Digit Span (WAIS)			+*	+*		+°			
Sternberg's test									V
Memorization test (UC)		+*							
Progressive matrices	Cognitive processes Orientation		+*						
Numeral repetition				+*		+*			
Addition test (or Pauli)					V	+*			
d2 test					V	+*			
Word recognition		+*							
Trail-marking test						+*	+*		
Labyrinth test						+*			
Mosaic (WAIS)						+°			
Reaction time, simple choice	Psychomotor performances					V*			
Reaction time, multiple choice						V°			
Color-reaction test									
Visual pursuit test						V			
Flicker-fusion	Cortical reactivity					V			V
EEG						V*	+*	+*	V*

+ = test used; +* = statistically significant results; +° = results tending toward significance; V = studies in healthy volunteers; (2) = Arrigo; (3) = Augustin; (10) = Dieli; (12) = Gessner; (16) = Kugler; (17) = Leroy; (20) = Pidoux; (24) = Subhan, Hindmarch.

The possible activity of EGb on visual disturbances was examined in 38 patients.(5),(6),(29) The good or very good results recorded in 65% of the patients agree with those of Saracco and Estachy.(23)

The same is true of patients complaining of tinnitus, with good or very good improvements being obtained in 27 of the 37 patients tested.

Vertigo and instability are among the major symptoms of which elderly persons complain. These symptoms were present in 212 patients; 81% obtained good or very good results. This is also in agreement with the study of Guerrier et al., who concluded to an improvement in 73% of the patients presenting with a dizzy or vertiginous syndrome.(13)

Another major symptom was improved in the same proportions: headache. The conclusions of a specific study on migraine were that the drug was highly efficient in patients presenting with a recent syndrome.(9) In the course of pharmacoclinical studies, this symptom was studied in 145 patients by Wackenheim; here again, 80% good and very good results were found with EGb.(29)

In summary, EGb was therefore shown to be remarkably effective in other signs and symptoms which are often associated with dementia in addition to intellctual function disorders.

Dosage

The dosage used in the different tests varied from 120 mg EGb per day(1-6),(10),(11),(16-20),(28) up to a single dose of 600 mg,(24) ranging through the dose of 360 mg.(9) The high acute doses of 600 mg improved cerebral efficacy and cognitive performances in healthy volunteers, but therapeutic efficacy in elderly persons and patients suffering with chronic cerebral insufficiency was obtained with a much lower dosage of 120 mg per day. There seems to be no therapeutic advantage in using doses higher than 160 mg per day in long-term treatments.

The duration of treatment varied considerably from one study to the other, from two to 52 weeks. Several studies were devoted to the problem of treatment duration. It seems that the longer treatment is continued, the more obvious and lasting the result. Even at the end of a year, it was found that improvement was continuing and that adherence to the treatment was good.(28) At least eight days are necessary before the first clinical effects are manifested, and it was only at the end of 18 days that the optimal effects were recorded in most of the indications of chronic cerebral insufficiency. Convincing results could therefore not be expected from treatment for a week or less.

Tolerance

Clinical efficacy having been established, it was important to study all adverse effects recorded in the course of EGb treatments in senile subjects that have occasionally caused interruption of the treatment. The possible side effects could not be attributed routinely to EGb.

EGb was found to be remarkably devoid of any toxic effect during its clinical use. The most common alleged side effects were gastric malaise and nausea, and it is well known that vague gastrointestinal disturbances are usual in the course of any treatments given orally. It should be noted that a much larger number of these intolerances was reported in an exhaustive analysis involving 2,855 patients treated with EGb. Tolerance was excellent in 2,701 of the patients (94.25%). Among the 5.75% alleged side effects, 3.7% were digestive disturbances labeled by the patients as "gastric malaise" or "nausea". Choussat's analysis revealed some rare evidences of adverse effects such as headache, dizziness and vertigo, paradoxical manifestations in view of the high level of success of EGb in this type of symptom.

In contrast with cerebral vasodilators (for example, papaverine) EGb does not modify cardiac work and therefore does not inrease oxygen consumption by the myocardium. In normotensive individuals, blood pressure remains completely stable, whereas in hypertensives, a very slight decrease in the pressure readings is observed. The patient has thus been protected from sensorial ischemia consecutive to the sudden loss of blood flow in a fragile parenchyma. The data communicated do not mention any change in hepatic or renal functions, or any variation in the hematological and ionic constants, regardless of duration of treatment or the dose used. Neither was any variation in weight or appetite recorded.

Discussion of the therapeutic results

Mechanisms of effect

The clinical pharmacology data clearly plead for a therapeutic effect of EGb in dementia of vascular etiology. This clinical efficacy of EGb on memory and intellectual efficiency is closely correlated with the activity in mood disturbances. This correlation leads us to ask whether the improvement in memory was not due solely to improvement of mood and attenuation of the depression. Thus, for example, for Shader et al., the improvements in memory following treatments with hydergine resulted from the improvement in mood. According to another interpretation, there would be no cause-and-effect relationship, but this dual result was due to the fact that memory and mood would depend on the same type of intracerebral neurochemical transmission.

One study on this subject was found to be interesting; it analyzed the effects of EGb on the intellectual processes in healthy subjects.(24) A battery of psychometric tests was used at the same time as a mood-evaluation scale. A single dose of 600 mg EGb increased the rate of memory exploration, but the subjective evaluation scale showed no effect on mood; this supports the hypothesis according to which the results on intellectual performances are independent of those which affect mood.

Such beneficial effects on memory without an influence on mood or the waking state in healthy subjects suggest that EGb could effectively prevent the deterioration related to age by acting on different neurochemical systems, thus improving intellectual efficacy and mood, although the transmitter system might be the same. For example, a relationship has been established between mood and serotonin, and thus the catecholaminergic systems (dopamine and noadrenalin), whereas the consolidation of memory has not been attributed to acetylcholine. The pharmacological data having shown that EGb acts on the catecholaminergic systems, such a mode of activity on the mnesic processes is a very real possibility.

Target population

As we have stated in detail above, dementia can result either from degenerative changes in the cortex (as in senile dementia and Alzheimer's disease), or from vascular lesions as in atheromatous dementia or dementia due to multiple infarctions; the two etiologies can occur together. The majority of the patients treated with EGb belong to these categories. In these patients, the experimental data lead us to believe that the clinical effect of EGb lies in ameliorating intellectual dysfunction rather than in slowing deterioration.

Two arguments suggest that EGb may be useful in the early stages of dementia. First of all, Egb is active in healthy volunteers on both mnesic functions(24) and cerebral electrical activity.(16) Then, the results obtained on the capacity for binding acetylcholine to the receptors in rats tends to show that EGb can slow the progress of the deterioration.

These data are important, since they demonstrate that patients should be treated in the early stage of dementia in order for the therapeutic effect to be maximal before the deterioration has become too advanced. Too often the dementia syndrome is concealed by the family and by the patients themselves, either intentionally to avoid hospitalization or because of the alteration in their judgment.

An early diagnosis requires exact classification of the patients in such a way as to be able to decide upon the eventual drug therapy. A precise differential diagnosis is essential before any prescription, and thorough behavioral investigations, using different techniques, should be undertaken before a serious therapeutic attempt can be considered. This is necessary in order to avoid confusing different types of mental dysfunction: depression, thyroid insufficiency, alcoholism, etc.

Scales making it possible to quantify the behavioral disturbances in the activities of daily life and therefore of postulating an early diagnosis, are limited in number. An attempt to construct such a scale has just been made. Designed for thorough investigation of the lifestyle of elderly persons, it takes into consideration intellectual activities, physical conditions, and social life. A scale of this type could be useful in detecting the first symptoms of intellectual decline.

Conclusion

Many categories of elderly patients should benefit from the therapeutic properties of EGb. In addition to its frequent use in patients suffering with vascular disorders, the data collected indicate that EGb should be effective in dementias in general, cerebral deficits of organic etiology, and even in patients in whom the decrease in intellectual function is related to a depressive state, because of its beneficial effects on mood. One category appears to be particularly concerned: these are the subjects who are just beginning to experience the first signs of deficit in their intellectual functions. The research on EGb leads us to believe that this compound could retard deterioration and permit them to continue to lead a normal life while avoiding hospitalization. Lastly, EGb is a very well-tolerated medication, even at much higher dosages than those which are ordinarily recommended.

References

1. Agnoli A.: Clinical and psychometric aspects of the therapeutic effects of GBE. *In*: Effects of GBE and Organic Cerebral Impairment, Paris, London, *John Libbey*, 1985.

2. Arrigo A., Cattaneo S.: Clinical and psychometric evaluation of Ginkgo biloba extract in chronical cerebro-vascular diseases. *In*: Effects of Ginkgo biloba on Organic Cerebral Impairment, Paris, London, *John Libbey*, 1985.

3. Augustin P.: Le Tanakan en gériatrie; Etude clinique et psychométrique chez 189 malades d'hospice. *Psychologie Médicale*, 1976, *8*, 123-130.

4. Boismare F.: Etude de l'action hémodynamique de l'extrait concentré de Ginkgo biloba comparée à celle du gaz carbonique chez le sujet jeune et chez le sujet sénile. *Ouest Médical*, 1976, *29*, 747-749.

5. Bono Y., Mouren P.: L'insuffisance circulatoire cérébrale et son traitement par l'extrait de Ginkgo biloba. *Med. Med.*, 1975, *3*, 59-62.

6. Boudouresques G., Vigouroux R., Boudouresques J.: Intérêt et place de l'extrait de Ginkgo biloba en pathologie vasculaire cérébrale. *Médecine Practicienne*, 1975, *598*, 75-78.

7. Chaterjee G.: Effects of Ginkgo biloba extract on cerebral metabolic processes. *In*: Effects of Ginkgo biloba extract on organic cerebral impairment, Paris, London, *John Libbey*, 1985.

8. Choussat H., Beloussoff T., Dartenuc J.Y., Emeriau J.P.: Essai clinique d'un extrait végétal concentré en gériatrie. *Gériatrie*, 1977, *2*, 370-375.

9. Devic M.: Le Tanakan dans le traitement de fond de la migraine. *Lyon Médical*, 1978, *239*, 735-738.

10. Dieli G., La Mantia V., Saetta M., Costanzo E.: Studio clinico in doppio cieco del Tanakan nell'insufficienza cerebrale cronica. *Il Lavoro Neuropshiatrico*, 1961, *68*.

11. Eckmann F., Schlag H.: Etude contrôlée, à double insu, de l'activité de l'Extrait de Ginkgo biloba chez des malades atteints d'insuffisance cérébrale chronique. *Fortschritte der Medizin*, 1982, *31/32*, 1474-1478.

12. Gessner B., Volp A., Klasser M.: Study of the long-term action of a Ginkgo biloba extract on vigilance and mental performance as determined by means of quantitative pharmaco-EEG and psychometric measurements. *Arzneim. Forsch/Drug Res.*, 1985, *2*, 35.

13. Guerrier Y., Bassères F., Artières J.: Le Tanakan dans le traitement des vertiges. A propos de 26 observations. *Cahiers d'ORL*, 1978, *13*, 421-428.

14. Heiss W.D., Zeiler K.: Medikamentöse Beeinflussung der Hirndurchblutung. *Pharmakotherapie*, 1978, *3*, 137-144.

15. Israel L., Ohlman T., Delomier Y., Hugonot R.: Etude psychométrique de l'activité d'un extrait végétal au cours des états d'involution sénile. *Lyon Méditerranée Médical*, 1977, *13*, 1197-1199.

16. Kugler J., Krauskopf R., Hauser B.: Increased performance and vigilance changes in cerebrovascular insufficiency after 60 days of treatment with Rökan or with dihydroergotoxin methanesulphonate (DHETM); an electroencephalographic and psychometric study. *Documents I.P.S.E.N.*

17. Leroy H., Salaun P., Chovelon R., Bouilloux E.: Approche clinique et psychométrique en gériatrie. Méthodes d'études et choix d'une thérapeutique. *Vie Médicale*, 1978, *19*, 2513-2519.

18. Moreau Ph.: Un nouveau stimulant circulatoire cérébral. *Nouv. Presse Méd.*, 1975, *4*, 2401-2402.

19. Pidoux B., Bastien C., Niddam S.: Clinical and quantitative EEG double-blind study of GBE. *J. Cerebral Blood Flow Metabolism*, 1983, *3*, 5556-5557.

20. Pidoux B., Bastien C., Niddam S.: Normalization of electroencephalographic activity in ageing brain by an extract of Ginkgo biloba; *In*: Bes. A. Braquet P., Paoletti R., Siesjö B.K. Eds., Cerebral Ischemia, Amsterdam, *Excepta Medica*, 1984, 385-388.

21. Rapin J.R., Le Poncin Lafitte M.: Modèle expérimental d'ischémie cérébrale. Action précentive de l'extrait de Ginkgo. *Semaine des Hôpitaux de Paris*, 1979, *55*, 42-43.

22. Safi N., Galley P.: Tanakan et cerveau sénile. Etude radiocirculographique. *Bordeaux Médical*, 1977, *10*, 171-176.

23. Saracco J.B., Estachy G.: Etude du Tanakan sur la microcirculation oculaire. *Médecine Practicienne*, 1980, *4*, 67-72.

24. Subhan Z., Hindmarch I.: The psychopharmacological effects of Ginkgo biloba extract in normal healthy volunteers. *Internat. J. Clin. Pharmacol. Res.*, 1984, *4*, 89-93.

25. Taylor J.E.: The effects of chronic, oral Ginkgo biloba extract administration on neurotransmitter receptor binding in young and aged Fisher 344 rats. *In*: Effects of Ginkgo biloba extract on organic cerebral impairment, Paris, London, *John Libbey*, 1985.

26. Tea S., Celsis P., Clanet M., Marc-Vergnes J.P.: Effets cliniques, hémodynamiques et métaboliques de l'extrait de Ginkgo biloba en pathologie vasculaire cérébrale. *Gazette Médicale de France*, 1979, *86*, 4149-4152.

27. Terrasse J., Morin B.: Expérimentation du Tanakan par voie parentérale. *Lyon Médical*, 1976, *245*, 841-842.

28. Vorberg G.: GBE – long term study concerning the major symptoms of age-related cerebral disorders. *Clinical Trials Journal*, 1985, *22*, 149-157.

29. Wackenheim A.: Essai clinique du Tanankan dans le syndrome fonctionnel des traumatisés du crâne et l'insuffisance vasculaire cérébrale. *Médecine du Nord et de l'Est*, 1977, *1*, 73-78.

30. Warburton D.M.: Brain, Behavior and Drugs, *Wiley*, London, 1975.

Subject Index

348